Benia

Guide to Coronary Angioplasty and Stenting

Guide to Coronary Angioplasty and Stenting

Peter J.B. Hubner

*Consultant Cardiologist, Glenfield Hospital
Leicester, UK*

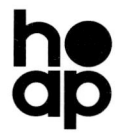

harwood academic publishers
Australia • Canada • China • France • Germany • India • Japan
Luxembourg • Malaysia • The Netherlands • Russia • Singapore
Switzerland • Thailand

Copyright © 1998 OPA (Overseas Publishers Association) Amsterdam B.V. Published under license under the Harwood Academic Publishers imprint, part of The Gordon and Breach Publishing Group.

All rights reserved.

No part of this book may be reproduced or utilized in any form or by any means, electronic or mechanical, including photocopying and recording, or by any information storage or retrieval system, without permission in writing from the publisher. Printed in Singapore.

Amsteldijk 166
1st Floor
1079 LH Amsterdam
The Netherlands

British Library Cataloguing in Publication Data

ISBN: 90-5702-278-8

To my wife Sandra and our children Timothy, Richard, Sarah, and Philip, for helping me to remember the important things in life, to my mentor Dr Monty Goldberg and in memory of my parents.

Contents

Acknowledgements		ix
Abbreviations		xi
Introduction		1
1	Guide Catheters	5
2	Balloon Catheters	13
3	Guide Wires	27
4	Radiographic Views	41
5	Intravascular Ultrasound and Angioscopy	59
6	Patient Selection and General Care	67
7	Review of the Diagnostic Angiogram	79
8	Routine PTCA Case	89
9	PTCA from the Arm	99
10	Stents (History and Types)	103
11	Indications for the Use of Stents	121
12	Complications with Stents	127
13	Routine Stent Case	147
14	Abrupt Closure – 1 (Risks and Causes)	155
15	Abrupt Closure – 2 (Vessel Dissection)	167
16	Emergency Surgery	177
17	Ad Hoc PTCA	183
18	Primary Angioplasty	189
19	PTCA of an Occluded Coronary Artery	201
20	PTCA Post CABG	209
21	LIMA PTCA	221
22	Osteal Lesions, Lesions on Bends and Undilatable Lesions	227
23	Bifurcation Lesions	237
24	Restenosis	249
25	PTCA Quotes	259
26	Angioplasty Formulary	263

Further Reading	**267**
Manufacturers of Equipment	**271**
Index	**275**

Acknowledgements

Many people have helped directly or indirectly with the production of this book. I am very grateful to them all. If I have omitted anybody, I offer my sincere apologies. The list of those I wish to acknowledge includes:

Julie Amos, David de Bono, Menko Jan de Boer, Chris Brown, Nick Byrne, Jeff Chandler, Brian Chapman, Debbie Coleman, Peter Cook, David Cumberland, Helen Dangreaux, Neil Farmer, Nina Gale, Tony Gershlick, Sue Greasley, Cindy Grines, Mike Harris, Mark Hickey, Phillipa Hill, Sarah Hooper, Enid Hutchinson, Roman Mychajluk, Richard Myler, David Porter, Kate Radford, Christine Reek, Julian Relf, Tony Rickards, Robin Robinson, Mike Simpson, Ulrich Sigwart, Gary Slack, Tom Spyt, Lawrence Swan, Stephen Terry, Martyn Thomas, Neal Uren and Judy Warrillow.

Abbreviations

Most will be well recognized. Some will be less well known. Some are peculiar to this book.

ACE Inhibitor	Angiotensin Converting Enzyme Inhibitor
ACT	Activated Clotting or Coagulation Time
AL2	Left coronary artery catheter of the left Amplatz shape, size 2 (or II)
AMI	Acute Myocardial Infarction
Angio	Angiogram
APTT	Activated Partial Thromboplastin Time
AR1	Right coronary artery catheter of the Amplatz right shape, size 1 (or I)
A-V Branch	Atrio-Ventricular Branch of RCA = Posterior Left Ventricular Branch
aVL	Augmented left arm lead of the electrocardiogram
CABG	Coronary Artery Bypass Grafting
CAD	Coronary Artery Disease
CVA	Cerebrovascular Accident
ECG	Electrocardiogram
EmCABG	Emergency Coronary Artery Bypass Grafting
F	French size
GC	Guide Catheter
GI	Gastrointestinal, e.g. bleed
GP	Glycoprotein, e.g. IIb-IIIa antagonist
GTN	Glyceryl Trinitrate
GW	Guide Wire
IABP	Intra Aortic Balloon Pump
I/C	Intra Coronary
ICU	Intensive Care Unit
IM	Intramuscular injection
INR	International Normalised Ratio
ISDN	Isosorbide Dinitrate
ITU	Intensive Therapy Unit
IV	Intravenous
IVUS	Intravascular Ultrasound
JL4	Left Judkins shaped catheter, size 4
JR4	Right Judkins shaped catheter, size 4
LAD	Left Anterior Descending Artery
LAO	Left Anterior Oblique (Radiographic Projection)
LAST	Left Anterior Small Thoracotomy procedure

LCA	Left Coronary Artery
LCX	Left Circumflex Artery
LIMA	Left Internal Mammary Artery
LMS	Left Main Stem
LV	Left Ventricle, or Left Ventricular Function
MI	Myocardial Infarction
OTW	Over-The-Wire Balloon Catheter
PDA	Posterior Descending Artery (a branch of the RCA)
POBA	Plain Old Balloon Angioplasty
PTCA	Percutaneous Transluminal Coronary Angioplasty (Alternatives to note:- Put That Catheter Away, or Professional Tennis Coaches Association!)
PTTK	Partial Thromboplastin Time with Kaolin
QCA	Quantitative Coronary Angiography
RAO	Right Anterior Oblique (Radiology Projection)
RCA	Right Coronary Artery
RIMA	Right Internal Mammary Artery
SK	Streptokinase
SVG	Saphenous Vein Graft
TPA or tPA	Tissue Plasminogen Activator

Introduction

In November 1977, a remarkable paper was read by Dr Andreas Grüntzig to the American College of Cardiology meeting held in Miami, Florida in the USA. The title was 'Non operative treatment of coronary disease'. The paper was greeted with a mixture of astonishment by most of the 86 people present, and by delight from others such as Dr Mason Sones, who had introduced coronary angiography two decades earlier at the Cleveland Clinic. There was applause both *during* and at the end of the presentation. The abstract was published in Circulation in 1977, and as a Letter to the Editor in the Lancet in 1978.

The work was not a sudden one-off 'daring' procedure as many of the initial cardiac transplants had been. Rather it was the culmination of a decade of study. This had included work in the peripheral arteries, experimental work in the post mortem room, and trial work during cardiac surgery prior to coronary artery bypass.

The idea of blowing a balloon up in the coronary artery did certainly seem incredible to many when they first heard about it. However, the principle of passing a fine collapsed balloon across a narrowing, inflating it and then deflating it, was, as with many inventions, so simple and yet such an advance. The older and traditional method of reducing a narrowing in a tube was to pass a series of increasingly larger dilators along the tube and across the narrowing. This method had been used by Dr Charles Dotter in the peripheral arteries. The new balloon technique applied pressure in a radial manner to relieve the narrowing. Grüntzig gave the name to the new procedure of *percutaneous transluminal coronary angioplasty* or *PTCA* for short.

Grüntzig's final contribution to angioplasty was to nurture the new technique to ensure that those who performed it did so as safely as possible. From the start of his own practice he held courses in angioplasty, first in Zurich and then later at Emory University, Atlanta, USA. Many thousands of cardiologists received training from the live demonstrations at these courses.

Through the widespread performance of coronary angioplasty a new subspeciality of cardiology was born, that of *interventional cardiology*.

In 1987, Dr Ulrich Sigwart of Lausanne, Switzerland, reported the first use of an intracoronary stent to reopen a vessel which had become occluded at the time of angioplasty.

Whilst at the start stents were mainly used for this bail-out purpose to avoid emergency bypass surgery, Dr Richard Schatz of San Diego, USA, and Professor Patrick Serruys of Rotterdam in the Netherlands, showed that stents could reduce the risk of renarrowing or restenosis after angioplasty. Dr Antonio Colombo from Milan, Italy led the way in devising a safe and simple anticoagulation regime to prevent clotting or thrombosis within the stent. Stenting has been described as 'the second wind of angioplasty'. For this reason, coronary artery stenting has become an integral part of angioplasty. The types of stents are under active development and the ones currently in use may well later be replaced.

Readership

This book is offered as an introduction to the practice of coronary angioplasty and stenting. It presumes a basic knowledge of cardiac anatomy and coronary angiography. The techniques, equipment and management of the patient is continuously changing and improving. Hence the principles of PTCA will be considered. It is hoped that this book may be useful to doctors starting training in PTCA and the nurses, physiological measurement technicians and radiographers who play important roles in the management of these patients. Medical students, doctors in other fields, and staff in coronary care units and intensive care units, may find browsing through relevant sections to be helpful in the treatment of their patients. Finally, for the many colleagues in Industry, who manufacture and promote angioplasty equipment, this book will explain the principles of PTCA, and give some insight into how at least one doctor 'thinks' and approaches the procedure.

Exclusions

Two topics will not be described that some might expect to find in the book. These are *atherectomy* and *rotablation*. The author has limited personal experience, and at present neither are in regular use by many operators performing PTCA. These techniques at present can be described as having 'niche roles' and though helpful in these specific indications, have a relatively limited application. Put another way ... the great majority of PTCA cases can be done without their use. This situation may change for these and other technologies, as the field of PTCA is a rapidly moving one.

IVUS (Intravascular ultrasound)

Despite only a limited number of centres using IVUS at present, the topic is covered in the book. The author has experience of the technique and considers it very valuable. Its role during angioplasty may become larger.

Acknowledgement

I am very grateful to Dr Richard K Myler, who kindly provided details of the original presentation of PTCA in humans by Andreas Grüntzig.

References

Grüntzig A, Myler R, Hanna E, Turina M. *Circulation* **84**, Abstracts III55–56 (1977).
Grüntzig A. Transluminal dilatation of Coronary Artery Stenosis. *Lancet* **1**, 263 (1978).
Sigwart U, Puel J, Mirkovitch V, *et al*. Intravascular stents to prevent occlusion and restenosis after angioplasty. *N Engl J Med* **316**, 701–706 (1987).

1 Guide Catheters

The equipment routinely used for PTCA, percutaneous transluminal coronary angioplasty, includes:

1. Guide catheter.
2. Guide wire.
3. Balloon catheter.
4. Inflation device.
5. Y-connector.
6. Stent (or 'coronary artery stent').

Guide Catheter (GC)

Guide catheters are similar to diagnostic coronary angiography catheters but usually differ from them by:

1. Teflon inner coating to ease passage of a balloon catheter along its lumen.
2. Non tapering tip.
3. Flexible tip (Figure 1.1): the final 2–3 mm is of a thin rubber-like compressible

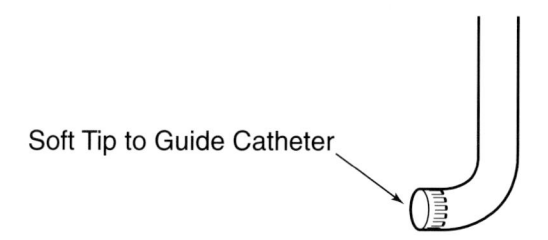

Figure 1.1. Guide Catheter (Judkins R-Shape).

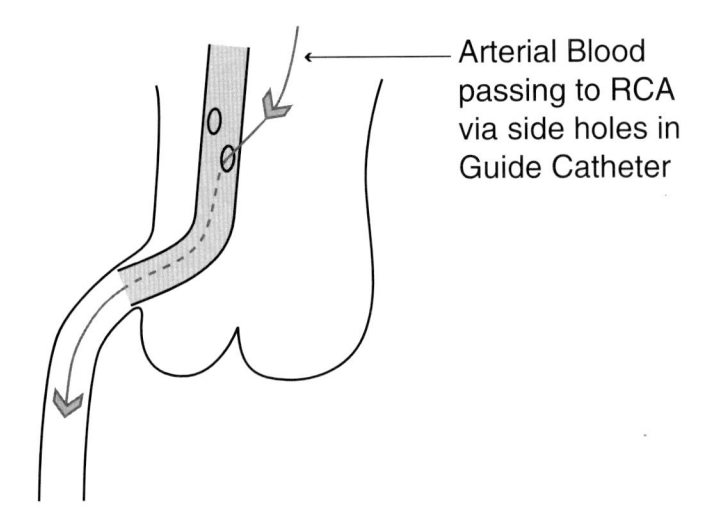

Figure 1.2. Guide Catheter with side holes.

material, so that when the tip is up against the wall of the mouth of an artery, it does not scratch it or damage the artery.
4. Side holes (Figure 1.2): Some catheters have these to allow flow of blood into the guide catheter and then out through the end of the catheter. This feature is useful when there is a tight fit between the catheter and the wall of the artery. This typically occurs with the right coronary artery. With a standard catheter when passed into the artery, there may be insufficient flow around the side of the catheter. The pressures may damp off and ischaemia may ensue. A catheter with side holes allows the distal artery to supplied with blood via the side holes which are outside the artery. There is a potential snag which it is important to recognise. The pressures recorded are those of the aorta, i.e. **not** within the lumen of the artery. Sometimes with a balloon catheter, especially one on which is mounted a stent, there is very little space to allow adequate flow of blood. The myocardium supplied by the artery may become ischaemic … *but the pressures may well still be satisfactory, showing a normal pattern which is not damped off.*

Guide Catheter Shapes

1. Judkins Shape (Figure 1.3)

Most operators use the Judkins shaped catheters, Right 4 cm, 3.5 cm and 3.0 cm, abbreviated to JR4, JR3.5 and JR3 respectively, for the right coronary artery (RCA). For the left coronary artery (LCA), they are JL4, JL3.5 and JL3 catheters.

For RCA, changing from JR4 to JR3.5 or JR3 catheter rarely seems to be helpful and operators usually stick to one of these sizes (JR4 probably the commonest) and if this is not successful in cannulating the RCA, then another shape is selected.

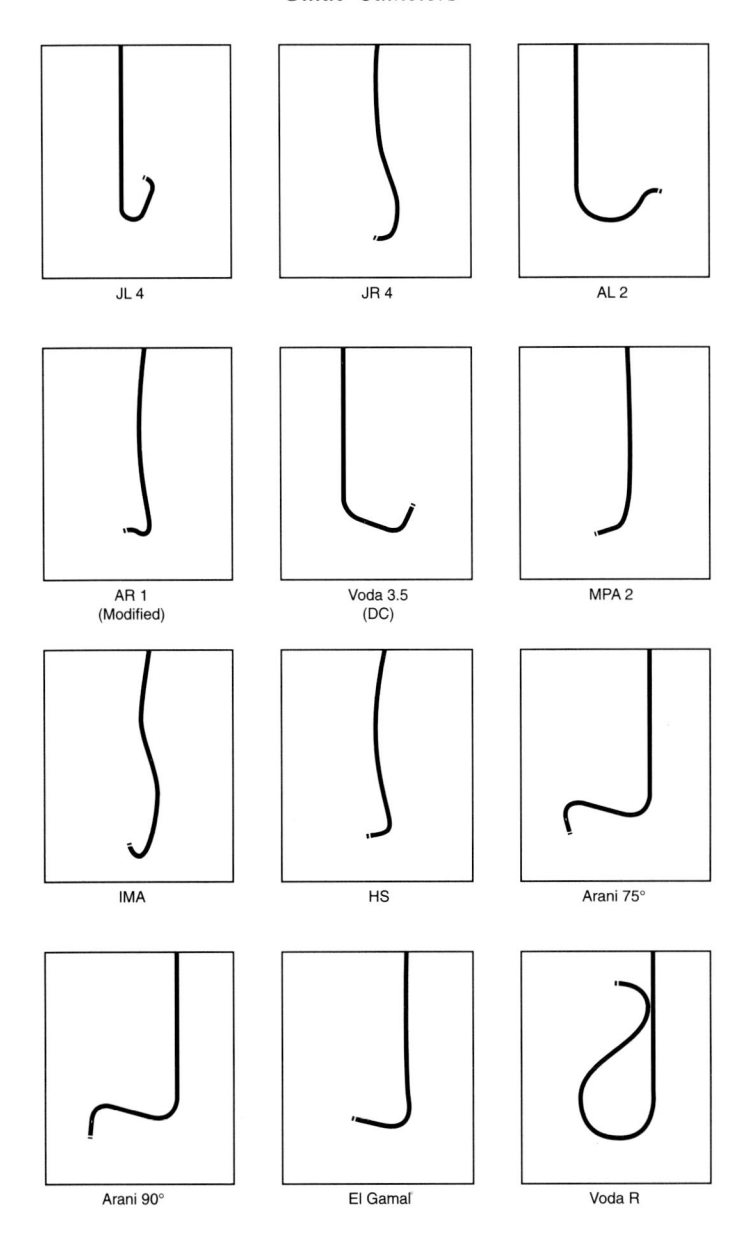

Figure 1.3. Guide Catheter Shapes.
JL4   Left Judkins
JR4   Right Judkins
AL2   Left Amplatz 2 or II
AR1   Right Amplatz 1 or I
Voda 3.5   Left Voda 3.5   DC = Doctor's choice, a similar shaped catheter
MPA2   Multipurpose A 2
IMA   Internal mammary artery catheter
HS   Hockey stick
Arani   75° or 90°
El Gamal
Voda R   Right Voda

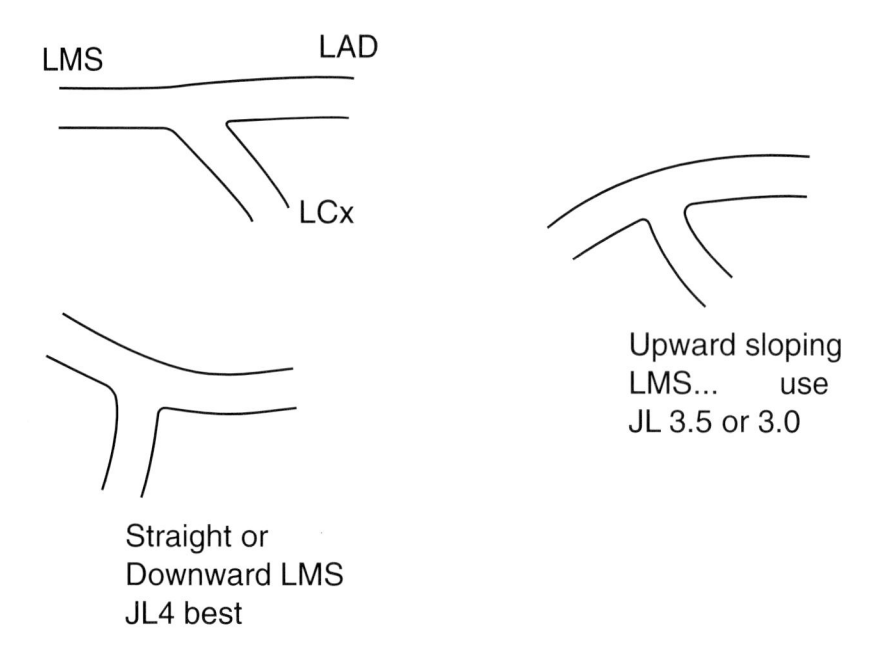

Figure 1.4. Varieties of left main stem: selection of appropriate size of left Judkins catheter.

For LCA, the course of the left main stem (LMS) governs which size of Left Judkins catheter is used (see Figure 1.4). For a straight or downward sloping LMS, the JL4 is suitable (see Angiogram 7.2, page 82).

For an upward sloping left main stem, JL3.5 or JL3 should be used. Note with JL3/3.5 catheters the tip of the catheter tends to point upwards to the left anterior descending artery (LAD) (see Angiogram 8.1, page 90), whilst with JL4 catheters the tip points more to the left circumflex artery (LCX).

2. Amplatz Shape (Figure 1.3)

This shape gives increased support or back-up when trying to pass a balloon catheter across a stenosis. Amplatz catheters are often more difficult to use than the Judkins catheters, both to cannulate the artery and also to withdraw the catheter from the vessel.

Right Amplatz or AR1 is usually a modified shape (see Angiogram 2.1 and 17.1 on pages 22 and 185). This is a very useful catheter especially with side holes.

Left Amplatz AL1, AL2 and AL3 (Angiogram 6.1 and 8.2 on pages 71 and 94). These are particularly helpful for lesions in the LCX artery, where increased support may be needed when this vessel comes off the left main stem at a right angle or even a more acute angle (see page 81). AL1 and AL2 catheters can *also be used in the RCA* as well as the LCA, but great care is needed to avoid dissection of the proximal RCA. For saphenous vein grafts JR4, AR1, AL1 and AL2 may all be used as the guide catheter.

Guide Catheters

The *withdrawal* of an Amplatz catheter from the coronary artery is potentially hazardous. As the catheter is pulled out, the tip tends to descend further into the vessel, instead of coming out of the artery. The tip may damage the LMS or the mouth or proximal portion of the RCA or vein graft. Dissection may ensue. This hazard can be reduced by the following measures:

1. Always treat Amplatz catheters with extra respect and know that they are potentially more dangerous to use than Judkins catheters (Angiogram 8.2, page 94).
2. Always withdraw Amplatz catheters under screening.
3. If the catheter is only just sitting in the orifice and during initial entrance or during the procedure the tip would easily come out, merely withdraw the catheter in the normal manner by pulling on the proximal end.
4. Withdraw the guide catheter over the balloon catheter and guide wire whilst these are still in the proximal vessel. The guide catheter tip then abuts onto the balloon catheter and will not scrape the vessel wall.
5. Gently advance the guide wire distally against 'obstruction' of the distal coronary artery. As you push against the vessel wall the GC will tend to prolapse out.
6. Advance GC gently into the artery and also rotate gently clockwise or anticlockwise. The catheter tip will tend to prolapse out. This particular manoeuvre has variable success and to the operator it may be 'uncomfortable' pushing in further a catheter known to be dangerous, in order to extract it from the artery.

3. Voda Shape (Figure 1.3)

There are left and right Voda catheters from SciMed, but the left is more often used. The left Voda is similar to JL4, but has a longer section in contact with the opposite aortic wall to the LCA. This gives increased back up intermediate between Judkins and Amplatz shapes (see Figure 1.5). This catheter is useful for both LAD and LCX lesions. Usually the Voda catheter is a half cm downsized, compared with the Judkins catheter, i.e. where JL4 or JL3.5 would have been used, for Voda catheters it would be 3.5 and 3.0 respectively. When judged correctly, the tip of the Voda catheter lies in line or is coaxial to the left main stem of LCA, as opposed to the tip pointing upwards and resting of the superior wall as often occurs with a Judkins catheter. The tip of a Voda catheter tends to point to the LAD, rather than the LCX.

The Voda catheter is advanced with the 0.035 or 0.038 inch guide wire retained inside until the tip is about an inch away from the LCA osteum. The GW is removed and if the tip of the catheter is below the LCA the catheter is withdrawn with a slight anticlockwise twist until it enters LCA. If the tip is above the osteum advance with a slight clockwise rotation to engage the osteum. To achieve this it is best to enter the LCA in the left anterior oblique (LAO) projection. Rotating the proximal end anticlockwise, the tip will tend to selectively enter or point to the LAD; rotating clockwise it will pass to the LCX. Sometimes it is possible with the Voda catheter to enter selectively the LCX or LAD and then advance over the balloon catheter for a short distance to give extra support or back up.

There are similar shaped catheters known as Extra Back Up (Cordis), Doctor's Choice (DC) (from Medtronic), Support (Cook Cardiology) and Champ (Bard/USCI) which perform in a similar way to the Voda catheter.

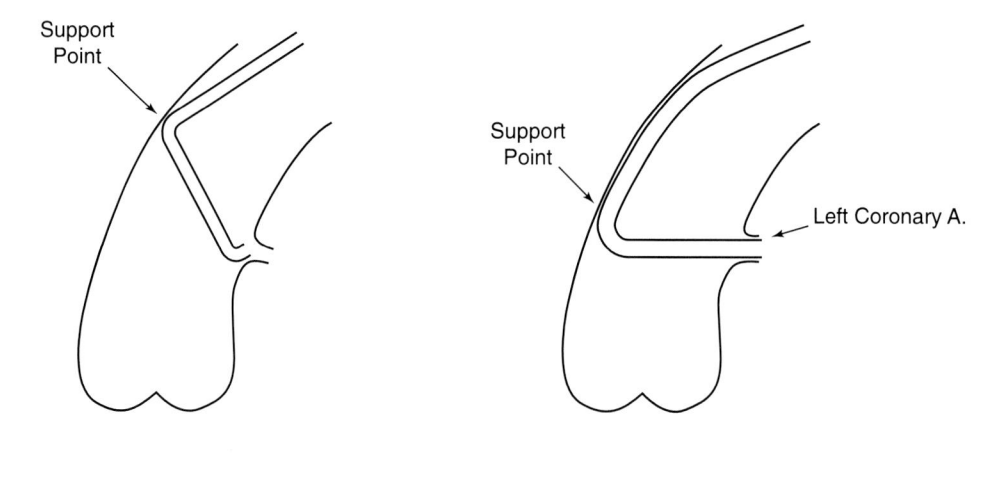

Left Judkins Catheter   **Voda Left Catheter**

The support point for the left Judkins catheter is high above the osteum, and tip of catheter points upwards.

With the Voda catheter, there is a longer length of of catheter support in contact with opposite aortic wall, giving increased catheter support. The support point is directly opposite the osteum of the left coronary artery (LCA). The tip of catheter is straight or coaxial with the LCA.

Figure 1.5. Comparison of Left Judkins and Voda Catheters.

4. Arani Shape (Figure 1.3)

This shape is useful for high take off RCAs, which then usually have a prominent U-shaped initial course or 'shepherd's crook'. The Arani shape allows the catheter to enter the RCA and then may provide good back up. The Arani catheter comes with 90° and 75° angles of the terminal tip from the preceding segment. The Arani 75° is for the more extreme upward pointing RCA. The *Voda Right* catheter has some similarities in shape to the Arani shape and also gives increased back up compared to the Judkins Right catheter. The *El Gamal* shape is similar to both Arani and Voda being used for RCAs, but does not have the initial looped segment to encourage support from the posterior aortic wall.

5. Hockey Stick Shape (Figure 1.3)

This shape is similar to Amplatz Right and to Judkins Right and may give some extra support.

6. Multipurpose Shape (Figure 1.3)

This catheter shape has a downward pointing relatively long final segment. It is useful especially the Multipurpose A2 for:

1. Downward pointing RCAs.
2. RCA grafts, which usually are also downward pointing as they come off the aorta (Angiogram 20.1, page 212).

With this shaped catheter it is possible to safely advance the catheter down into the artery or the graft to near the lesion to give very good back up.

7. Internal Mammary Artery Shape (Figure 1.3)

This is specifically designed to cannulate the left (or right) internal mammary artery. For a description of its use (see Chapter 21).

8. Other Shapes

There are many other shapes to guide and diagnostic coronary catheters as can be seen from any catalogue of catheters. However the other shapes are used infrequently and the standard ones usually suffice. With PTCA from the arm, the Sones shaped catheter may be used (see Chapter 9).

Catheter Sizes

The size or calibre of cardiac catheters is measured in units of French (F), where one unit French equals 1/3 of a millimetre. The usual sizes are 6, 7 and 8F. For some procedures such as atherectomy larger guides 9, 9.5 and 10F are needed. With the newer lower profile balloon catheters, they take up less space within the guide catheter. Smaller guide catheters i.e. 6 and 7F can be used and yet perfectly adequate contrast injections can still be made to visualise the coronary vessels. Most of the modern stents can pass down 6F guide catheters.

Diagnostic Catheters

Whilst not designed for angioplasty, diagnostic catheters can be used for example in an emergency, or if a particular shape is only available in the diagnostic form. The tip of a diagnostic catheter is tapered, so there will be very little space between the balloon and guide catheter wall. Despite hard pressure on the contrast syringe, injections will be slow and the vessel visualisation will be poor. Also ... the operator's right hand will not enjoy these contrast injections! After inflation and deflation of an angioplasty balloon at a lesion, it may not be possible to withdraw the balloon back into the catheter. Use the right tool for the job ... diagnostic catheters are not constructed for PTCA.

Conclusion

Manufacturers over the 20-year period of PTCA have considerably improved guide catheters, which now have larger lumens, safer tips and are less likely to buckle or become soft with use. The regular size used has fallen from 8–9F to 6–7F.

2 Balloon Catheters

Angioplasty balloon catheters are fine instruments which are manufactured with great care and engineering skill. Once doctors get at them, they are often rather maltreated!

Balloon catheters are often just called 'balloons'. They have five main sections (Figures 2.1 and 2.2):

1. the balloon itself.
2. the shaft.
3. the tip.
4. the central lumen for the guide wire.
5. the inflation port — passing to the balloon for its inflation.

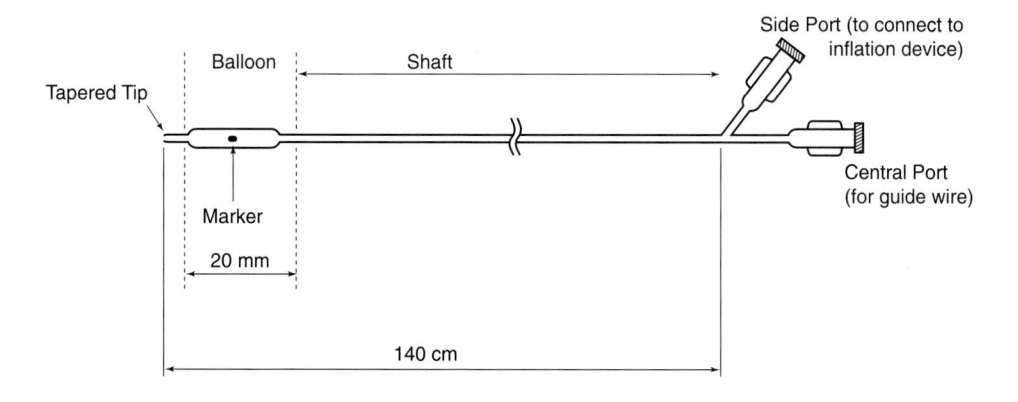

Figure 2.1. Angioplasty balloon catheter (over the wire type).

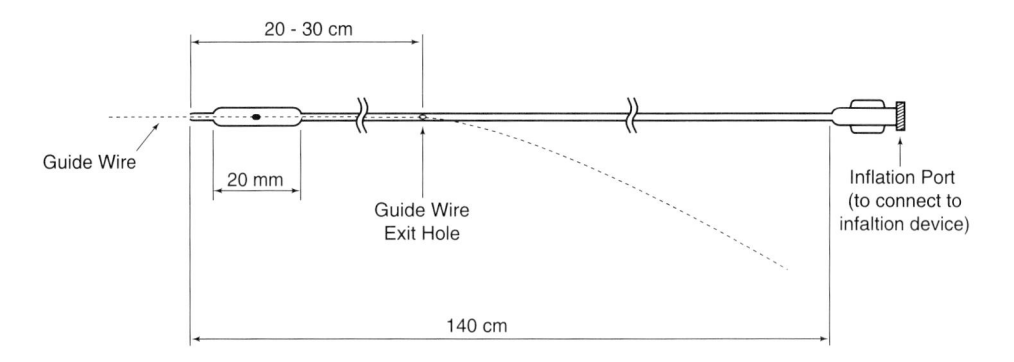

Figure 2.2. Angioplasty balloon catheter (rapid exchange or monorail type).

1. Balloon

This is constructed of a very *fine* but *incredibly strong* material. This allows the thickness of the collapsed balloon to be as low as possible, to make it easier for the balloon to cross a narrowing. The *profile* of a balloon, refers to the size of the smallest hole through which the deflated balloon can pass. Profiles of balloons have fallen considerably since angioplasty balloons were first made, e.g. for a 3 mm balloon from values of 0.045 of an inch to current values of 0.028–0.032 inches. The profile of a balloon is lowest when it is first removed from the package and before any inflation has occurred. After the initial (and subsequent) inflations, the balloon does not collapse and rewrap so tightly and so the profile is not as good.

Size of Balloon

This refers to the diameter of the balloon when it is inflated. The commonest size used in the coronary arteries is 3.0 mm. Usually balloon sizes have step-ups of 0.5 mm and range from 1.5–4.5 mm. Quarter sizes, i.e. step-ups of 0.25 mm are also available.

The size of the balloon depends on the amount of pressure used to inflate it. This is measured in atmospheres, where 1 atmosphere (or bar) = 15 lb per square inch. Usually the size of the balloon specified by the manufacturer, is reached at 5–7 atmospheres. This pressure, at which the balloon reaches the specified size is referred to as the *'nominal pressure'*. If the inflating pressure is further increased e.g. to 8–12 atmospheres a variable increase in the size of the balloon will occur from the stretching of the balloon material. The amount of stretching depends on the material used to construct the balloon. Virtually all materials will expand to some extent. However, some balloons are described as:

a) *Compliant*: The size of the balloon will definitely increase with greater pressure. This is usually of the order of 0.25 mm over the rated size, e.g. a balloon of 3 mm at 7 atmospheres, may increase to about 3.25 mm at 12–15 atmospheres.
b) *Non-Compliant*: The size of the balloon alters very little despite increasing to high inflation pressures.

Compliant materials include Duralyn, POC (polyethylene copolymer), PE (polyethylene), PE3, TPE and PMR. Compliant balloons are useful to allow a balloon to 'grow' to a slightly larger size. You therefore avoid replacing the balloon if after dilatation there is still a residual stenosis and the vessel appears slightly larger than the balloon size selected. However the *snag* of compliant balloons is that with a hard lesion resisting dilatation, if the inflating pressure is progressively increased, a portion of the balloon on either side of the lesion will more and more dilate the normal artery. The balloon will resemble a dog bone and the vessel may be dilated above its true size and be damaged by dissection (see page 235).

Non-compliant balloons are useful to allow high pressures (e.g. 15–20 atmospheres) to be applied to a stent mounted on the balloon to fully expand the stent. The commonest non-compliant material used is PET (polyethylene terephthalate).

Previously, whether a balloon material was compliant or non-compliant was considered of some importance. Non-compliant balloons were believed (on rather slim evidence) to be safer with a lower risk of dissection, especially on bends. Nowadays nearly all balloons are made of an ultrathin layer of a material which can withstand high pressures, often up to nearly 20 atmospheres. The material is 'semi-compliant' or has 'controlled compliance', i.e. will predictably expand at higher pressures, from a nominal size at about 8 atmospheres to an extra 0.25 mm–0.35 mm at about 15–20 atmospheres.

Coating of the Balloon

Virtually all balloons have a slippery or lubricious coating to reduce friction and enable the balloon to cross a lesion more easily. Often the shaft of the catheter has the same or similar coating to aid its passage along the guide catheter and the proximal coronary vessel, i.e. to improve the *trackability* of the balloon catheter. Examples of the coatings are Microglide (ACS), Pro/Pel or Hydro/Pel (Bard), SLX (Cordis) and Enhance (Medtronic). Sometimes the wall of the central lumen along which the guide wire passes is also given a lubricious coating which aids tracking of the balloon catheter over the wire.

Length of Balloon

The standard length of an angioplasty balloon is 20 mm (2 cm). Shorter 9–10 mm balloons e.g. the 9 mm Schneider 'Chubby', or the SciMed 10 mm Non Compliant Viva balloon and longer 30–40 mm balloons are also available (Angiograms 22.2 and 23.1 on pages 233 and 246).

Balloon Marker

There is a radiopaque marker on the shaft of the catheter within the balloon to allow accurate positioning of the balloon at the lesion. Usually there is one central marker. Most balloons on which stents are mounted have markers at each end to aid accurate placement of the stent. Long balloons i.e. 30–40 mm versions also have a marker at both ends.

2. Shaft

This is the section of the angioplasty catheter from the balloon to the hub of the catheter. It is typically 125–160 cm long. As with balloon profile, the diameter or calibre of the

Guide Wire   Balloon Marker

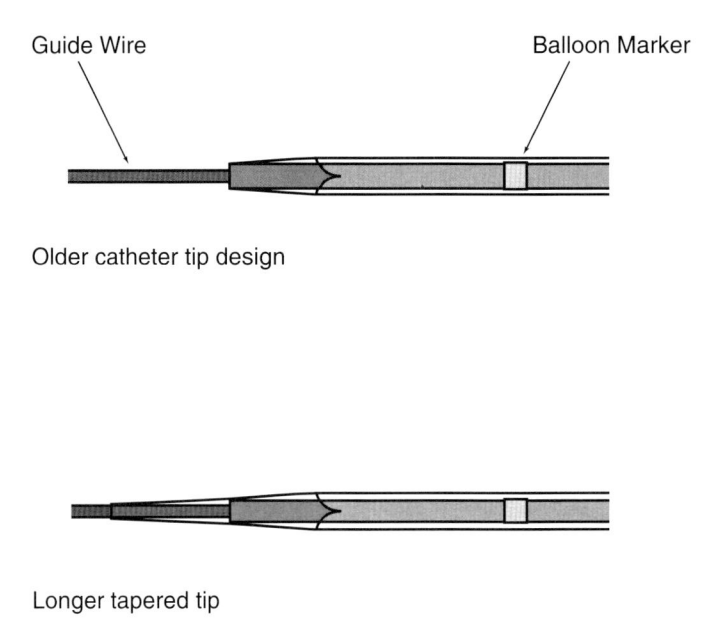

Older catheter tip design

Longer tapered tip

Figure 2.3. Tapered tip of modern balloon catheter.

shaft has become progressively smaller over the years, from about 4.3 F to now 2.6–3.3 F. The shaft takes up less space within the guide catheter allowing better injections of contrast and improved vessel visualisation.

The shaft needs two features which tend to oppose each other. On the one hand it needs to be *rigid and firm* to aid pushing a balloon across a stenosis. But it also needs to be *flexible and trackable* to allow the balloon to pass easily down and round the bends of the coronary arteries. Some balloons are more *pushable* and less *trackable*, whilst others are the reverse. With several manufacturers' modern balloon catheters, the main length of the shaft is quite rigid and stiff, sometimes being made of a thin hypodermic metal tube. The final 20–30 cm is softer and makes it easier for the balloon to track down to the lesion. Unfortunately when outside the body on the catheter table, this type of balloon catheter is very springy and has a knack of landing on the floor which does not amuse those in charge of finances!

Generally, the lower the profile of the balloon, the smaller the size of the shaft and the more rigid the proximal shaft, the easier it will be for a balloon to track to the lesion and to cross it.

3. Tip of the Balloon Catheter (Figure 2.3)

This is the short segment of the shaft beyond the balloon through which the guide wire emerges (Figure 2.3). It is the first part of the catheter to pass across a lesion. Usually this section is about 2–5 mm long and is tapered down to just above the size of the guide wire to assist the balloon crossing.

4. Central Lumen for the Guide Wire

This passes from the proximal end or hub down the length of the catheter to its tip (Figure 2.1). The guide wire passes down this channel to emerge from the catheter. The calibre is sufficient to allow a 0.014 or 0.018 inch size guide wire. The Schneider Magnum balloon allows a 0.021 inch guide wire for crossing of a chronic occlusion.

With the guide wire removed, the central lumen allows the recording of pressures from the distal coronary artery and the injection of contrast to this site. Both these techniques are now rarely used.

If it is necessary to change a balloon catheter e.g. to go up to a larger size, the guide wire is left in place and a *second extension wire* is attached to its proximal end. The balloon catheter is withdrawn and the new one is advanced along the extended guide wire (see page 31). This procedure is relatively lengthy and awkward.

In 1988, Tassilo Bonzel from Fulda, Germany, introduced a modification where the guide wire exits a short distance (about 10–30 cm) back from the balloon (Figure 2.2). This allows the removal of a balloon catheter without the need to extend the guide wire. The central lumen no longer extends down the length of the shaft which can be smaller. This type of balloon catheter is referred to as *Rapid Exchange* or *Monorail*, as opposed the original form of catheter known as '*over the wire*' or *OTW*.

Rapid exchange is the commonest form of balloon catheter used in Europe. It allows the operator to hold and manipulate the guide wire and the balloon, rather than relying on an assistant to secure and manipulate the guide wire as with OTW catheters.

Over the wire catheters are the dominant type in the USA. They probably offer more support and back-up for crossing a lesion than the rapid exchange versions. If it is necessary to change the guide wire, e.g. to a stiffer one, the balloon can be left in position whilst the guide wire is removed and replaced. This is not possible with a rapid exchange catheter as the guide wire does not traverse the length of the catheter.

5. Inflation (or Balloon) Port and Lumen

This is the channel running from the proximal end of the catheter to the balloon along which diluted contrast is passed and withdrawn under negative pressure to fill and empty the balloon. With OTW balloons there is a separate side channel and hub at the proximal end. With rapid exchange balloons there is only one proximal hub which is for the balloon (Figures 2.1 and 2.2).

Inflation Device (Figure 2.4)

This is connected to the inflation port of the balloon catheter and allows diluted contrast under pressure to pass to the balloon to inflate it. On withdrawal of the contrast under negative pressure, the balloon is deflated. The simplest variety has a syringe and a pressure gauge. The syringe usually of 10 or 20 ml capacity has a lock and ratchet arrangement to aid a controlled increase of pressure and then to fix or maintain it at a given level for half to two minutes whilst the balloon is inflated. Deflation of the balloon is the reverse procedure. Most operators use a disposable version such as the Indeflator (ACS), the Wizard (Bard), the Everest (Medtronic), or the Encore (Scimed).

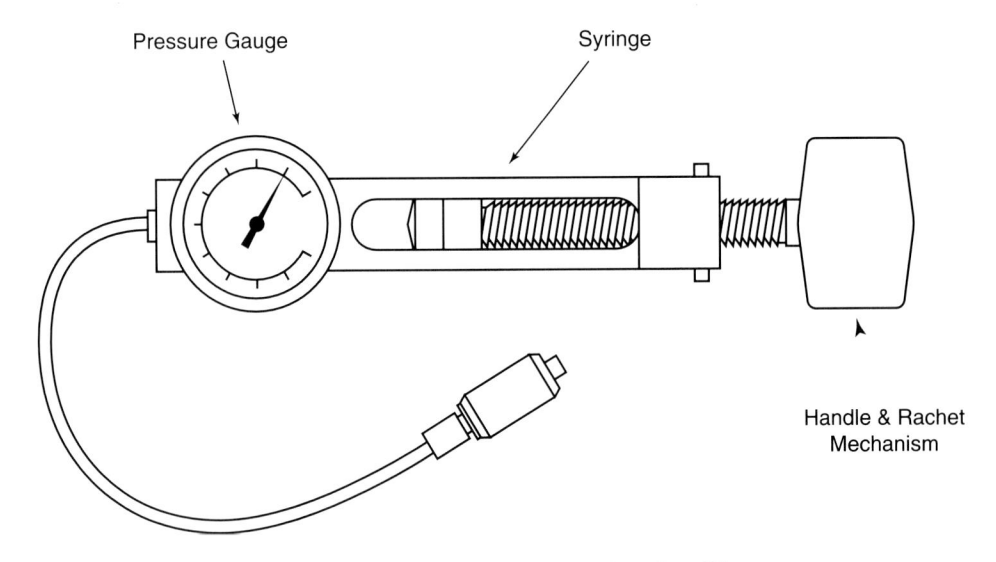

Figure 2.4. Inflation device ("Indeflator", ACS).

Y-Connector or Haemostatic Valve (Figures 2.5 and 2.6)

This is a simple but important item of equipment; its distal end is connected to the hub of the guide catheter. Through its proximal end which has a screw valve, the balloon catheter and guide wire are passed to reach the guide catheter and eventually the coronary

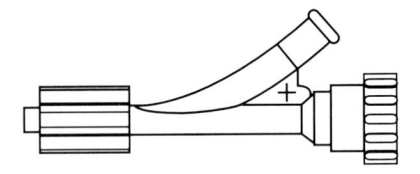

Figure 2.5. Y-Connector (Gateway Plus Y-Adapter, SciMed Products).

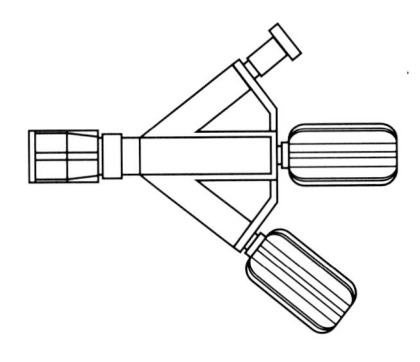

Figure 2.6. Double Y-Connector (Duostat, ACS).

Balloon Catheters

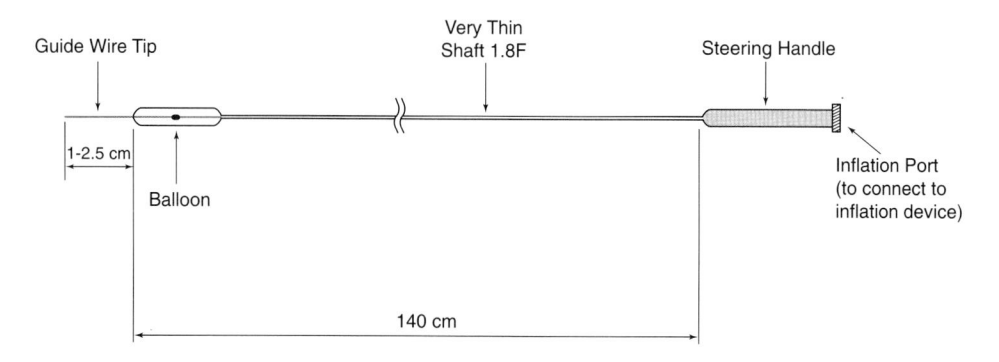

Figure 2.7. Fixed-wire balloon.

artery. The screw valve is adjusted to allow free passage of a balloon, but still maintain adequate pressure recording of the arterial pressure at the tip of the guide catheter. To the side arm or infusion port is connected the pressure and contrast double tap. Sometimes a *double Y-connector* is used. This has two side arms, with the second one also having a screw valve. This allows for two guide wires to be introduced, one along the central channel and a second via the side arm. This type of Y-connector is needed where two wires are used for bifurcation lesions, typically LAD and a diagonal branch (see Chapter 23).

In the USA, Y-connectors are also known as Tuohy Borst adaptors.

Fixed-Wire Balloon Catheter

These balloon catheters have a short length (1–2.5 cm) of floppy guide wire protruding from the distal end of the balloon. The wire is fixed and is part of the balloon catheter itself. There is no guide wire on which the balloon passes along to and from the lesion. This type of balloon catheter looks very like a guide wire onto which a balloon has been grafted near the tip (see Figure 2.7).

A bend is fashioned on the short guide wire tip to allow it to be turned to the desired direction. The proximal end of the shaft has a handle similar to a torquer to facilitate manipulation of the guide wire tip.

The Advantages of the fixed-wire balloon are:

1. *Very Thin Shaft*
   The shaft is often merely a very thin hypotube to allow inflation of the balloon. The size of the shaft may be as small as 1.4–2F and takes up very little room in the guide catheter. This can be useful if two balloons need to be passed up the same guide catheter as in PTCA of a bifurcation lesion (see page 240).
2. *Good Trackability*
   The balloon behaves much more like a guide wire than a conventional balloon.
3. *Low Profile Balloon*
   As the balloon is wrapped on a very narrow shaft, the profile of the collapsed balloon is very small.

The Disadvantages of the fixed-wire balloon are:

1. *Very Short Distance of Guide Wire across the Lesion*
   This is a major problem, as it is very easy to come back across the lesion in error.
2. *Inability to Change the Balloon*
   As the guide wire tip is part of the balloon catheter, it is not possible to change the balloon without withdrawing the whole system. It may not be able to recross the lesion.
3. *Difficulty to Dilate a Long Lesion*
   The guide wire tip comes in varying lengths (see above), but may be insufficient to cross the length of a long lesion or a dissection, which makes dilatation more difficult.
4. *Difficulty to Use this type of Balloon Catheter*
   Whilst this catheter behaves more like a guide wire than a balloon catheter, it is actually more difficult to manipulate than a routine guide wire.

Examples of fixed-wire balloons catheters are the Probe (Bard), the Ace (SciMed) and the Lightning (Cordis).

The fixed-wire balloon catheter was the original form of PTCA catheter used by Grüntzig at the start of coronary angioplasty. This design was soon overtaken by the 'steerable' system, with a balloon running over a separate guide wire, introduced by Professor John Simpson of San Francisco. The modern OTW and monorail balloon catheters now have shaft sizes and balloon profiles very similar to those of the fixed-wire versions; these modern balloons have the benefits but not the disadvantages of their fixed-wire cousins.

Perfusion Catheter (Figure 2.8)

This type of balloon was introduced by Dr Richard Stack of Duke University, Durham, North Carolina, USA and subsequent versions are still often known as *Stack Balloons*.

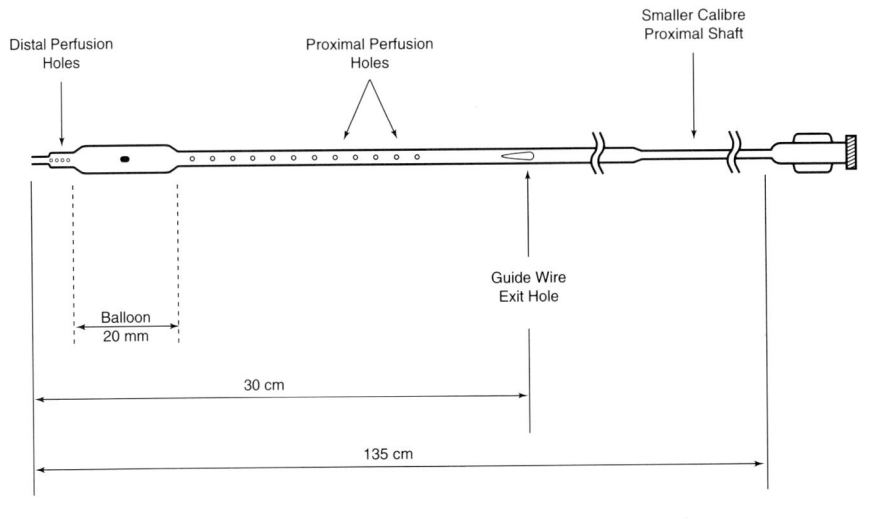

Figure 2.8. Perfusion balloon. (Rapid exchange type).

Two modern versions are the ACS Rx Lifestream Balloon and the Monorail Speedflow (Schneider).

The aim of this balloon is to permit a prolonged balloon inflation of 5–30 minutes by allowing blood to flow into the distal vessel during balloon inflation. This is achieved by blood flowing via a series of holes in the wall of the catheter shaft, tracking past the balloon and exiting through a further set of holes along the catheter tip (see Figure 2.7).

The flow to the distal artery varies with:

1. *Number and Size of Proximal and Distal Holes.*
   The Monorail Speedflow has 13 proximal and 3 distal sideholes. The ACS Rx Lifestream has 15 proximal and 8 distal sidcholcs of 0.013 inches diameter, i.e. just smaller than an 0.014 inch guide wire, which is thereby prevented from exiting from these holes.
2. *The Size of the Central (Guide Wire) Lumen.*
   The larger this channel the greater will be the flow; but the larger the catheter shaft, the less trackable the catheter becomes.
3. *Presence or Absence of the Guide Wire.*
   This an important factor influencing flow. If the guide wire is withdrawn past the start of the proximal holes, the channel will be larger and the flow greater (see Angiograms 2.1 and 24.1, on pages 22 and 254). For example with the Monorail Speedflow balloon:
   With guide wire pulled back, the flow of blood is approximately 40 ml/minute.
   With guide wire retained, the flow of blood is approximately 25 ml/minute.
4. *Systemic Blood Pressure.*
   If this is low, then the flow of blood into and out of the catheter will be less and the perfusion of the distal artery will be inadequate.

Use of the Perfusion Balloon Catheter

1. *Dissection*
   A perfusion balloon with a prolonged inflation of 10–30 minutes, may be able to tack up the vessel wall. There is about a 30% success rate, but this role has been largely superseded by stents (see Angiogram 15.2, page 173).
2. *Elective Use*
   Especially for more complex lesions, an inflation of 7–10 minutes will often give a very satisfactory result (see Angiograms 2.1 and 13.2 on pages 22 and 152). There may be very little time difference between several dilations with a routine balloon and a prolonged inflation with a perfusion balloon. Screening time and contrast used will usually be lower with a perfusion balloon.
3. *High Risk for Ischaemia from Balloon Inflation*
   With a high risk angioplasty e.g. on the last remaining coronary artery especially with poor left ventricular function, a perfusion balloon may be used to minimise the ischaemia produced by a short (one minute) inflation of the balloon (see page 156 and Angiogram 6.1, page 71). It may similarly be used for a very proximal LAD lesion to protect a large area of myocardium during balloon inflation.
4. *Lesion with Recoil*
   Occasionally a balloon will fully inflate, but as soon as it is let down the lesion is seen to persist. The lesion has prominent elastic recoil. A prolonged inflation for

22   Guide to Coronary Angioplasty and Stenting

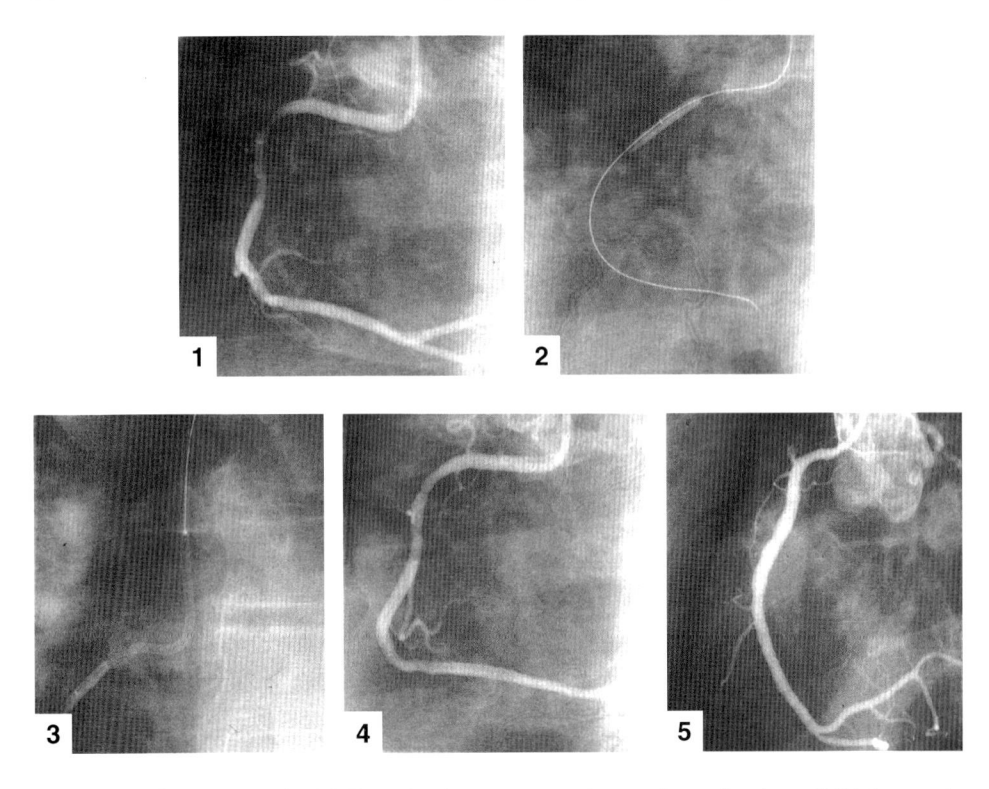

Angiogram 2.1. *PTCA of RCA Stenosis.* A severe stenosis on a large dominant RCA is seen in LAO 25° projection (1). Using 7 French right Amplatz I (ARI) guide catheter (3), the lesion was pre-dilated with 2.5 mm. balloon over 0. 014" Bard Hi-per flex guide wire. As considerable improvement in the stensosis was achieved, instead of stenting the lesion, a 3mm. ACS Lifestream perfusion balloon was used (2). The guide wire was withdrawn to the proximal marker at the start of the proximal perfusionholes, and the balloon inflated at 6 atmospheres for 7 minutes (3). The result was very satisfactory and is almost 'stent-like' as seen in Figure 4, and also in the RAO Caudal projection (RAO 20°, Caudal 25°) (5).

20–30 minutes may fully relieve the stenosis. Some circumflex lesions are in this category (see page 233).

5. *As a Perfusion Bridge to Emergency Coronary Artery Surgery*
   This was the original role for a perfusion catheter/balloon, which was also known as a 'bail-out' catheter. The catheter was placed across a dissected region and the guide wire was withdrawn (Angiogram 15.2, page 173). The catheter was left *in situ* as the patient was taken to surgery. However, the small perfusion holes tend to easily become clogged up by thrombus, despite heparinization. Merely keeping a guide wire across a dissected region is usually sufficient to splint the segment and partially maintain patency and a variably adequate distal flow.

Disadvantages of Perfusion Balloons

1. *Poor Trackability and Balloon Profile*
   To have sufficient flow rate the shaft needs to be relatively large which makes it stiffer and less trackable. The larger the shaft on which the balloon is mounted, the greater

the size or profile of the collapsed balloon. With some of the earlier versions it is was very difficult or impossible to advance the perfusion catheter into the circumflex artery or down a tortuous RCA. The two modern perfusion balloons have smaller shafts and lower balloon profiles, leading to much improved trackability and ability of the balloon to cross a lesion.

2. *Inadequate Distal Perfusion*
   Sometimes even with the guide wire removed the distal myocardium becomes ischaemic and balloon inflation can only be maintained for a short period time (2–4 minutes only).
3. *Side branch Ischaemia*
   If a side branch arises at or near the lesion it will not be perfused and ischaemia may limit balloon inflation.
4. *Withdrawal of the Guide Wire*
   When used for dissection, if the guide wire is withdrawn it may later not be possible to pass it back out of the perfusion balloon into the true lumen to reach the distal artery. This is a serious situation and unless the dissected segment can be recrossed further dilatation with a balloon and or use of a stent will not be possible. For elective cases (with a non-dissected lesion), this concern does not usually arise unless the distal artery is also diseased or very tortuous.

Balloon with Differential Materials (The CAT Balloon)

The Controlled Angioplasty Technology or **CAT** balloon (Cardiovascular Dynamics) is constructed with two materials (Figures 2.9 and 2.10):

a) central section — compliant material (PE, polyethylene)
b) end sections — non compliant material (PET, polyethylene terephthalate).

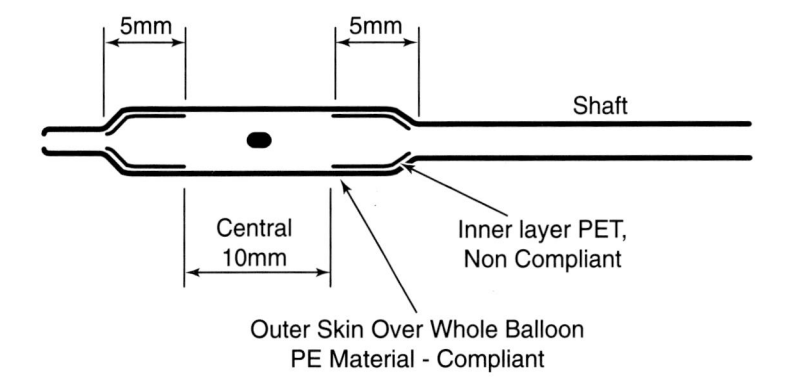

PE - Polyethylene
PET - Polyethylene Terephthalate
(Two Materials Bonded Together)

Figure 2.9. Balloon with differential expansion (CAT Balloon).

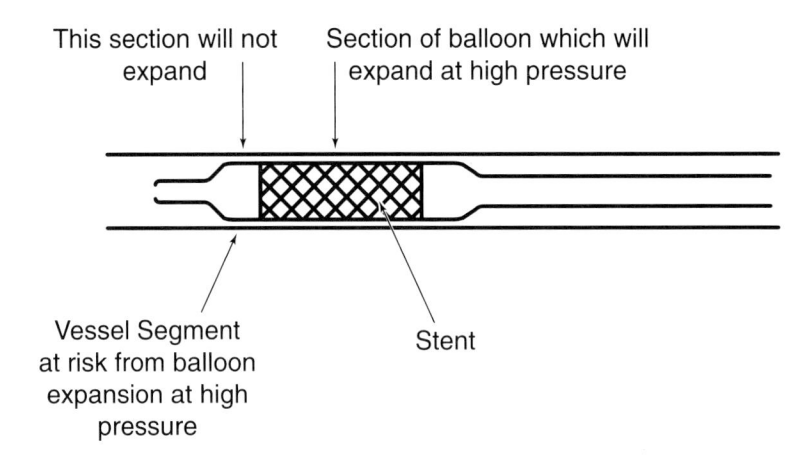

Figure 2.10. Use of balloon with differential materials to deploy/expand stent to high pressures.

With inflation pressure of 5–7 atmospheres the whole balloon expands to nominal size. With higher pressures of 15–20 atmospheres the central section will expand by approximately 0.25 mm, but the two end sections will not enlarge to any extent. This type of balloon is potentially useful in coronary stenting. For example a hand crimped Palmaz-Schatz stent mounted on the central section of the balloon can be expanded to high pressure. The balloon protruding from each end of the stent will not progressively expand, reducing the risk of damage and dissection to the vessel at either end outside the stent, especially at the distal segment (Figure 2.10). Likewise, it may be used after the delivery of any type of stent, if redilatation at high pressures is needed.

Double Balloons

Instead of one there are two balloons, with the distal balloon being of a small calibre and the second balloon being larger. The distal balloon first crosses the stenosis and 'predilates' the lesion for the second balloon which is the correct size for the vessel. With modern low profile balloons, it is rare for the balloon not to cross whatever the size chosen.

Drug Delivery Balloons

There are a variety of such catheters which will allow a drug be delivered locally to the vessel wall at the time of angioplasty. Usually the drugs are to inhibit thrombosis at the site and or to reduce restenosis. At present this type of catheter is a research tool only.

Laser Balloon

Incorporated within the balloon is a laser facility which can be applied to a lesion. The catheter was found to be helpful to tack up a dissection. However the energy acts in a similar way to heat and intense scarring as with a burn ensued. This led to a high rate of restenosis of about 50%.

Cutting Balloon (InterVentional Technologies)

When inflated this balloon displays blades which incise the lesion. It is claimed that dissection is less common than with routine balloon angioplasty. The cutting balloon is relatively rigid, which limits its trackability. Once it has been inflated and used for a lesion, full retraction of the blades is not possible, so that the balloon cannot be used to track down to another lesion for its dilatation too.

Conclusion

Balloon catheters are the central item of equipment of PTCA. Since their introduction in 1977 they have undergone remarkable improvements and developments. Angioplasty manufacturers have considerably reduced the profile of the balloon and the calibre of the shaft of catheters. The great majority of lesions can be crossed at the first attempt with a balloon of the correct size for the calibre of the artery. The smaller shaft takes up less space in the guide catheter and the proximal coronary artery, allowing better visualization of the coronary vessels with contrast injections.

The second major development has been the introduction by Bonzel of the monorail or rapid exchange balloon catheter. This design greatly simplifies and speeds up exchanges of balloon catheter; it also improves the control of the guide wire by the operator.

The third ongoing improvement is of the balloon material, which can sustain increasingly higher inflation pressures, without tearing and balloon rupture. Some materials are relatively non-compliant and despite high pressures stretch only to a minor degree, so that the balloon enlarges only by a small amount above its nominal size. This reduces the risk of dissection with high pressure inflations, such as with stent deployment.

3 Guide Wires

These form the 'third man' of angioplasty, i.e. guide catheter, balloon catheter and then guide wire. Often the abbreviation GW will be used for guide wire(s).

Construction of Guide Wires

Like the balloon catheters, guide wires are wonderfully engineered pieces of equipment (Figures 3.1–3.4). Guide wires are usually 175–180 cm long and have a:

1. Flexible coil
2. Shaft
3. Docking end — for extending the GW.

The *shaft* consists of a solid stainless steel *core wire* about 150 cm in length. The core wire gives the firmness, stability and steerability (torque) to the GW from its proximal end to the distal tip.

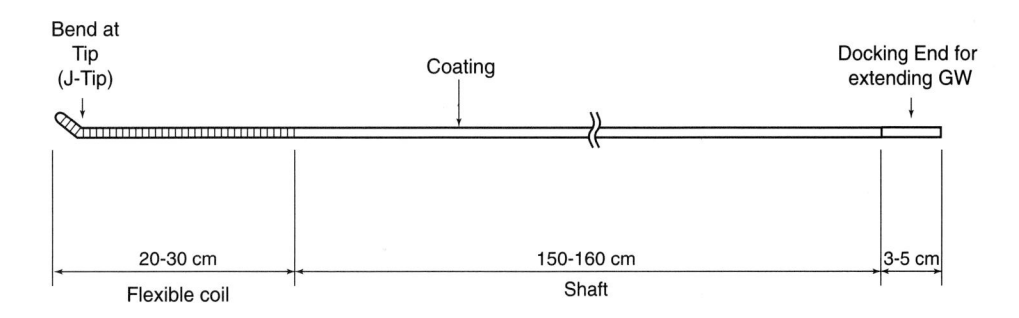

Figure 3.1. Guide wire (GW).

28   *Guide to Coronary Angioplasty and Stenting*

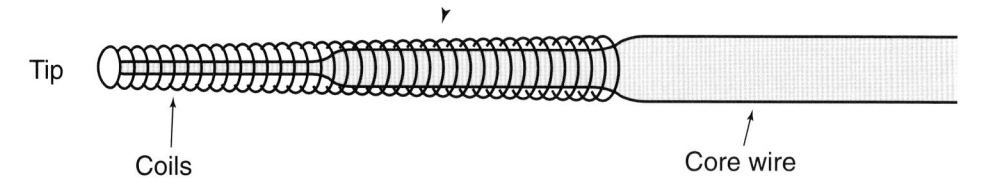

Figure 3.2. Flexible Coil Section of a GW.

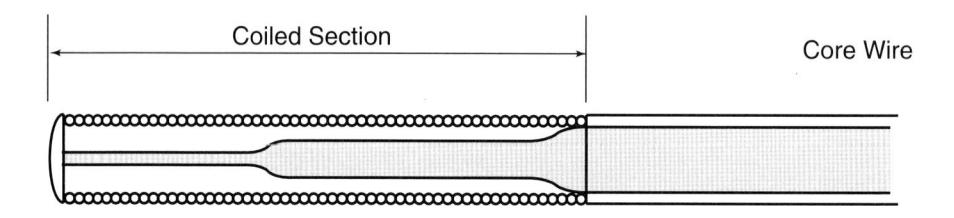

Figure 3.3. High Torque Floppy GW.

Core wire extends to about 1/2 length of Terminal section and then becomes much thinner.

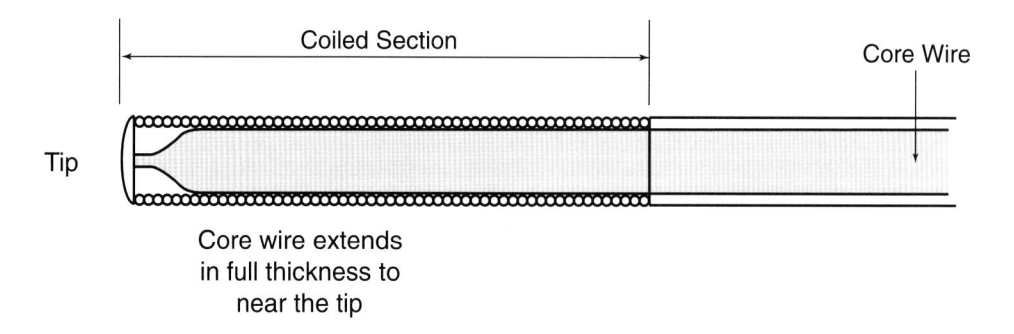

Figure 3.4. Standard GW.

Core wire extends in full thickness to near the tip

The *flexible coil* which is about 20–30 cm long, consists of a spring of stainless steel wound over the core wire, forming a tube or cylinder. The core wire within this cylinder tapers to become softer and more flexible. The tapering may be a series of 3–4 steps or as a smooth progression. Stiffer GWs have a thick core wire extending to the distal tip of the GW, whereas with softer GWs the core wire becomes thin near the start of the flexible coil. If the core wire does not extend to the tip of the GW there is a short *safety wire* (known as the *forming ribbon* or *mandril*) between the two. This prevents the spring coil from unwinding.

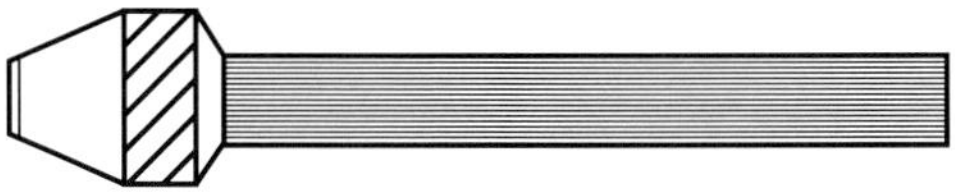

Figure 3.5. Torquer/Torquing Device.

The final 2–3 cm, or the whole of the flexible coil, is made of a radiopaque metal such as platinum or gold, so that it is visible under fluoroscopy. The flexible coil is coated with a hydrophilic lubricant such as Microglide, ICE and Propel for ACS, SciMed and Cordis guide wires respectively.

The *Docking end* is about 3–5 cm long at the proximal end of the GW. It allows an extension wire to be connected to the GW, thereby doubling its length. This is necessary when an over the wire (OTW) balloon catheter (see page 17), needs to be withdrawn and replaced by another balloon catheter (see below on page 31).

Torquer or Torquing Device (Figure 3.5)

This is a small pencil-like tool which is slipped over the proximal end and screwed down onto the guide wire. By turning the torquer between thumb and index (and middle) finger(s), the GW tip can be rotated. This facilitates manipulation of the GW, but some operators prefer to rotate the bare GW between thumb and index finger.

When passing a GW along a vessel, rotating the tip clockwise and anticlockwise as you go helps to prevent the tip catching on side branches and small plaques. As a general principle it is also wise to pass the GW as far distally as possible. This reduces the risk of the wire accidentally coming back across the lesion. With the softer section of the GW distally, more of the stiffer proximal part of the wire will be in the proximal portion of the artery, which will aid tracking of the balloon catheter to and across the lesion.

Wire Introducer

This is a hollow needle-like probe through which an uncovered (by a balloon) guide wire is passed safely into the Y-connector and the guide catheter.

Size of Guide Wires

Guide wires come in different *sizes*, or calibre or thickness. The commonest size is 0.014 inches; 0.018, 0.016, 0.012 and 0.010 inch wires are also used.

Firmness of Guide Wires (Figures 3.3 and 3.4)

The wire coils on the tapered core wire, give the flexible coil its soft, floppy and flexible features. They allow the GW to pass along the often tortuous course of the coronary artery and then to cross the lesion. The flexible coil will buckle or bend when the tip meets resistance, rather than passing into the wall or lifting a plaque of atheroma and causing dissection.

Manufacturers have specific names to indicate the firmness of the GW. For ACS/Guidant guide wires:

High Torque Floppy (HTF)	is the softest and most flexible.
Intermediate	is of moderate firmness.
Standard	is the stiffest version.

For Bard guide wires:

Hi-Per Flex	is the softest.
Flex and Veriflex	are of moderate flexibility.
Standard	is the stiffest or firmest wire.

Other manufacturers have guide wires of varying stiffness and use similar terms. The *standard* GW is used mainly to attempt crossing of a chronic occlusion of a coronary artery, where a firm wire is needed to cross the lesion. The danger with a standard GW lies in its ability to push the wire not through the occlusion, but instead into and along the wall producing a dissection of the vessel wall. It is even possible to perforate the wall, which is virtually unknown with the softer GWs.

The firmness of a GW, especially its shaft, may be used to aid tracking of a balloon catheter. With a circumflex artery arising at a 90° or greater angle to the left main stem (see page 81), it may be difficult to pass a balloon into and down the circumflex vessel; instead the GW may prolapse and loop into the proximal LAD. Changing to a stiffer GW may get over this problem by giving more support and also by partly straightening the out the bend(s) along the vessel. This often happens in the RCA where a tortuous proximal vessel can be clearly seen to be straightened out by the GW.

This aid to tracking is useful for delivering a balloon mounted stent, or an intravascular ultrasound (IVUS) catheter to a lesion. There are specific GWs produced for stent delivery which are similar to the *standard* GWs with a firm central core wire, but have a final 2–3 cm which is similar to that of a High Torque Floppy or Hi-per Flex wire. These GWs are known as '*Extra support or Extra back-up Wires*'. Examples of these wires are Extra-support Platinum Plus from SciMed and the Extra Support High Torque Floppy from ACS. The *S'port* GW from ACS has a distal 3 cm flexible coil of platinum. There are no proximal coils of stainless steel and instead the core wire is reduced over this 20 cm segment to 0.010 inches, whereas the platinum tip is 0.014 inches diameter.

Extra back-up wires may induce spasm of a segment of a coronary artery, especially in the RCA. New 'lesions' may appear away from the target lesion and be worrying. Their benign nature can be confirmed by their relief after intracoronary nitrate injection e.g. 0.1–0.3 mgm of GTN or 1–3 mgm of isosorbide. On withdrawal of the GW at the end of the procedure the lesion(s) also disappear (see Angiograms 11.1 and 13.2, on pages 122 and 152, and page 139).

Radiopacicity of Guide Wires

The common form of GW has the final 2 cm made of coils of platinum or gold, which are radiopaque. The remainder of the flexible coil which has stainless steel coils is poorly

Routine J-Shape

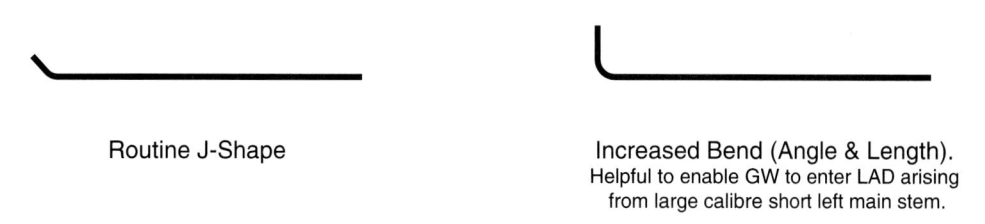

Increased Bend (Angle & Length).
Helpful to enable GW to enter LAD arising
from large calibre short left main stem.

Figure 3.6. Shapes to tip of guide wire.

or non radiopaque. This type of GW will not interfere with assessment of the lesion during the PTCA procedure. Deployment and indentification of a stent is also easier.

Some GWs have the whole of the floppy terminal section (i.e. final 20 cm) radio opaque. This type shows the course of the GW down the coronary artery. It will show any tendency of the GW to buckle on itself if the balloon is having trouble tracking to the lesion. Usually the radiopacicity does not interfere to any extent with assessment of the lesion. One possible exception of this view is when dilating a bifurcation lesion using two wires. With two radiopaque GWs the lesion may be difficult to asses. On the other hand with both GWs radiopaque it is easier to detect if the two GWs become entwined (see page 243 and Angiogram 23.1 on page 246).

Shape of Guide Wire Tip (Figure 3.6)

A bend at the tip of the GW allows it to be manipulated to face a given direction to enter a coronary vessel and pass down it avoiding small side branches. Most operators prefer a straight GW and to fashion their own bend at the tip. Others use a preshaped J-tip, where the final 2–4 mm is bent at a small angle of about 20–30° from the remainder of the terminal section. Preparing the tip and the amount of angle, is part of the 'mystique' of angioplasty and the techniques used vary widely with operators. Basically the wire tip may be drawn over a needle or a finger/thumb nail. The wire may be nipped or bent over a thumb nail. Care is needed to avoid damaging the wire. Sometimes it is necessary to increase the bend from 30° to 60° or even 90° and also to increase the length of the bent section from 3 mm to 5–10 mm. This type of bend may be needed to enter the LAD arising at a right angle off a large and short left main stem (see page 52).

Extension Wires and Exchange Guide Wires

With a GW across a lesion it may be necessary to change the balloon catheter. This is simply done with a rapid exchange balloon, by withdrawing it along the wire and out of the patient. For an OTW (over the wire) balloon catheter the GW runs down the whole length of the catheter and there is only a small amount of GW protruding out of the proximal end of the catheter. This is insufficient and needs to be *extended* to allow the balloon catheter to be withdrawn along the wire and out of the body. An *extension wire* is connected and approximately doubles the length of the GW. Extension wires are 120–140 cm long and have a tapered front end which fits into a hollow hypotube at the docking

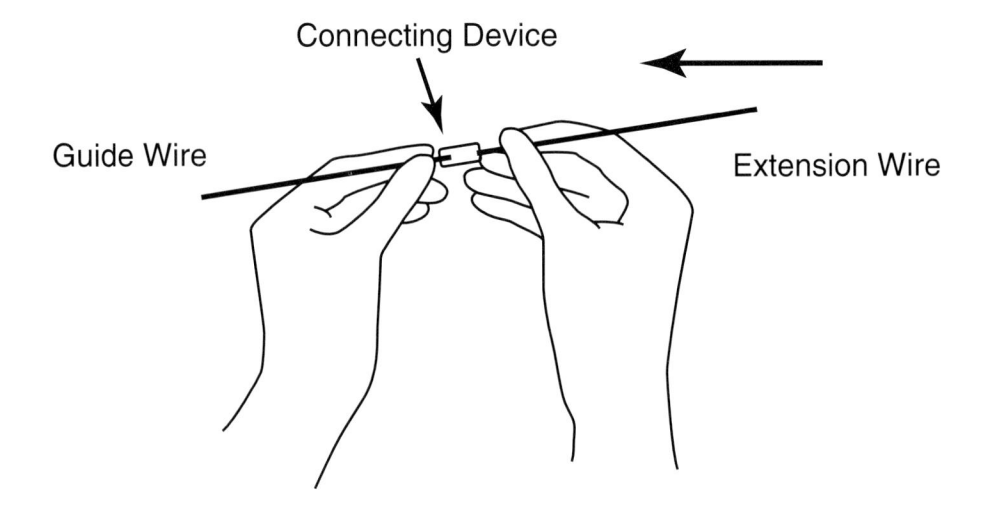

Figure 3.7. Extension wire.

end of the GW, or vice versa, i.e. the proximal end of the GW slips into the start of the extension wire. There is a short sleeve or 'connecting device' to assist the process, which is slipped off the extension wire once the process is complete (Figure 3.7).

An extension wire is very cleverly designed so that once the tapered section is fully within the hypotube, it is locked safely into the GW and will not easily come apart. However once the balloon catheter has been changed, it also possible to separate the two wires, allowing the GW to be more easily manipulated. With the Bard *Linx EZ* (Figure 3.8) system, there are a series of rings on the tapered section of the extension wire, which lock within the hypotube of the GW. To separate the wires the extension wire is unscrewed whilst applying gentle traction. With the Cordis *Cinch* wire (Figure 3.9), the rings are along the wall of the hypotube, into which the 'male' extension wire locks. The docking end section of an ACS GW (Figure 3.10), has a series of snake like curves which are sufficient to lock it within the hypotube port of the *Doc* extension wire. If they need to be separated, slow firm pulling on both wires releases the extension wire. Usually, one manufacturer's extension wire will only work with its own GW.

Before extension wires became available, if a balloon needed to be replaced it was left in position at or near the lesion, the original GW was taken out and replaced by an *exchange guide wire* 300 cm long and then the lesion recrossed. The balloon catheter was withdrawn and finally the new balloon catheter passed to the lesion. This process is slow, tedious and fiddly and runs the risk that the exchange GW may not recross the lesion. The distal end of an exchange GW has the same soft flexible coil of 20–30 cm length possessed by the routine GWs.

Some operators use an exchange GW as their routine GW so that any OTW balloon catheter can easily be replaced. However this leaves over 150 cm of GW outside the balloon which tends to spring about and may become desterilized. Also manipulation of the GW tip of an exchange GW is more difficult than a routine GW. Exchange GWs may be used as the primary GW when deploying coronary stents especially with a stent delivery system using an OTW balloon.

Guide Wire

Extension Wire

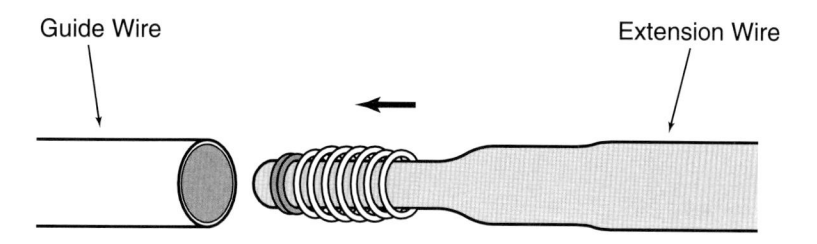

To connect, slide extension wire into hypotube.

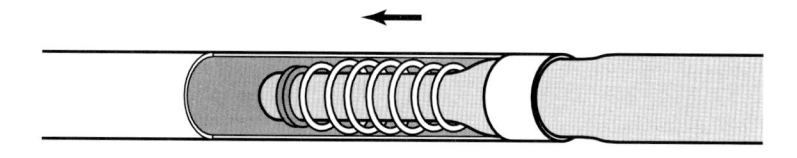

Spring coils elongate when inserted into hypotube.

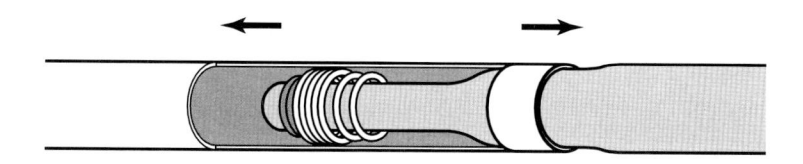

Pullback causes springs to expand, which locks the extension wire against the hypotube wall of the GW.
To disconnect, simultaneously rotate the extension wire counter clockwise and pull.

Figure 3.8. Extension wire (LINX System, Bard).

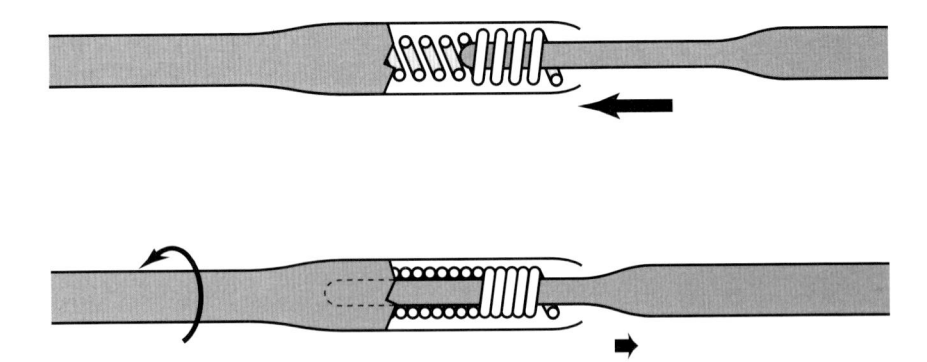

Figure 3.9. Extension wire (Cordis Cinch System).

Alternatives to Extension Wires

Using an extension wire can be slow and fiddly and the tip of the extension wire may become bent and the system then not work. Alternative equipment can secure the GW in position as the balloon catheter is withdrawn.

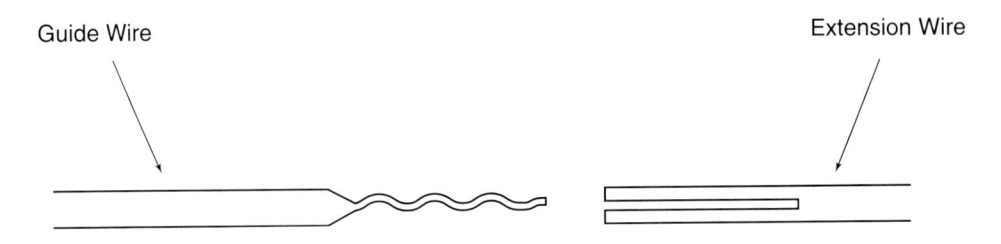

Figure 3.10. Doc extension wire (ACS).

The Trapper (SciMed)

The balloon catheter is withdrawn into the guide catheter as far as possible. A very small second balloon is passed up the guide catheter to beyond the end of the PTCA balloon, but still *within* the guide catheter (Figure 3.11). It is then inflated, trapping the GW against the wall of the guide catheter and allowing the PTCA balloon catheter to be withdrawn.

The Anchor (ACS)

Inside a fine tube made of nitinol, is an even finer wire whose distal end is hook-shaped (Figure 3.12). The proximal end of the wire is connected to a ratchet system. The balloon is withdrawn as much as possible. The anchor system is advanced into the guide catheter and passed to beyond the end of the balloon catheter to reach the GW within the guide catheter. The ratchet is advanced extruding the wire from the tube which then wraps itself

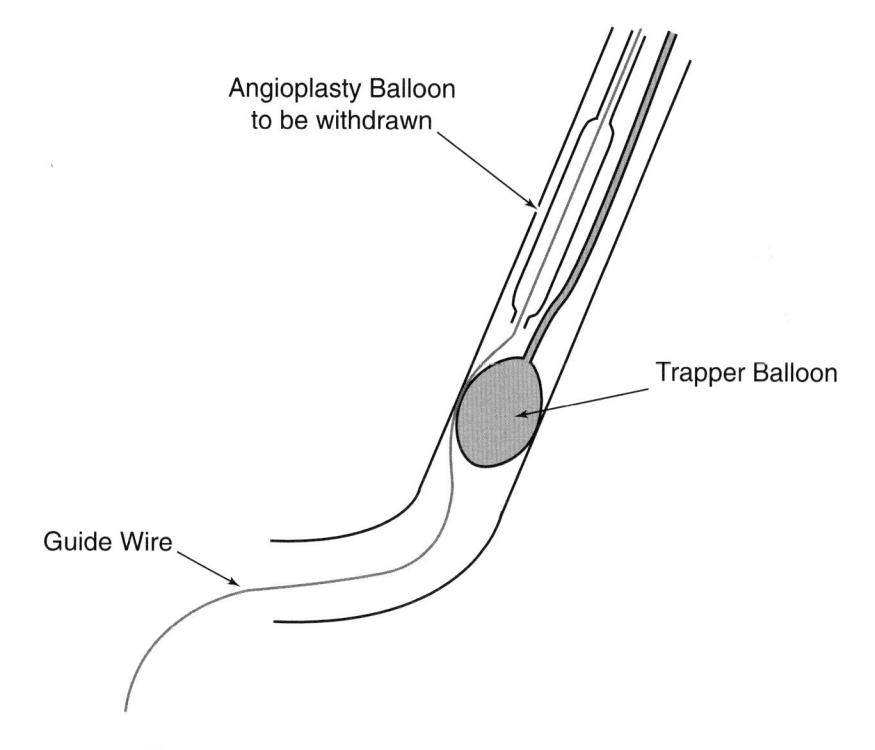

Figure 3.11. The Trapper balloon exchange device (SciMed).

around the GW about 25 times. The GW is anchored and the balloon catheter may be withdrawn.

The Magnet Exchange Device (SciMed)

This device needs a special guide wire which has a magnetic proximal section, such as the SciMed wires, of Graphix, Septor, Transend EY, Choice Plus and Choice PT Plus.

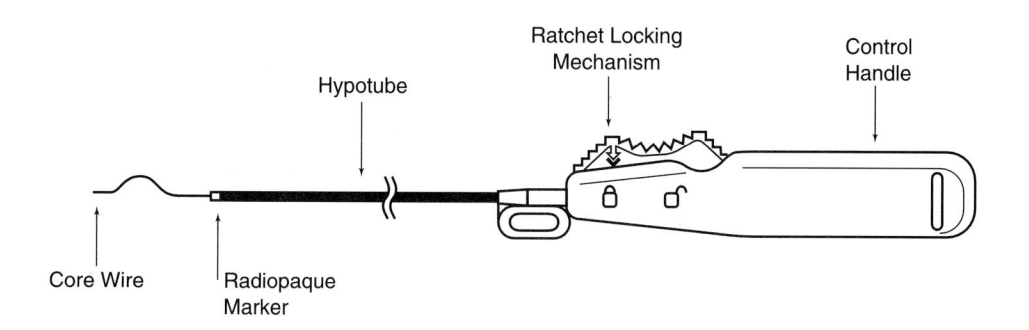

Figure 3.12. Anchor exchange device (ACS).

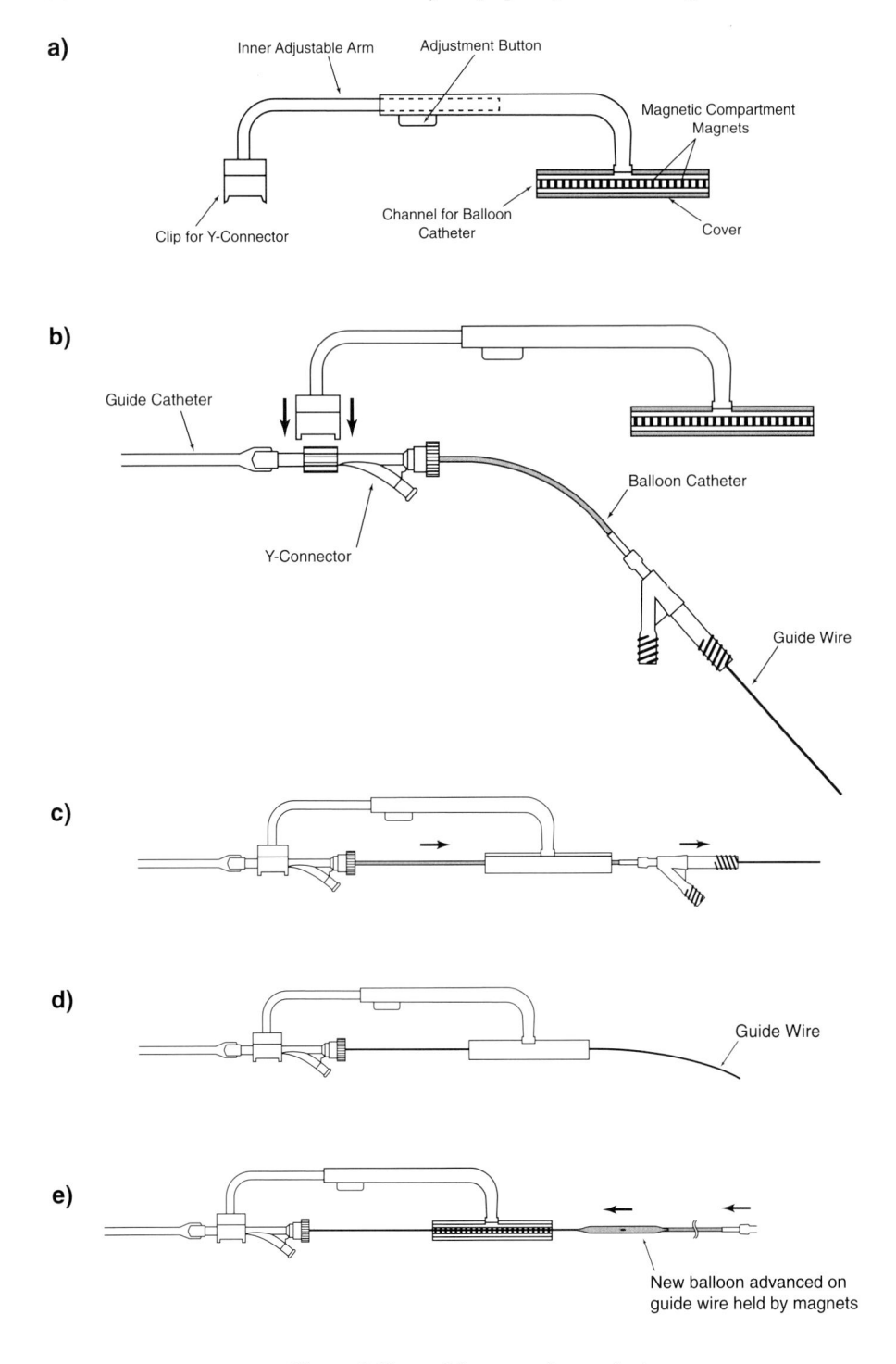

Figure 3.13a–e. Magnet exchange device.

Guide Wires

The device clips onto the Y-connector and the proximal end of the balloon is inserted into the magnetic compartment and the cover closed. The guide wire is then fixed allowing the balloon catheter to be withdrawn and another to be passed back along the wire (Figures 3.13a–e).

The Cumberland technique

This technique has been demonstrated by Professor David Cumberland of Sheffield, England. The GW is advanced as far distally as possible and the balloon catheter withdrawn until the GW end is just within the hub of the balloon catheter. A one ml hypodermic syringe filled with saline is connected to the balloon catheter and the ring of the Y-connector is undone. The saline is injected with moderate force, as the balloon catheter is gently pulled back. Initially there may be some resistance, but after about half the balloon catheter has come out, the remainder will almost whip out with the injection. Incredibly, the GW remains in position, or may come back somewhat. It may be necessary to refill the syringe during the manoeuvre which should be done under screening to check that the GW is not being pulled back. The balloon catheter must be able to run freely along the GW and an 0.014 inch GW in a balloon catheter that can take an 0.018 inch GW (e.g. *Schneider Speedy* balloon) is ideal. With modern lower profile balloons where the GW channel is smaller and will only allow an 0.014 inch (or smaller) GW, this technique rarely works.

Nitinol Wire (*Microvena*)

Instead of stainless steel, the core wire is made of nitinol. The guide wire has very good torque control, even after traversing several bends, e.g. along a tortuous LIMA graft. The size for PTCA is 0.014 inch diameter. The floppy tip (2 or 4 cm length), is radiopaque as it is gold coated.

Magnum Wire (*Schneider*)

This wire was designed by Professor Bernhard Meier of Bern Switzerland to cross chronic occlusions (Figure 3.14). It is a large (0.021 inch) and relatively stiff guide wire. The coiled

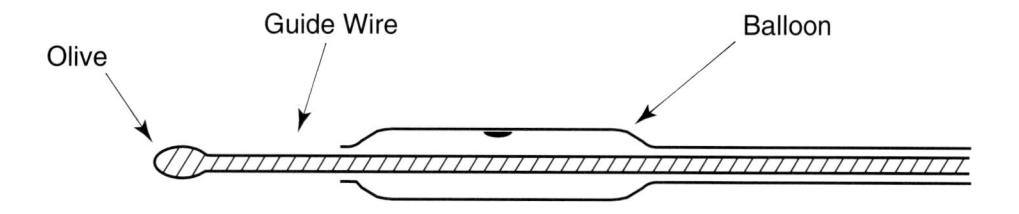

Figure 3.14. Magnum wire and balloon.

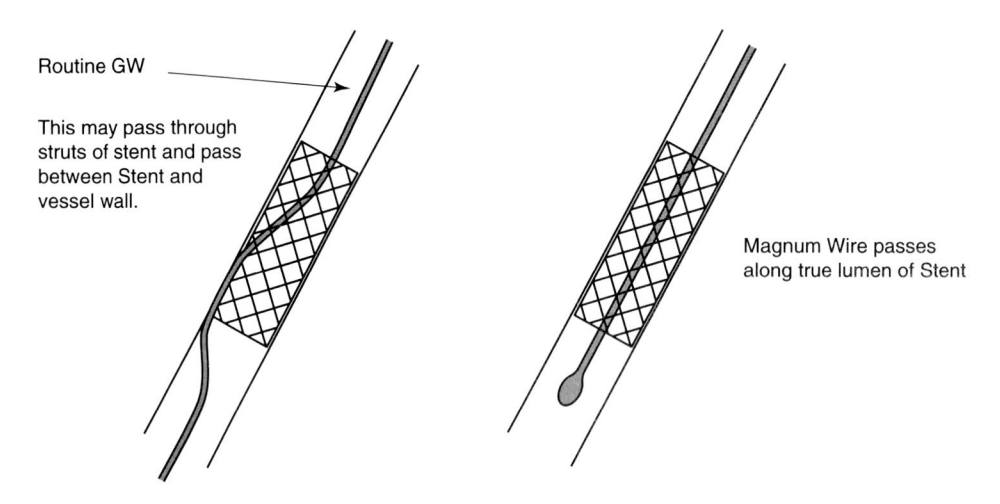

Figure 3.15. Magnum wire used to recross a stent.

section is made from gold plated tungsten and has an expanded olive-shaped tip, one mm in diameter. Special balloons are needed (Magnum, Magnorail) to be compatible with the wire's large diameter. With a chronic total occlusion, firm pressure can be applied to the olive tip, which because of its shape and size tends to pass along the true lumen rather than creating a false channel in the wall. In practice vessel dissection may occur, but the wire will often re-enter the true lumen.

Smaller Magnum wires with diameter of 0.014 and 0.018 inch are also available for use with a wider range of angioplasty balloons. The Magnum wire is useful to recross a stent e.g. after stent thrombosis, as its olive tip is less likely to snag on the struts or pass through the struts between the stent and the vessel wall (Figure 3.15 and see Angiogram 12.1, page 128).

Terumo Wire (*Terumo*)

This GW has two special features:

1. *Core wire of nitinol (nickel-titanium).*
   This gives very good torque control to the GW.
2. *An extremely slippery surface.*
   This is due to a special hydrophilic surface which once in contact with blood (or water) the wire becomes so slippery that it becomes difficult to hold and may slip out of one's hand on to the floor! The wire needs to be soaked before use, by injecting 20 ml of saline into the coiled plastic GW holder and leaving it there for about 3 minutes.

The GW is 0.014 inch in diameter and it has a radiopaque terminal segment made from a platinum-iridium coil.

The GW is useful:

1. To cross chronic occlusions, as it is so slippery.
2. To negotiate very tortuous vessels, e.g. the LIMA artery.

The special problems with the GW are:

1. *Risk of dissection.*
   The GW may easily pass into the vessel wall and along a false channel. This is especially true when used for crossing total occlusions. When used to cross a stenosis, ensure that the distal GW tip is not abutting up against the vessel wall especially in a branch.
2. *Increased risk of fracture of the core wire.*
   Nitinol is more brittle than steel and repeated flexion and rotation movements, especially with the tip stuck in a chronic occlusion, may lead to fracture of the GW.
3. *GW moving forwards with contrast injections.*
   This may occur despite a closed 'O' ring on the Y-connector. This can be prevented by attaching the torquer firmly to the wire just outside the Y-connector.

Pilot Wire *(Bard)*

This wire has a tip which can be deflected or straightened by a device at the proximal end (Figure 3.16). It allows the degree of bend to be varied without removing and reshaping the GW tip. The controlling device (called the commander) is attached to the GW. By sliding the collar away from (or towards) the handle the GW tip is deflected (or straightened). The commander unit can be removed and the GW can also be extended if needed. This GW may be helpful in very tortuous vessels and where the LAD comes off at right angles from a large calibre left main stem. Entry into the LAD may be difficult and frustrating. To enter LAD a large 90° deflection or bend is used. Once in the LAD the bend is reduced to allow the GW to pass easily along the course of the vessel.

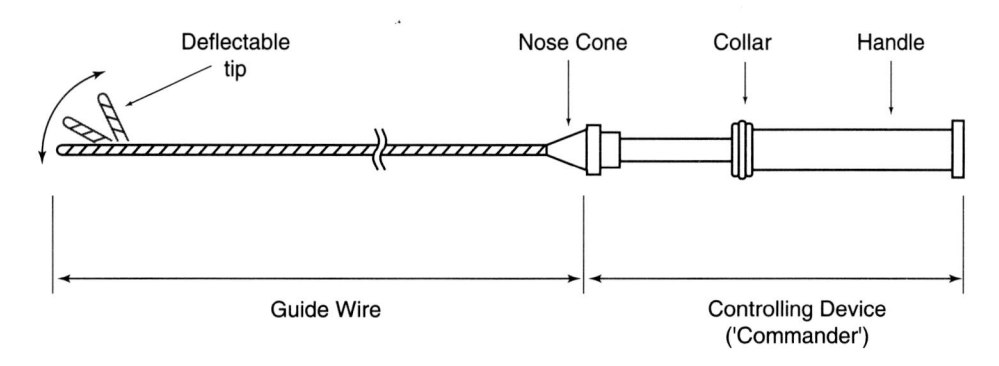

Figure 3.16. Pilot wire (Bard).

Dual Use Guide Wires

The primary use of a GW is to act as a rail along which the balloon catheter will pass to and across the lesion. Some GWs can also perform other functions.

1. **Pressure wire**
   This has a pressure manometer a short distance back from its tip, which allows recording of the pressure beyond the lesion. A number of versions are under development.
2. **Doppler wire** (*FloWire, Cardiometrics*)
   This allows the recording of doppler ultrasound to give a measurement of coronary blood flow. The recording can be done at rest and after a vasodilator to increase coronary flow. After intracoronary adenosine in the normal vessel, coronary flow should increase by a ratio of 2:1 or more, compared to the control value. The ratio is termed the *coronary flow reserve*.
3. **IVUS (intravascular ultrasound) wire**
   A number of research projects to produce these are in progress. One version consists of a hollow tube which slips over the routine GW acting as a fine IVUS catheter sleeve.

Other Interventional Equipment

There are specific GWs as part of the equipment for atherectomy, *Rotablator*, *Rotacs* and some *laser* systems. These GWs are usually firmer and less easy to manipulate than the routine GWs.

Conclusion

The great majority of PTCAs can be done with a routine 0.014 inch soft tip GW. Become familiar with one or two wires, which will be your 'work horse' wire(s). Since the advent of stents, extra support wires have become popular but are more likely to induce coronary artery spasm. Firmer wires are needed to cross chronic occlusions.

Rapid exchange balloon catheters have simplified the use of guide wires so that extension and exchange wires are no longer needed to change a balloon catheter. Rapid exchange balloons also allow the operator to manipulate and be 'in charge' of the GW at all times ... if the wire comes back or is displaced, the operator has only himself, or herself, to blame!

4 Radiographic Views

To obtain good results from PTCA, the following are needed:

1. *Good radiographic equipment:*
   usually single plane is sufficient.
2. *Competent catheter room team:*
   of nurses, radiographers and physiological measurement technicians. Don't forget to thank them, and remind them of their valued important role.
3. *Good radiographic views:*
   to see the lesion well.

Radiographic Views

There are major differences between the approach and the detail needed for diagnostic angiography compared to that for PTCA. In the former, angiography is required to show the extent of disease to allow a decision on management by medical treatment, surgery, or angioplasty. For PTCA, the demands on angiography are greater. The aim of angiography for PTCA is to show a vessel or section of a vessel with a stenosis, so as to clearly define the severity, complexity and length of the stenosis. The lesion needs to be shown:

a) in two planes at right angles.
b) with the minimum of foreshortening.
c) with the least vessel overlap by other coronary artery branches.

Foreshortening (Figures 4.1 and 4.2)

This occurs when part of the vessel is not viewed at right angles to the X-ray beam. A lesion will often appear shorter and more severe. Using the radiographic projection which

42 *Guide to Coronary Angioplasty and Stenting*

X-Ray beam at 90°

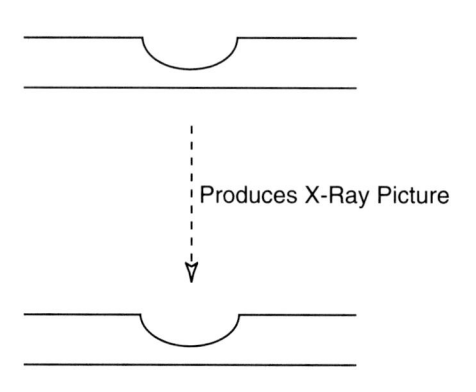

Produces X-Ray Picture

Satisfactory image.
Little or no foreshortening.

Figure 4.1. Direction of X-Ray beam, and amount of foreshortening.

X-Ray beam at an angle

Produces X-Ray Picture

Foreshortened view.
Lesion shorter, and more severe.

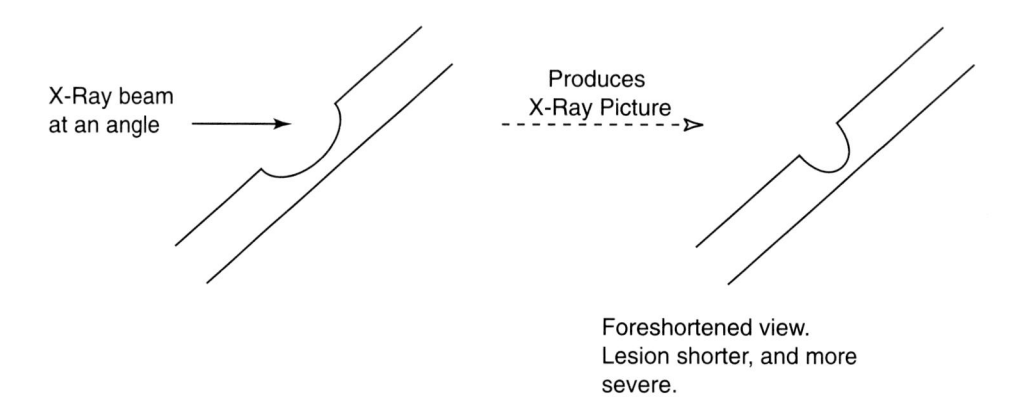

Figure 4.2. Direction of X-Ray beam, and amount of foreshortening.

has the least foreshortening, allows the best assessment of the lesion's severity, complexity and length.

Limitations of Angiography

It is increasingly appreciated that angiography has its limitations and may give a false impression of the lesion's severity, especially after angioplasty has been performed. Angiography studies the lumen, which is only a mirror of pathological events in the wall of the artery, which are better defined by intravascular ultrasound, IVUS. (See also Chapter 5 on IVUS).

Primary and Back-up Views

Often with PTCA, one projection or view is mainly used during the procedure. This *primary view* shows the vessel and the lesion well. The intensifier is moved to 1–3 *back-up views* to confirm satisfactory progress, particularly at the end of the procedure. One of the back-up views will usually be orthogonal (approximately at right angles) to the primary view.

Suggested Views

The recommended values, such as for LAO cranial (LAO 50°, cranial 25°) are average ones and sometimes 5 to 10° on either side, may give a better angiographic image. The image may be clearer or have less vessel overlay at the arterial segment of interest.

Right Coronary Artery

This is the easier vessel to assess, as unlike the LCA there is usually not a problem of overlying branches obscuring the lesion. Three or four views usually suffice and these may include:

1. *LAO 30°–50°*
   (LAO = Left Anterior Oblique)
   This shows the proximal and mid portions of the vessel (Figure 4.3). Using the shallower projection LAO 30°, rather than LAO 40°–50° the diaphragm is well below this part of the RCA and will not obscure it. It is not necessary for patient to take repeated deep inspirations to clear the diaphragm.
   With the shallow LAO view the patient can usually have both arms by the side, which is more comfortable than keeping them above the head.
2. *LAO Cranial (LAO 50°, Cranial 25°)*
   This view (Figure 4.4) demonstrates the distal third of the main RCA, the bifurcation and the two terminal branches, posterior descending artery (PDA) and the atrio-ventricular branch (or posterior left ventricular branch). These parts of the RCA are

Atrial Branch

Marginal Branch

Diaphragm

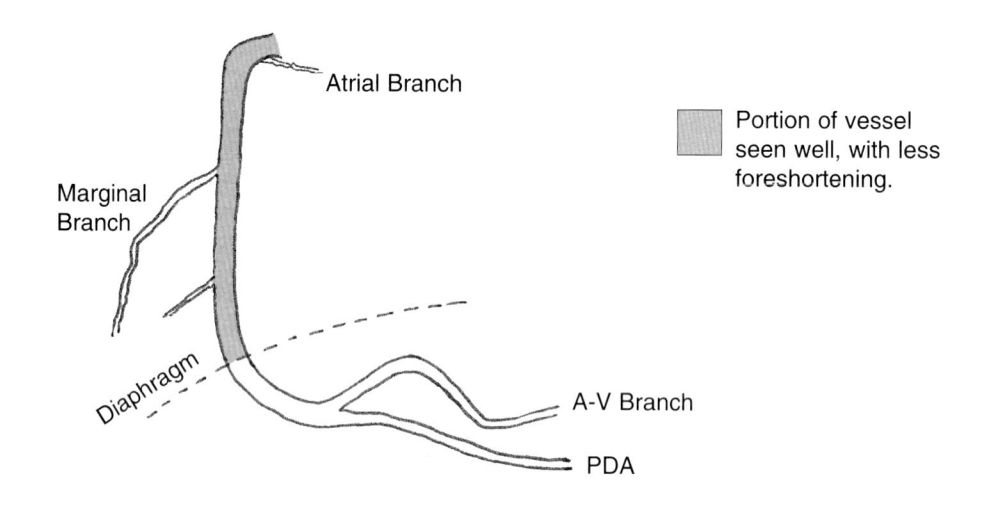

A-V Branch

PDA

Portion of vessel seen well, with less foreshortening.

A-V Branch = Atrio-Ventricular Branch

PDA = Posterior Descending Artery

Figure 4.3. RCA, LAO 30° (shallow LAO) projection.

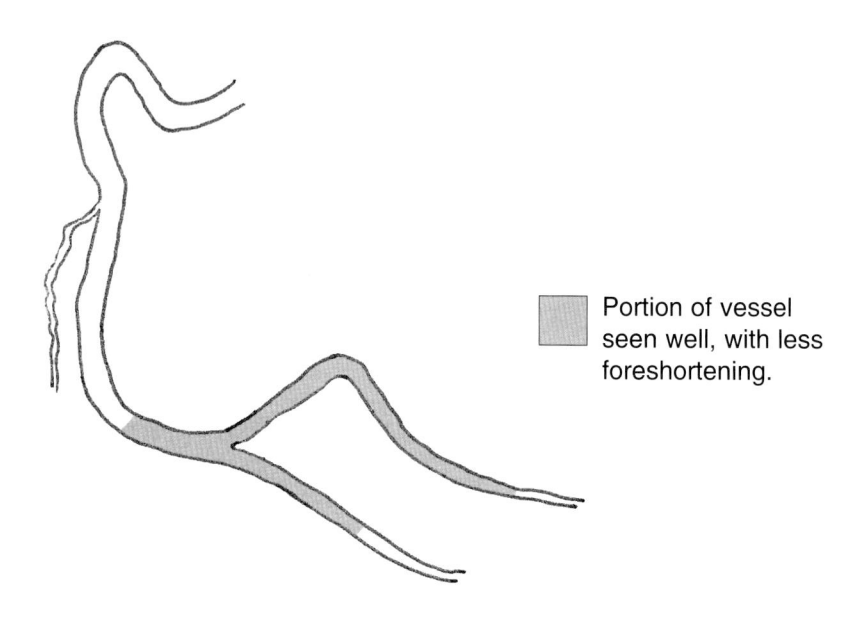

Portion of vessel seen well, with less foreshortening.

Figure 4.4. RCA, LAO Cranial view.

Radiographic Views 45

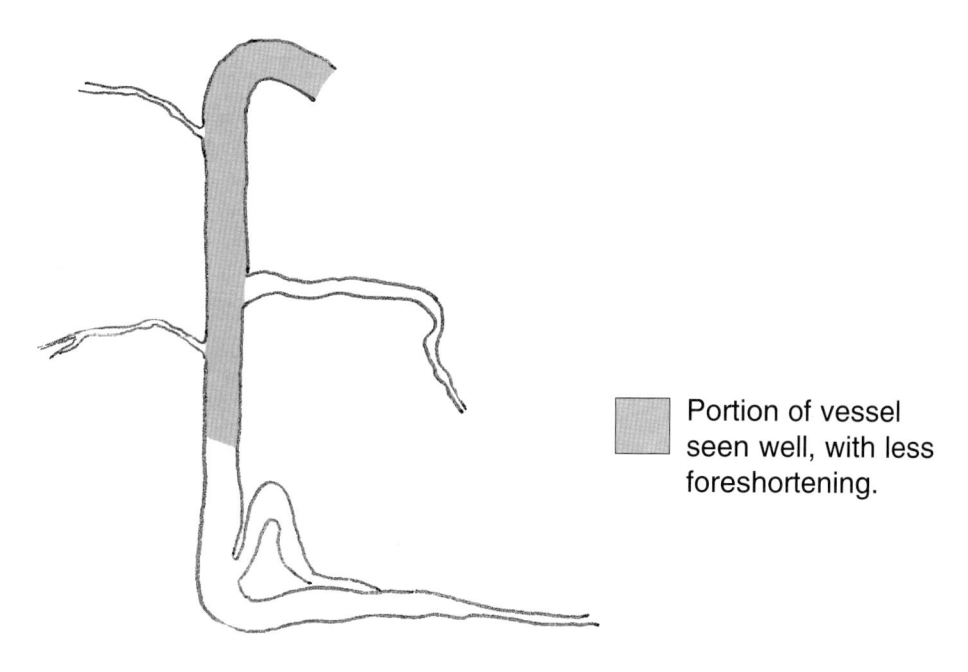

Figure 4.5. RCA, RAO 30° projection.

Portion of vessel seen well, with less foreshortening.

usually below the diaphragm, even when a deep inspiration is taken. Sometimes it is better to screen with the patient breathing quietly when all the distal part of the RCA is below the diaphragm. There is less glare from the X-ray equipment recording above and below the diaphragm. However the radiation dose to the patient will be slightly greater.

3. *RAO 30°, PA, or RAO Caudal (RAO 40°, Caudal 20°)*
   (RAO = right anterior oblique. PA = postero-anterior)
   These views all show the RCA, but usually less clearly than the LAO projection. The RAO 30° shows well the mid-portion or body of the RCA (Figure 4.5). The RCA caudal may show the bifurcation clearly. On X-ray screening these views, especially the RAO 30° have considerable side-to-side movement as the RCA runs down the atrio-ventricular groove. This makes lesion assessment and passage of the guide wire and balloon more difficult. The operator may even begin to feel sea sick, especially if magnified or zoom fields are used!

   For RCA the LAO is the primary view where most of the PTCA procedure is done, with RAO and PA as back-up views.

Left Coronary Artery

Difficulties in Demonstrating LCA Lesions:

The LCA divides into LAD and LCX arteries, with the LAD passing along the front of the heart and the diagonal and circumflex artery passing along the back. Sometimes the left main stem (LMS) trifurcates with an intermediate artery passing to the back of the heart, equivalent to a very early obtuse marginal branch. The vessels often overlie each other obscuring the lesion to be dilated. When reviewing the *diagnostic angiogram* select the view(s) which should be the most suitable. With the *control angiogram* at the start of PTCA try first your selected view. However it will often be necessary to experiment to find the best view, a compromise between avoiding vessel overlap and foreshortening.

The radiographic views for the LCA will be considered separately for each of the branches of the LCA:

1. *Left main stem.*
2. *Circumflex artery.*
3. *Intermediate artery.*
4. *Left anterior descending artery.*

1. Left Main Stem (LMS)

The LMS curves downwards, forwards and to the right which makes it difficult to show. The PA, RAO caudal (RAO 40°, Caudal 20°), LAO caudal (LAO 60°, Caudal 20°) and LAO cranial (LAO 50°, Cranial 25°) views are the best ones to show the LMS. Sometimes the LAO 70°–80° and left lateral projections may show it well.

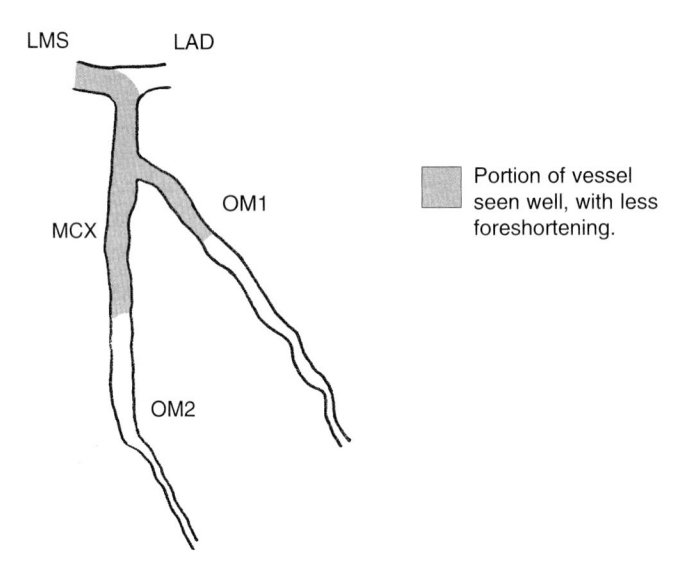

LMS = Left Main Stem
LAD = Left Anterior Descending Artery
MCX = Main Circumflex Artery
OM = Obtuse Marginal Branch

Figure 4.6. LCX, PA view.

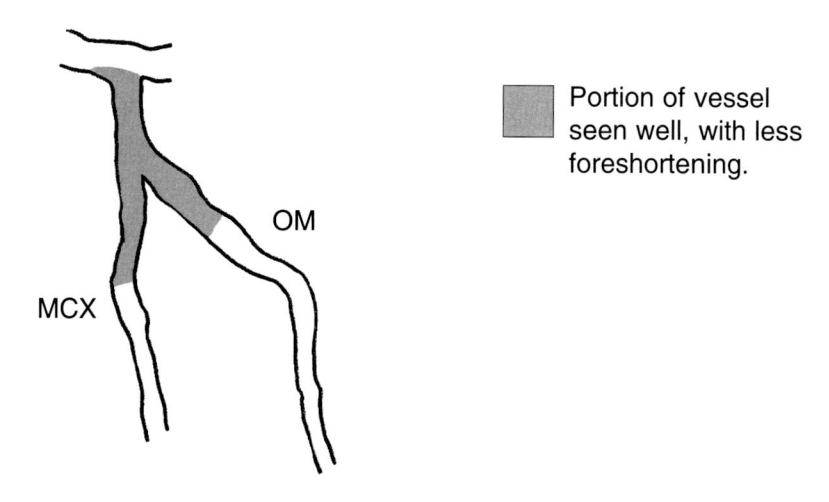

Figure 4.7. LCX, RAO Caudal view.

2. Circumflex Artery (LCX) (Figures 4.6 – 4.9)

The main circumflex and obtuse marginal branches are shown well in RAO caudal (RAO 30°–40°, Caudal 20°), PA and LAO caudal (LAO 60°, Caudal 20°) views. Sometimes a shallow RAO caudal (RAO 20°, Caudal 10°) may be very satisfactory.

The LAO caudal view (Figure 4.8) is less easy to work in, as the x-rays pass through the liver and the picture on fluoroscopy is relatively darker, more hazy and less clear, (see Angiograms 6.1 and 8.2 on pages 71 and 94). LAO 70°, LAO cranial (LAO 50°, Cranial 25°) and left lateral views may all sometimes show the LCX Artery.

The RAO caudal or PA is usually the primary view, with the others as back-up views for the LCX artery, (see Angiogram 13.2, page 152).

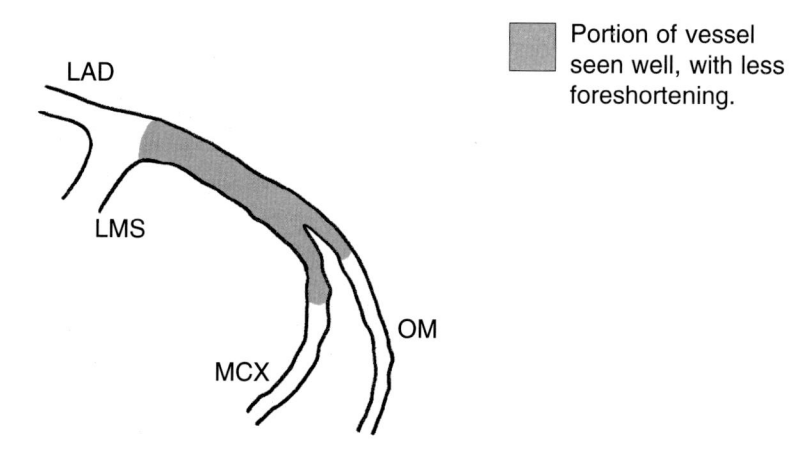

Figure 4.8. LCX, LAO Caudal view.

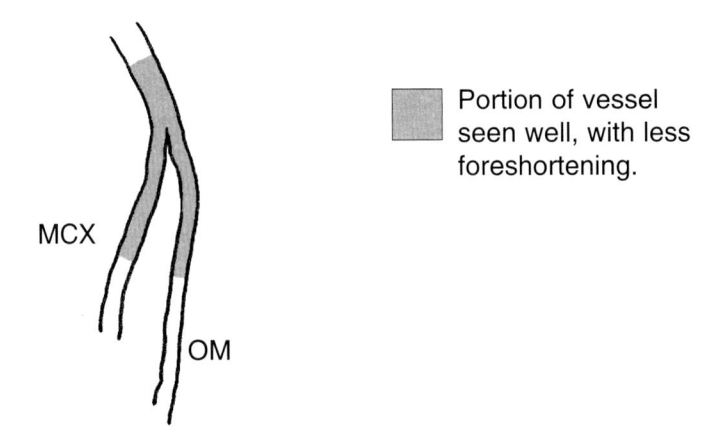

Figure 4.9. LCX, Lt. Lateral, or LAO 70° projection.

With a very dominant LCX passing all the way down the atrio-ventricular groove, the terminal branches are equivalent to the atrio-ventricular branch or the posterior descending artery of RCA. The LAO cranial view may show these vessels best.

3. Intermediate Artery (Figure 4.10)

Circumflex artery views are satisfactory, i.e. RAO caudal, PA, LAO caudal and LAO 70°. Usually there is good visualization of the intermediate artery.

4. The Left Anterior Descending Artery (LAD)

The LAD is the commonest artery to be dilated and lesions on it are often well seen in several views. However in about a third of cases, there is a problem of overlap of the lesion by the diagonal or obtuse marginal branches. Sometimes it can be a considerable challenge to demonstrate a LAD lesion adequately for PTCA and some compromise may be needed.

The views to show the LAD will be divided into the RAO, LAO and PA.

RAO Views (RAO = right anterior oblique)

RAO Caudal (RAO 40°, Caudal 20°) [Figures 4.11 and 4.12]

This view is often very helpful for the LAD, especially to show its proximal and middle thirds with minimal foreshortening. The LMS is also well seen and the RAO caudal view will show if the guide catheter starts to back out, when there is resistance to cross a lesion with the balloon catheter.

Radiographic Views 49

LAD
Intermediate A
LMS
LCX
LAO Caudal

LAD
LCX
Intermediate A
RAO Caudal

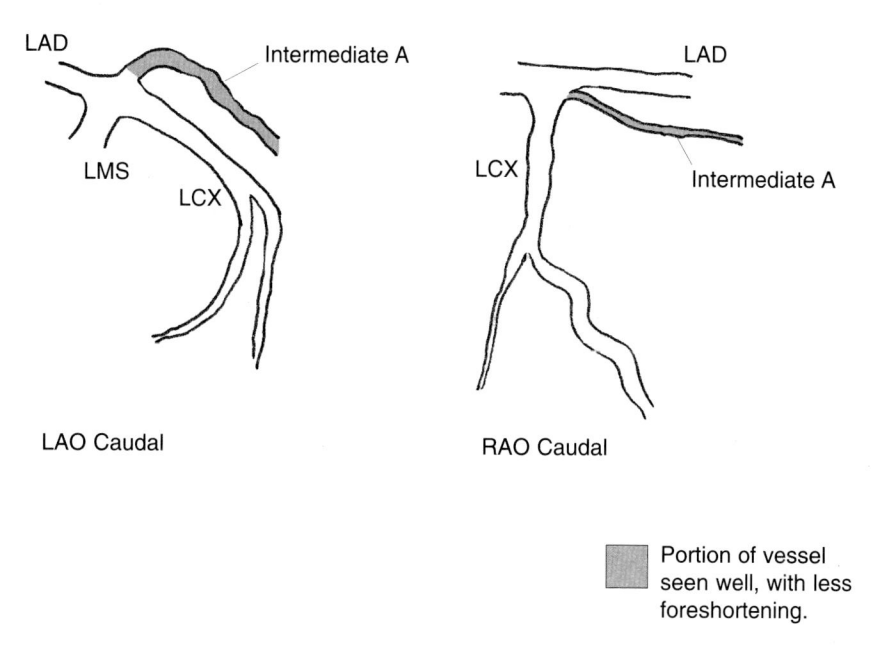

▨ Portion of vessel seen well, with less foreshortening.

Figure 4.10. Intermediate artery.

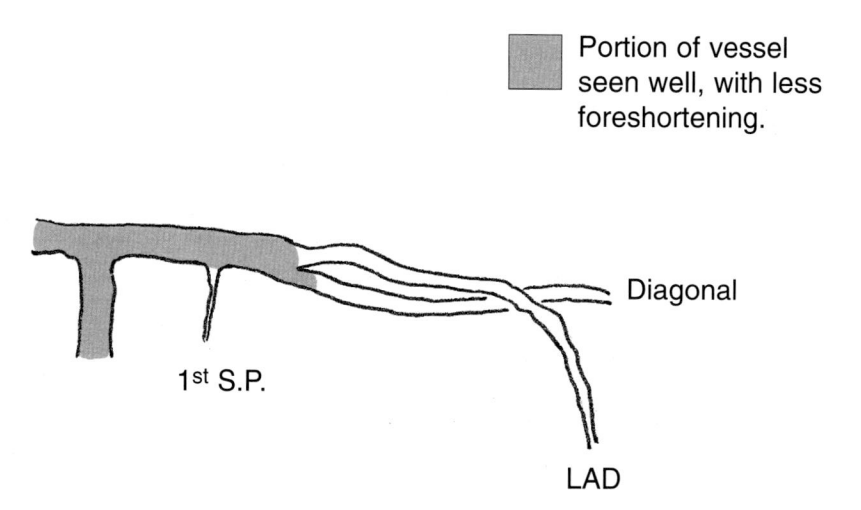

▨ Portion of vessel seen well, with less foreshortening.

Diagonal
1st S.P.
LAD

1st S.P. = First or Major Septal Perforator

Figure 4.11. LAD, RAO Caudal view.

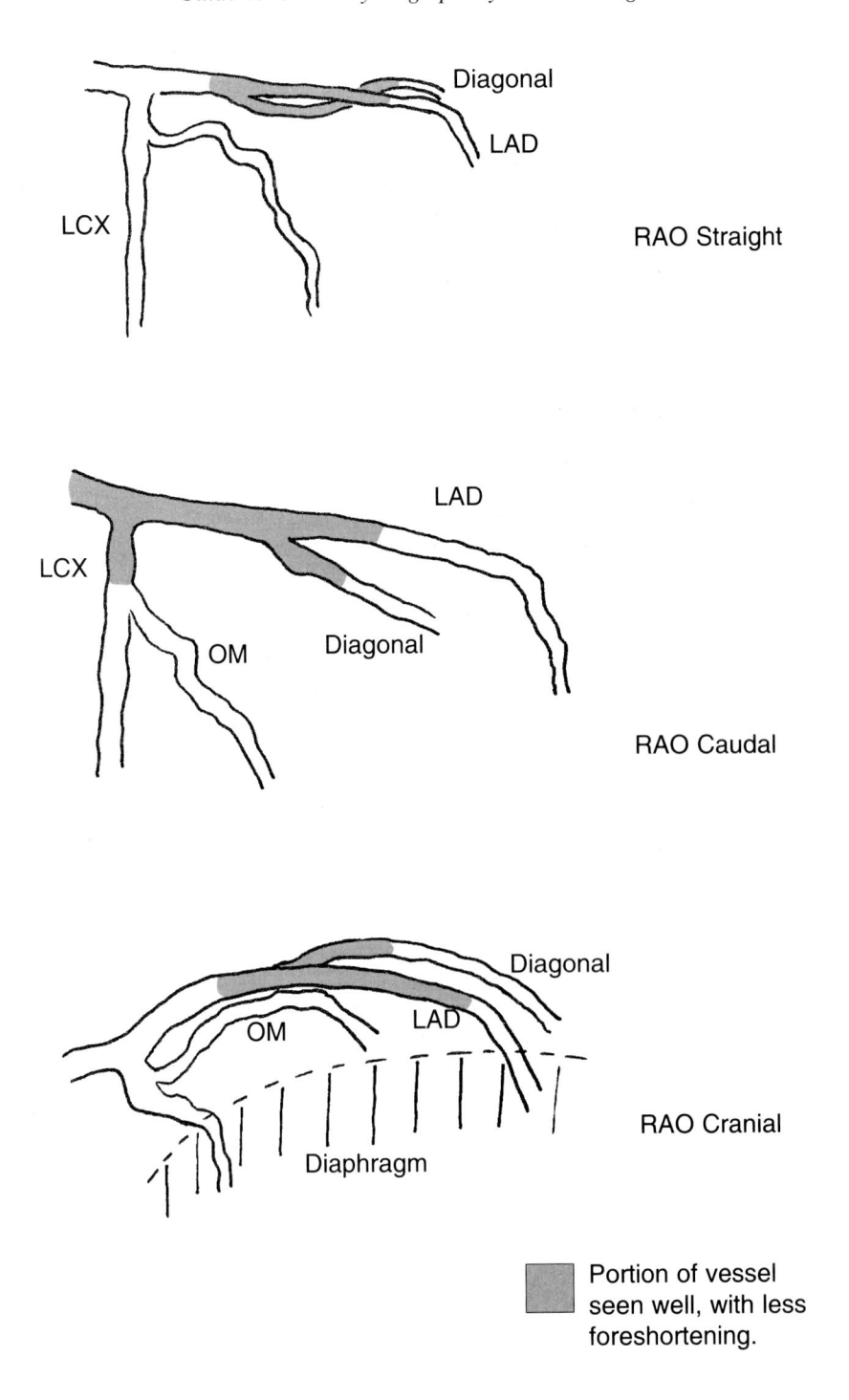

Figure 4.12. Relation of Diagonal and OM branches to LAD in RAO views.

Radiographic Views 51

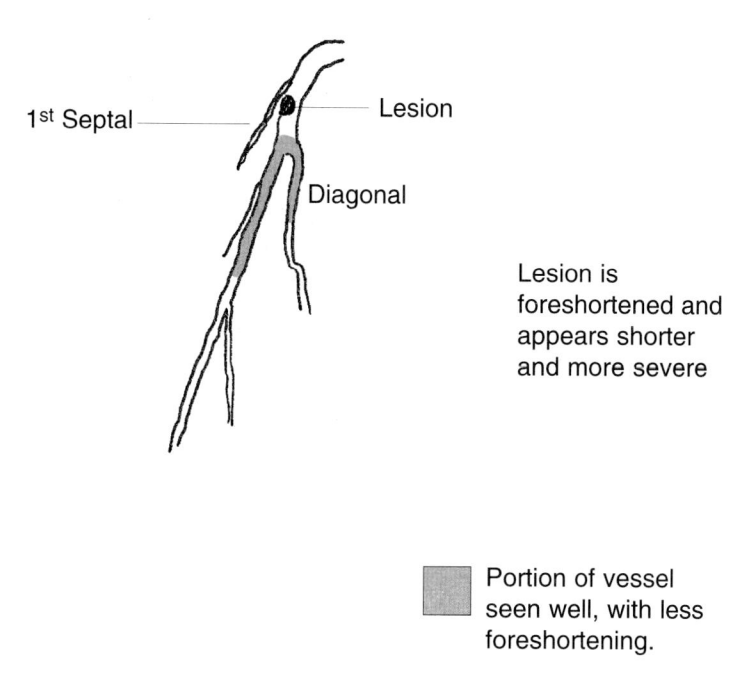

Figure 4.13. LAD, LAO Cranial view.

[Labels in figure: 1st Septal, Lesion, Diagonal. "Lesion is foreshortened and appears shorter and more severe". "Portion of vessel seen well, with less foreshortening."]

The guide catheter can be observed whilst it is advanced further along the LCA and even into the proximal LAD, to give more guide catheter support to cross the lesion with the balloon. The view shows well the origin of the LAD allowing an osteal lesion to be assessed. The projection will usually allow a guide wire to be seen to enter LAD as opposed to the circumflex artery.

Compared with the RAO 30° (i.e. a straight RAO without caudal or cranial angulation):
the RAO caudal view tends to *lower* OM and diagonal branches *below* the LAD,
the RAO cranial view tends to *raise* OM and diagonal branches *above* the LAD (see Figure 4.12 and Angiogram 23.1 on page 246).
The RAO caudal view shows the proximal 1/3rd of the LAD with minimal foreshortening.

RAO Straight (RAO 30°) [Figure 4.12]

This view is used less often. OM and diagonal branches frequently overlie the LAD.

RAO Cranial (RAO 40°, Cranial 25°)

This view shows well the more distal section of the proximal LAD and the middle third of the vessel. It is particularly helpful to show the origin of a diagonal branch when it arises in the proximal third of the LAD (Figure 4.12). The RAO cranial view is valuable to assess the extent of a 'bifurcation lesion' i.e. whether or not the lesion involves each of the LAD and diagonal branches. Similarly, if a 'two wire technique' is needed, then this view can be used to pass one guide wire into each of the branches (see pages 242 and 245 and Angiogram 23.1 on page 246).

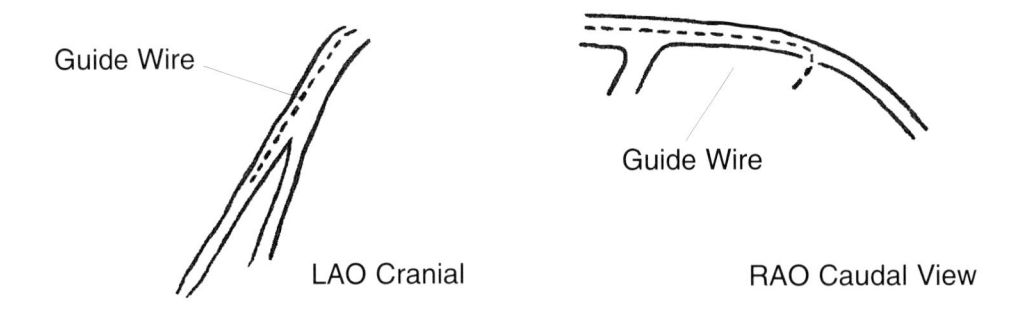

Figure 4.14. Guide wire passing into septal perforator instead of along LAD.

The snag of the RAO cranial view is that the diaphragm often overlies the heart and the patient needs to take a deep inspiration each time to view the vessels clearly.

LAO Views

LAO Cranial (LAO 50°, Cranial 25°)

This view shows most of the LAD, especially its proximal half. The diagonal branches are posterior, and the septal perforators are anterior to the LAD, and their origins are well seen. Usually this is the best view to pass a guide wire into a diagonal branch. It is a very helpful projection for a bifurcation lesion when using a 'two wire technique' to pass a guide wire into each of the LAD and diagonal branches.

The disadvantages of the LAO cranial view are:

1. Considerable foreshortening for the proximal LAD, so that a lesion appears shorter and more severe.
2. The origin and first 1–2 cm of the LAD are poorly seen, or not seen at all. The behaviour of the guide catheter cannot be assessed during attempted balloon crossing of the lesion (see RAO caudal view).
3. The diaphragm crosses the vessels so that the patient usually needs to take a deep inspiration to see the vessels clearly.
4. Sometimes confusion can occur between the LAD and a septal perforating branch running parallel or in the same plane as the LAD. A guide wire may seem to have passed along the LAD and then get stuck. By changing to an RAO view the guide wire can be seen to have passed (usually at right angles) down and below the LAD into the interventricular septum (see Figure 4.14).

LAO Caudal view (LAO 60° Caudal 20°) [Figure 4.15]

This view is also known as the '*spider view*' or '*up the barrel*' (of a gun) view. The LAO caudal view clearly shows the LMS and its bifurcation into LAD and LCX. The LAD passes to the left, the circumflex to the right. It can be a very helpful view if there is difficulty passing the guide wire from LMS into the LAD (see page 31). The diagonal

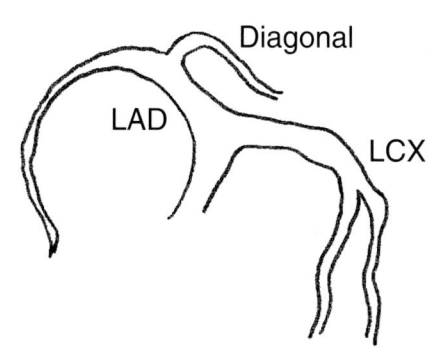

Figure 4.15. LAD, LAO Caudal view.

branch courses backwards and to the right. There is considerable foreshortening of the LAD and also haziness as X-rays pass through the liver to give this view. The LAO caudal view is not a primary view for LAD lesions, but can be a useful backup one.

Left Lateral (sometimes with Cranial 5–15°)

This view (Figure 4.16 and see Angiograms 8.1, 10.1, and 23.1, on pages 90, 106 and 246) is useful to show the:

1. Very early part of LAD, which is often shown better than on the LAO cranial view.
2. Proximal and mid portions of LAD. Often there is less foreshortening than the LAO cranial view.

The diaphragm tends to obscure the LAD and it is usually necessary for the patient to

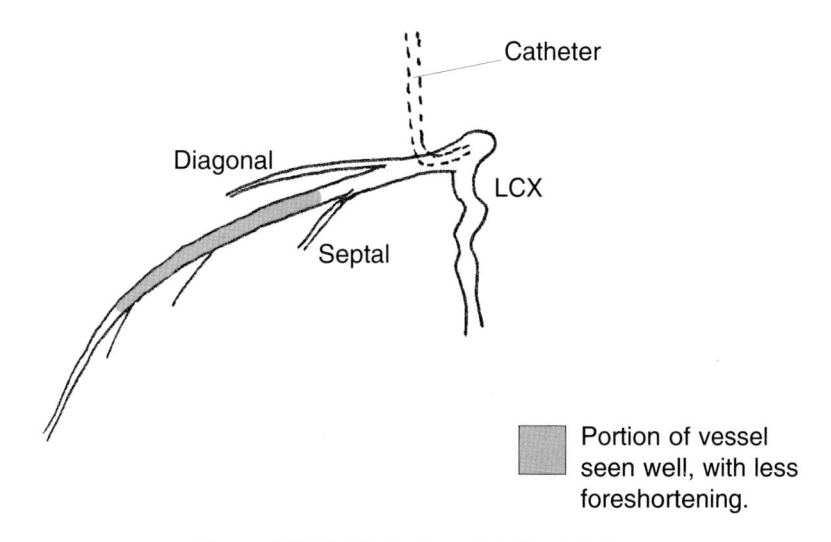

Figure 4.16. LAD, Lt Lateral ± Cranial view.

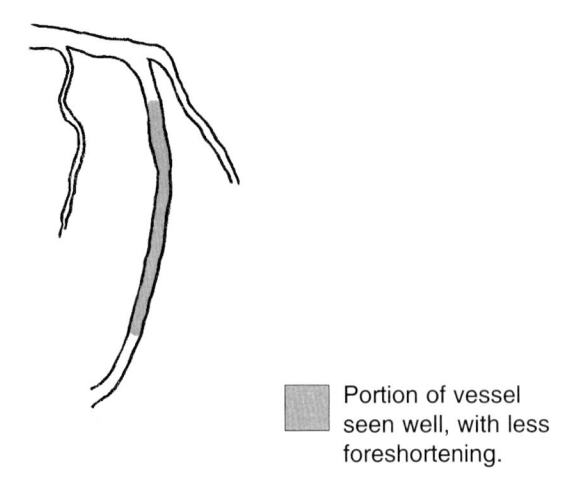

Figure 4.17. LAD, PA view.

(legend: Portion of vessel seen well, with less foreshortening.)

take a deep inspiration with this view.

PA View (Figure 4.17)

This is a very useful backup view to confirm that the vessel entered with a guide wire is indeed the LAD. In the PA view, the LAD runs straight down the centre of the heart. *No other vessel does this.*

There is moderate foreshortening of the proximal LAD in this view.

Other Views for the LAD (Figure 4.18, see Angiogram 8.1, page 90)

Shallow LAO Cranial (LAO 20°–35°, Cranial 35°), PA Cranial (Cranial 20°–30°) and shallow RAO Cranial (RAO 15°, Cranial 15°–25°).

These views are used less commonly and are tried when the standard views are unsatisfactory, with overlap of an LAD lesion by other vessels. By trial and error, a view may be found which shows the LAD lesion or a diagonal branch clearly.

With each of these views there is moderate foreshortening and sections of the LAD will be obscured by other vessels crossing it. The shallow LAO cranial and the AP cranial can be relatively dark as the LAD overlies the spine.

Summary of the Radiographic Views for RCA and LCA during Angioplasty

The radiographic projections used are to some extent personal preferences and most operators have one or more 'favourite' views. Sometimes a view can be either a primary or back-up one, depending on local anatomy. Remember that the recommended values,

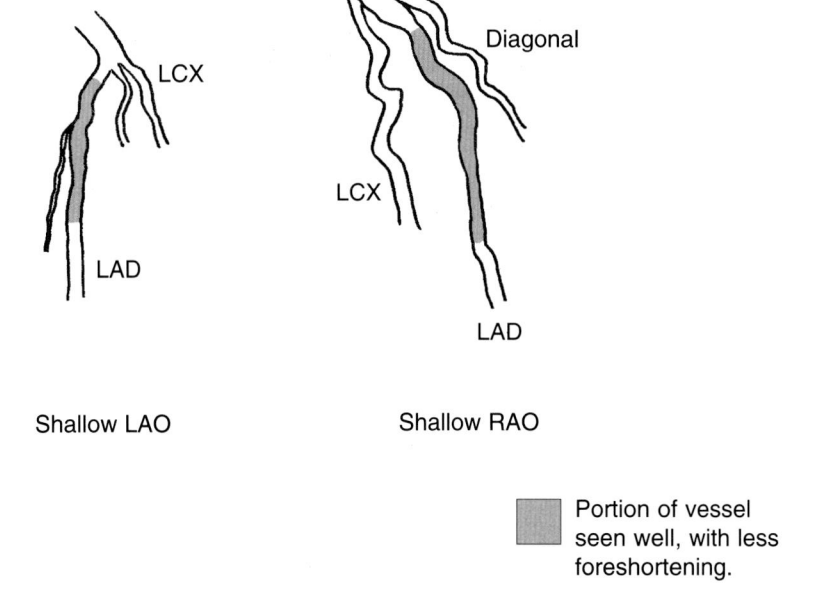

Figure 4.18. LAD, shallow LAO & RAO Cranial views.

such as RAO Caudal of RAO 40° and Caudal 20°, are average ones. With individual cases the projections may vary by 5–10° to obtain the clearest picture. The radiographic views for angioplasty may be summarized as:

Left Coronary Artery:

	Primary Views	**Back-up Views**
Left Main Stem	RAO Caudal LAO Caudal PA	Left Lateral
LAD/Diagonal	RAO Caudal LAO Cranial Left Lateral ± Cranial	LAO Caudal RAO Cranial LAO Cranial Shallow LAO Cranial Shallow RAO Cranial PA Cranial
LCX/Intermediate	PA RAO Caudal LAO Caudal	LAO Caudal LAO 70° LAO Cranial Left Lateral
Right Coronary Artery	LAO 30–50° LAO Cranial	RAO 30° PA RAO Caudal

The Projections for the Radiographic Views are:

RAO Caudal	RAO 40°	Caudal 20°
RAO Cranial	RAO 40°	Cranial 25°
RAO (straight)	RAO 30°	
Shallow RAO Caudal	RAO 20°	Caudal 10°
Shallow RAO Cranial	RAO 15°	Cranial 15°–25°
LAO Cranial	LAO 50°	Cranial 25°
LAO Caudal	LAO 60°	Caudal 20°
Shallow LAO Cranial	LAO 20°–35°	Cranial 35°
LAO (straight)	LAO 30°–70°	
Left Lateral ± Cranial	LAO 80°–90°	Cranial 5°–15°
PA Cranial	PA	Cranial 20°–30°

Saphenous Vein Grafts (Figures 4.19–4.22, see Angiograms 20.1 and 20.2 on pages 212 and 217)

A vein graft can usually be entered and the osteum shown in LAO 40°–70° and RAO 30°–40° projections. Take careful note, when assessing a previous diagnostic angiogram, of the relationship between the origin of vein grafts and sternal wires, which can be helpful landmarks to find the grafts again. The initial part and body of vein grafts are usually well seen in LAO 40–70°, RAO 30–50°, RAO caudal and PA views. It is often necessary to experiment to find a view that shows the graft lesion well with the minimum of foreshortening. At least with vein grafts there is not a problem of overlying vessels!

The anastomosis site between graft and native coronary artery is a common site for early graft stenosis, 1–6 months after CABG (see Chapter 20). The standard views of the coronary artery concerned should be used to view the anastomosis.

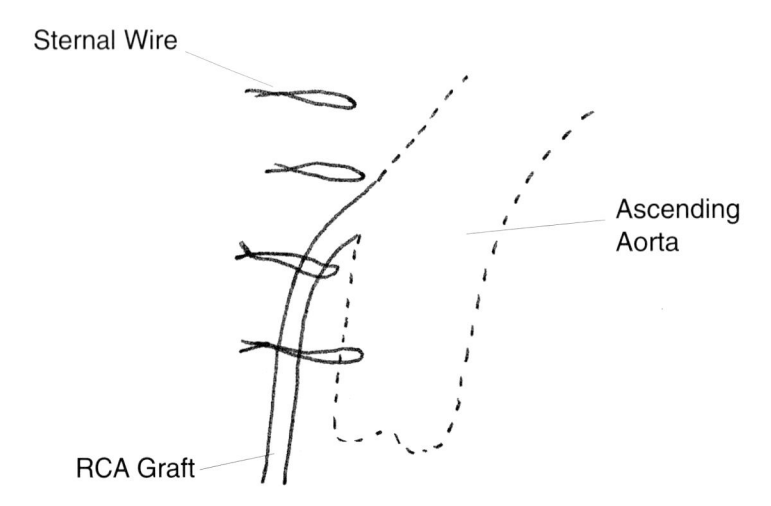

Figure 4.19. RCA Graft, LAO projection. Note sternal wires which can be helpful to locate osteum of saphenous vein graft.

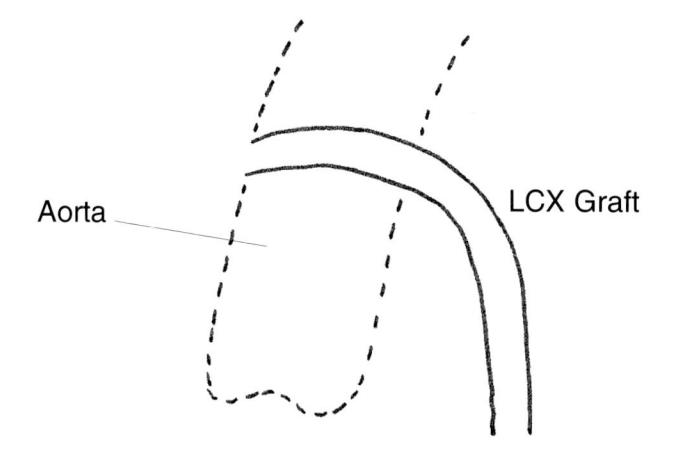

Figure 4.20. LCX Graft, LAO view.

LIMA and RIMA Grafts (Left and Right Internal Mammary Artery Grafts)

PTCA is relatively infrequent for these grafts, except for an early post CABG (1–6 months) stenosis at the anastomosis site with the native coronary artery. The lesion, usually a surgical technical problem, responds well to PTCA. The anastomosis is viewed using the standard projections for the coronary artery involved. For the LIMA and LAD, the left lateral, LAO cranial and RAO caudal projections are usually helpful views.

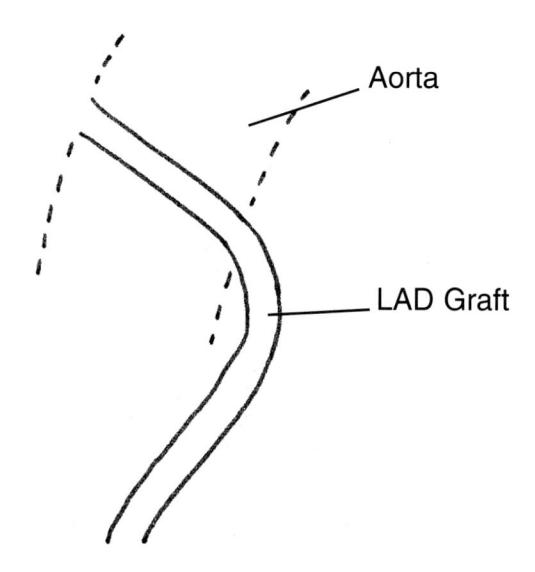

Figure 4.21. LAD Graft, LAO view.

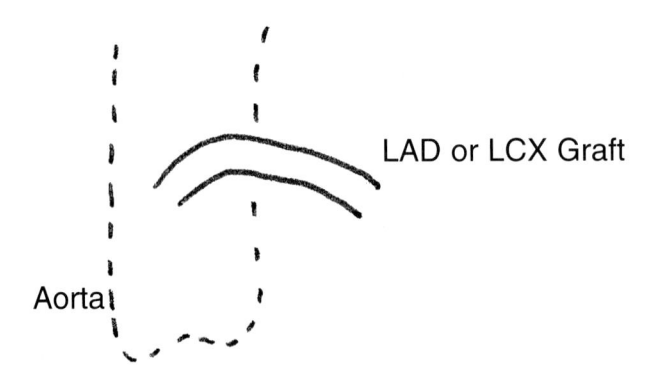

Figure 4.22. LAD or LCX Graft, in AP or RAO projection.

The course of the LIMA or RIMA may be viewed in LAO 40°–70°, RAO 30°–50°, RAO caudal, Left Lateral and AP views. For cannulation of LIMA or RIMA (see Chapter 21).

Other Arterial Conduits

Newer arterial grafts such as the gastro-epiploic artery are now being used. If angiography or angioplasty is needed, it is wise to seek assistance from a vascular radiologist.

Radiation Exposure and Selection of Radiographic Views

Some radiographic views expose the patient and the operator to a greater radiation dose. The larger doses for the patient occur with those views where the X-rays pass through the spine or the liver, e.g. the PA and RAO caudal views. For the operator, larger doses come from scatter of the rays off the patient, when the X-ray tube is on the same side as the operator. These include the LAO cranial, left lateral and LAO caudal views. The steeper the LAO view, the greater is the irradiation to the operator. The LAO cranial and left lateral views give the operator about seven times the irradiation of the PA or RAO caudal views.

Interventionists work many hours using X-ray equipment. Ensure that all practical measures of radiation protection are taken by yourself, your assistant(s), the nurses, the physiological measurement technicians and the radiographers.

Conclusion

Angioplasty requires the lesion and its vessel to be shown as clearly as possible and experimentation with the views may be needed to achieve this. To some extent the radiographic views depend on the local anatomy and on the personal preferences of the operator.

5 Intravascular Ultrasound and Angioscopy

Intravascular Ultrasound or IVUS

This form of imaging has great potential to assist during angioplasty and to aid in the assessment of coronary artery disease. IVUS studies the *wall* of the vessel and can give accurate measurements of the size the lumen, the amount of atheroma (plaque) and the true size of the vessel. Angiography assesses the *lumen* of the vessel and the features seen represent "a mirror" of the changes occurring in the wall of the artery. IVUS compliments the results obtained by angiography.

Why is IVUS then not used routinely?

The answer includes the following reasons, which are all becoming less valid:

1. Increased costs, as an IVUS catheter costs about the same price as a balloon catheter.
2. Prolongation of the procedure, by about 5–15 minutes.
3. A small risk of vessel damage and dissection. Segmental coronary artery spasm may be induced by an IVUS catheter. This is promptly relieved after an injection of intra coronary nitrate.
4. Lack of operator experience.

IVUS is particularly helpful in:

1. *The use of stents.*
   IVUS is superior to angiography to confirm full expansion of a stent. IVUS can assess inflow and outflow stenosis or dissection. It is useful to assess *stent restenosis*, as it may show incomplete stent expansion or intimal hyperplasia. The value of IVUS for stent deployment was first shown by Dr. Antonio Colombo of Milan.
2. *Measurement of vessel lumen and wall size.*
   This is a very valuable role to judge the correct size of the balloon or the stent that

may be used for the vessel. In about a third of cases the IVUS size of the vessel is significantly larger then the calibre shown on angiography. A larger sized balloon or stent can be used than the diagnostic angiogram suggested. This may be helpful for *restenosis* lesions (see page 253).
3. *Assessment of a lesion of uncertain severity.*
   The lesion is often found to be more severe than shown at angiography.
4. *Assessment of bifurcation/trifurcation lesions.*
   More disease may be detected which may be hidden at angiography by overlying vessel branches.
5. *Assessment of the result of angioplasty.*
   IVUS can show how good (or otherwise) the result from PTCA has been, as it can measure the lumen size and the amount of residual plaque. It can show the type and severity of vessel wall splitting and dissection. Often a satisfactory result seen on angiography may be disappointing when assessed by IVUS. Improved lumen size seen on angiography may be shown to have been achieved by dissection and flow down a false lumen rather than the true lumen.
6. *Assessment of the lesion prior to angioplasty.*
   Often an IVUS catheter can cross a stenosis before PTCA and give information on the type of lesion and assist in the selection of angioplasty equipment.
7. *Detection of intravascular calcification.*
   Angiography is relatively poor and IVUS is more sensitive. If a lesion has a ring of calcification detected by IVUS, there is an increased risk of vessel dissection or inability to dilate with a balloon catheter, so that the Rotablator may be the instrument of choice.

IVUS is Relatively Poor at:

1. *Detection of thrombus within the lumen*
   Angioscopy is the best technique.
2. *Predicting the success of an angioplasty*
   When balloon angioplasty is to be used.
3. *Predicting the risk of restenosis*
   after balloon angioplasty.

Technical Aspects of IVUS

1. **System Types**
   These are still under development and improvement. There are two methods of generating and recording the images:-
   a) *Mechanical — rotating mirror:*
      The two main manufacturers of this type of IVUS catheter, Boston Scientific and CVIS have combined. Both Hewlett-Packard and CVIS manufacture console equipment to use with Boston Scientific IVUS catheters.
   b) *Phased array:*
      The main system available is called Oracle, manufactured by Endosonics and marketed by Cordis.

2. **IVUS Catheters**
   An IVUS catheter is passed to and down the coronary vessel over a routine guide wire. The catheter may be monorail (rapid exchange) such as Sonicath, Microrail, Microview and Ultracross catheters from Boston Scientific. For the phased array system the monorail catheters are Vision and Vision FX. The Megasonic catheter has a monorail balloon for PTCA, plus an ultrasound probe mounted together and is produced by Endosonics.
3. **IVUS Sheath**
   Some IVUS catheters pass along within a sheath which protects the artery. Once the guide wire and then the sheath have been passed distally, the IVUS catheter can be advanced and withdrawn along the vessel without difficulty or risk. A snag with some systems, such as the 2.9F Ultracross catheter, is the need to withdraw the GW proximally before the IVUS catheter may pass along the sheath. With the 3.2F Ultracross catheter, the guide wire does not need to be withdrawn which is simpler and safer.
4. **Pull Back System**
   An IVUS catheter within a sheath can be connected to a 'pull back device' which withdraws it at a slow constant speed. A smoother pull back is obtained, i.e. less jerky and less of a 'stop-start' ride. This produces a better record for analysis, including attempts at 3-D vessel wall reconstruction.
5. **Video Record**
   The IVUS study is recorded on video during the pull back, which allows areas of interest to be frozen and analysed. Typically, the size of the lumen, the amount of atheroma or plaque and the size or calibre of the vessel are recorded by measuring the maximum and minimum diameters and the cross-sectional area of the vessel at the sites of interest.
6. **Voice Record**
   This documents or 'signposts' the stage reached and the details of an IVUS study. It is particularly helpful when later reviewing an IVUS video record.
7. **Simultaneous Records**
   Simultaneous screening and IVUS records during an IVUS pull back study gives an ideal IVUS record. This is especially so for assessment of the lesion and vessel at a later date, but is currently difficult to achieve.
8. **Dedicated Screen for IVUS**
   It is helpful to have a separate screen dedicated for IVUS next to the angiographic and pressure monitors. This arrangement makes for speedy and convenient review of IVUS images.
9. **IVUS Colleagues and Staff**
   Ideally a colleague with a specific IVUS interest and an experienced ultrasound technician should be available. They can supervise the IVUS aspects of the case, especially the analysis and measurements of the records. This allows the PTCA operator to concentrate on the angioplasty with the benefits of IVUS findings.
10. **Archiving of IVUS**
    Storage and retrieval of IVUS studies requires a system comparable to angiography to allow review of recent and previous procedures by PTCA operators and surgeons.
11. **Heparin for Diagnostic Procedures.**
    If the IVUS study is purely a diagnostic one and not part of a PTCA procedure, heparin

5,000 units is given prior to passing the IVUS equipment along the coronary vessel. For PTCA procedures the routine heparin cover (usually 10,000 units) is sufficient for the IVUS study too.

Appearance of IVUS Images

Instructions on IVUS may be obtained from attending courses or visiting centres regularly performing IVUS. Also useful are reference books such as 'Intravascular Ultrasound Imaging' by Jonathan Tobis and Paul Yock, Churchill-Livingstone, New York, 1992, or 'An Introduction to Intravascular Ultrasound' by Neal Uren, Remedica, Oxford, UK, 1996.

The records below give a 'flavour' of the use of IVUS (see Figures 5.1–5.9).

5.1 Normal Coronary Artery
 The three layered appearance of intima, media and adventitia is seen. The circle in the centre of the picture is the transducer and ring shadows ('ring down') are seen around it. At 3 o'clock there are echoes from the guide wire in the coronary artery, along which the IVUS catheter tracks, which are described as the 'guide wire artifacts'.
5.2 Fibrous Plaque
 A plaque is present from 11 to 6 o'clock, with brightness (or 'echodensity') similar to that of the adventitia.
5.3 Focal Calcific Lesion
 Calcification is seen as bright echoes with an acoustic shadow behind or external to the lesion.
5.4 Ring Calcific Lesion
 The calcification extends round a wide arc of the vessel lumen.
5.5 Extensive Dissection
 From 2 o'clock passing anticlockwise to 7 o'clock there is a C shaped shadow ('sonolucent zone') representing the media. Internal to this from 7 to 12 o'clock there is a crescentic linear shadow of dissection of the plaque. This extends from media shadow to media shadow suggesting extensive dissection. Around the IVUS catheter with a tongue-like projection upwards at 11–12 o'clock, are soft echoes (less dense than the adventitia) suggesting thrombus formation.
5.6 Inadequately Deployed Stent
 There is extensive malposition of stent struts, which are not in contact with the intimal surface over a large section of the lumen.
5.7 Well Applied Stent
 The stent struts are well positioned up against the intima and are well expanded to give a large lumen for the artery.
5.8 Minor Dissection at the End of a Stent
 A small intimal flap is seen, which is not occluding the lumen.
5.9 Instent Restenosis
 The stent struts are well expanded out into the vessel wall. Internal to the struts there is extensive plaque, due to intimal hyperplasia. There is a small crescentic lumen from 1–5 o'clock.

These IVUS echo studies were kindly provided by Dr Neal Uren, from Edinburgh UK.

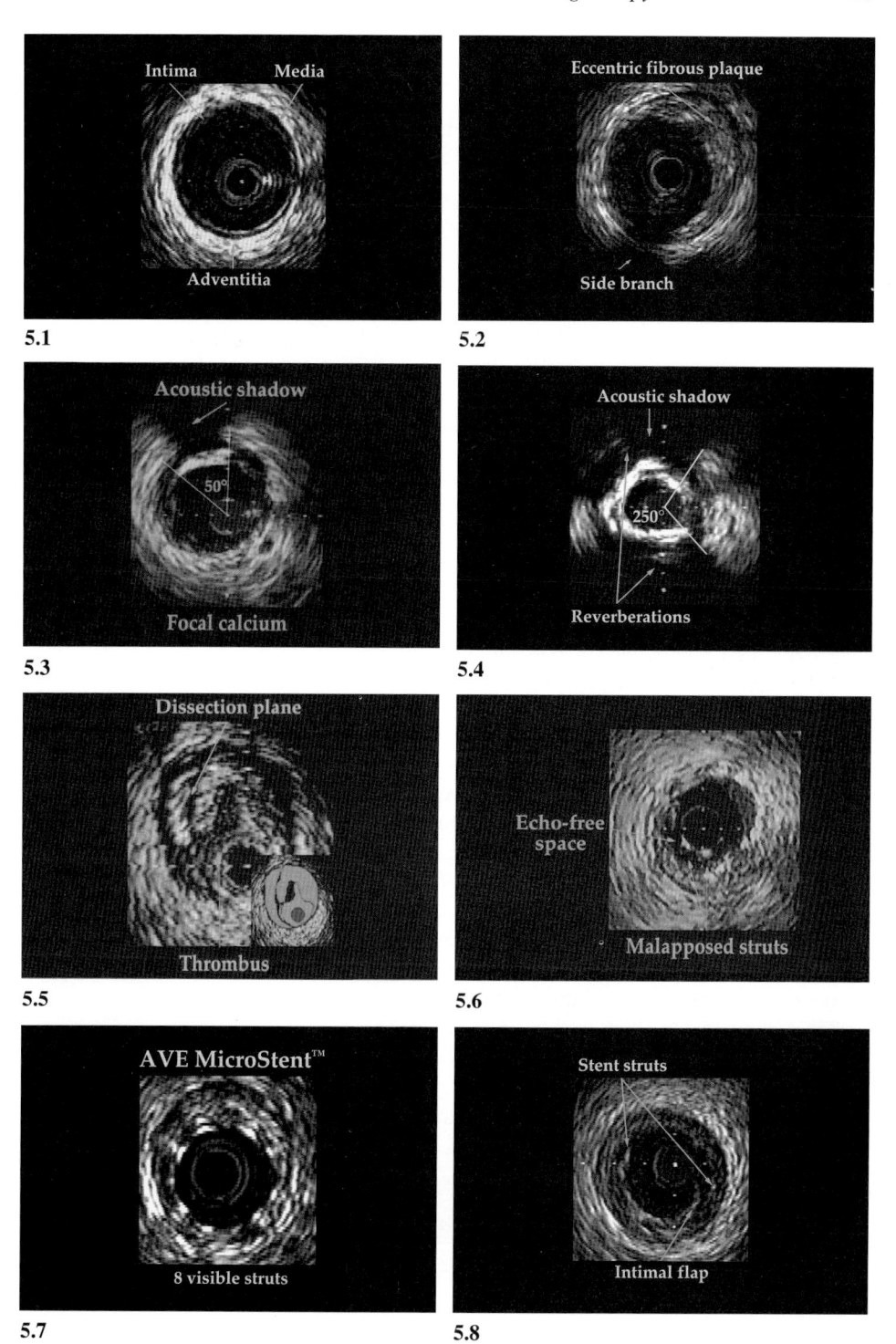

Figure 5.1–5.8. IVUS images.

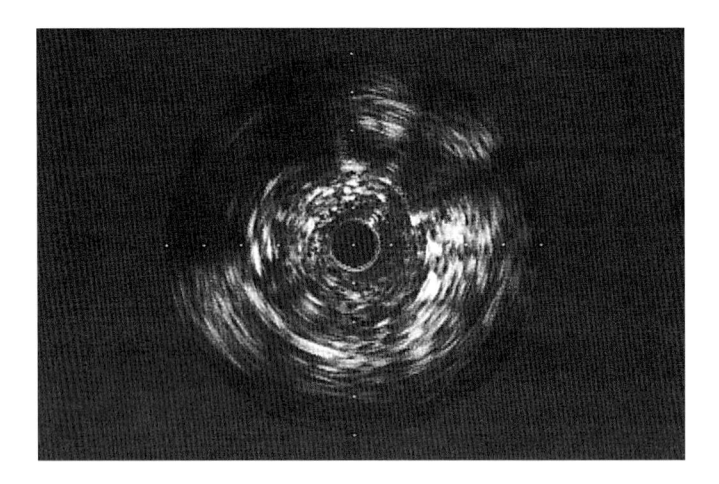

Figure 5.9. IVUS. Image of instent restenosis.

Conclusion

IVUS is not essential for PTCA. However once the technique is learnt the information obtained is very useful indeed. When used on a regular basis, an IVUS study takes only 5–10 minutes and is well worth the extra time and cost involved.

Angioscopy:

This involves passing a very small endoscope down a coronary vessel to directly visualize the lining to the vessel wall and any intraluminal material such as thrombus.

It may be performed using a monorail angioscopy catheter and equipment from Baxter Edwards. During angioscopic imaging, the distal artery is flushed with saline, which is injected at a rate of 30–40 ml per minute. Technically the catheter may not be able to cross or assess the lesion in about 30% of cases. The catheter is relatively inflexible and is not suitable to use in tortuous vessels. It is difficult to make measurements on the images, so merely descriptive recordings of the findings are usually done.

The technique can show whether a lesion is:

a) *Smooth*
   As in stable angina.
b) *Ulcerated with thrombus*
   As with unstable angina.
c) *Yellow lipid rich lesion*
   This type of lesion may be more liable to rupture leading to acute myocardial infarction.

Different types of thrombus can be identified:

a) *Greyish or white in colour*
   This is usually non occlusive, platelet rich and is seen in unstable angina.
b) *Red coloured*
   This thrombus which mainly contains fibrin and red blood cells, is found at occlusive lesions, such as acute myocardial infarction.

Angioscopy does not help with stent deployment, though it can demonstrate the type of thrombus present in subacute stent thrombosis (often grey/white, rather then red thrombus).

Conclusion

Angioscopy at present is well behind IVUS as the third player for imaging during PTCA. Its third position of usefulness is even under contention from the Doppler Flow Wire (see page 40).

6 Patient Selection and General Care

Any procedure or operation is more likely to be successful if there has first been careful planning and preparation. In the words of the SAS (Special Air Services) "The 7 P's of success are: 'Proper planning and preparation prevent piss poor performance' ". Time taken ensuring that patient is suitable for PTCA, discussing the procedure with the patient and relatives and planning the technique, will reap rich dividends during the procedure.

Patient Selection for PTCA

Patients fulfilling Grüntzig's original criteria are still the most suitable ones for PTCA and have very good results with low morbidity. Grüntzig's recommendations were that the patient should have:

1) *Angina*
2) *Documented ischaemia*
   On an exercise test, or exercise/stress radionuclear (Thallium) or echo scan.
3) *Single vessel disease*
   With a proximal subtotal discrete non-calcified lesion.
4) *Surgical candidate*
   To allow emergency CABG if the vessel occludes. This may exclude patients with malignancy, severe LV dysfunction or severe systemic disease especially pulmonary.

Stable angina, unstable angina, acute myocardial infarction and continuing ischaemia (pain) after acute MI, are all treatable by PTCA. The risks will be generally less in stable angina. Documented reversible ischaemia is usually available in stable angina. In the other patient categories an exercise test is often not possible, though the 12 lead ECG may confirm ischaemia or infarction.

Multivessel disease is often attempted as a single vessel dilatation, leaving the other diseased vessels which may not be severe or are of long standing duration. Alternatively, more than one vessel is dilated, at the same time, or as a staged procedure.

Some patients are offered PTCA, even though CABG will not be considered if the vessel does occlude during the procedure. The patient may have been turned down for cardiac surgery because of very poor left ventricular function, recurrent previous CABGs, or because of a poor general medical condition.

Preoperative Patient Assessment

It is not good practice to first meet the patient on the catheter room table! With urgent cases such as primary PTCA for acute MI and some with unstable angina, the initial meeting with the patient may be in the catheter room, which is reasonable as the they are emergencies. But for nearly all other situations, assessment of the patient, review of the tests and discussion with the relatives should be 'the order of the day'. Time spent properly assessing the patient may prevent hours of time in medical litigation.

The *history* should be recorded to determine severity of angina, past history of myocardial infarction, risk factors, current drug therapy and any other coexistent diseases and significant past illnesses. Also noted should be operations, including stripping of varicose veins.

On *examination*, assessment of anxiety, obesity, hyperlipidaemia, hypertension, other cardiac diseases such as valvular lesions, signs of cardiac failure, lung disease, the state of peripheral arteries in the neck and legs and the condition of the veins in the legs, should all be checked.

The *availability of a venous conduit* should be determined. Has the patient undergone previous stripping of varicose veins? Are there major varicose veins, or evidence of previous venous thrombosis?

The *ECG* should be reviewed for signs of previous Q wave, or non-Q wave infarction and evidence of heart block (suggesting the need for temporary pacing) (see page 70).

The *Chest X-Ray* is checked to asses heart size, signs of failure and for lung disease. Echocardiography is not needed routinely, but is very helpful if LV dysfunction or valvular disease is suspected.

The *Exercise Test* is reviewed to determine whether one has been done, when it was performed and whether the patient was on the current medical treatment. What stage of which protocol or work load, did the patient achieve? What was the reason for stopping, did the patient have angina and what was the amount of S-T segment change? If the patient has had a radionuclear (thallium) scan or echo stress test, these are reviewed.

The *pathology tests* are scanned, being on the look-out for raised lipids, anaemia, thrombocytopenia, renal impairment, diabetes and abnormal antibodies making cross-matching of blood difficult.

Discussion with Patient and Relatives

The importance of this matter cannot be emphasised too greatly. There are however many operators who consider this task less critical. Some patients are just not aware that they are having an operative procedure carrying risks. One patient for whom English was not his native language, believed that the proposed PTCA was to excise a sebaceous cyst on his back! When the true nature of the procedure was explained, he was not at all keen.

Patient Selection and General Care

After the son discussed PTCA with his father, he then returned and said, "my father — he will have the PTCA, but you doctor, you make sure you do a good job, or else ...!"

It is not enough to discuss PTCA with patient alone, as it will be the relatives who may have to bear the worry and the grief if a complication occurs. The patient *and the relatives*, must both understand the procedure, its benefits and risks of complications.

If a patient comes as an emergency transfer from another hospital, great efforts should be made to speak to the relatives, if necessary by telephoning them so that they can be forewarned of potential complications.

Routine Talk with Patient and Relatives (See also page 148)

The artery(ies) to be treated should be detailed and the basic mechanisms of angioplasty explained. The term 'angioplasty' is usually better understood and used with patients than the abbreviation 'PTCA'. The complications and risks should be described. A simple comparison of angioplasty with CABG can be helpful. Angioplasty is "mini" surgery or 'keyhole surgery', with the operation being within the artery, as opposed to by-pass surgery, where the chest is opened and a 'ring road' or 'by-pass' is made. Recovery is quicker but the procedure may need to be repeated. Any operation has a 'risk to life and limb' and angioplasty is no exception. Angioplasty has a mortality of about 0.5%, as opposed to CABG of 1–2%, though patient groups are different.

There are **3 complications** of angioplasty that patients need to know about.

Firstly, as the artery is stretched a spiral tear or dissection may occur and the vessel becomes *occluded*. This may require emergency coronary artery bypass surgery (CABG), or coronary artery stenting as a scaffold to support the wall and keep the channel or lumen open. The risk of emergency CABG is about 2%, i.e. about 1 in 50 patients. If agreeing to angioplasty, the patient also needs to agree to the small risk of emergency CABG. If the vessel occludes, there is about a 2% risk of M.I. and this may not be prevented by emergency CABG.

Secondly, after the procedure the vessel may *renarrow*, due to closing down by elastic recoil and scar tissue along the inner lining of the artery. There is 1 in 3 risk (30% chance), of renarrowing or 'restenosis' within 3 months. If the vessel renarrows usually angina will recur and a repeat angioplasty be performed. Suggest that *not one* angioplasty procedure but rather *a course* of angioplasty is being offered. Hopefully one angioplasty may be sufficient, but sometimes 2 or even 3 "bites at the cherry" may be needed.

Finally, any operation has a 'risk to life and limb' and as with a diagnostic angiogram, there is a small (1–2%) risk of a *groin complication*, which is slightly more common due to the use of heparin and the larger tubes (catheters) used for angioplasty.

Use simple approximations for the figures of the risks, as these will be easier for the patient and the relatives to understand and remember.

It is helpful having explained the above, to repeat the main facts for a second and sometimes even a third time, so that the message really is understood by the patient and the relatives. Do give out explanatory literature for patients from the PTCA manufacturers and others. The loan of a video of the procedure can be very valuable. Usually the more information the patient and relatives have, the better; to be forewarned is to be forearmed and less anxious.

Review of Previous Angiogram (See also Chapter 7)

If PTCA is to follow on directly from the diagnostic angiogram, this needs to be explained to the patient. More frequently for elective cases, a decision to perform PTCA will have been taken some weeks, or even months earlier. Check the angiogram with the patient's clinical status and confirm that PTCA is still appropriate. Is the lesion borderline, or very risky, or are the symptoms too mild? Is the anatomy and the disease perhaps better suited to CABG rather than PTCA? Is a PTCA really necessary? If there is a change of plan, go to the patient, apologise and explain that PTCA is not really the best solution for him or her at this time. Very few patients will mind you changing your mind before the procedure. All would prefer this, rather than have you deciding in the middle of PTCA that really it would have been better if you had never started!

Surgical Cover

During the early days of angioplasty, a surgical theatre and team would be free and standing by during a PTCA. One cardiac anaesthetist covering a PTCA in the private sector remarked, "that the only good PTCA was the one that went to surgery!". Another arrangement was for PTCA procedures to be scheduled between cardiac operations. Prior to all PTCAs, the diagnostic angiograms were reviewed jointly with the cardiac surgeon. With increased safety and numbers of PTCA, these practices have ceased in most cardiac units. PTCA and cardiac surgery now occur and it is hoped that the two don't meet!

The following cases should be discussed with a surgeon and arrangements for surgical cover agreed:

1) High risk case from whatever cause.
2) Unplanned or extra procedures starting late in the day's schedule, i.e. after 3–4pm.
3) Procedures outside routine hours, e.g. at the week-ends.
4) Procedures in the private sector — to ensure that surgical cover is at least as good, if not better, than with the routine 'Health Service' patients.

There has been much controversy and heated discussion on the topic of PTCA without cardiac surgery at the same hospital, so called *'off-site PTCA'*. Off-site PTCA can be performed safely, but emergency surgery is more complicated to arrange. Well rehearsed arrangements to allow speedy and safe transfer of a patient to the surgical unit are essential.

Cardiac Pacing

It is only necessary to insert a pacing catheter when heart block occurs, or when there is a higher risk of this problem developing, such as in the presence of a bundle branch block, complex higher risk RCA lesion (see Angiogram 11.1 on page 122), or with the use of the Rotablator.

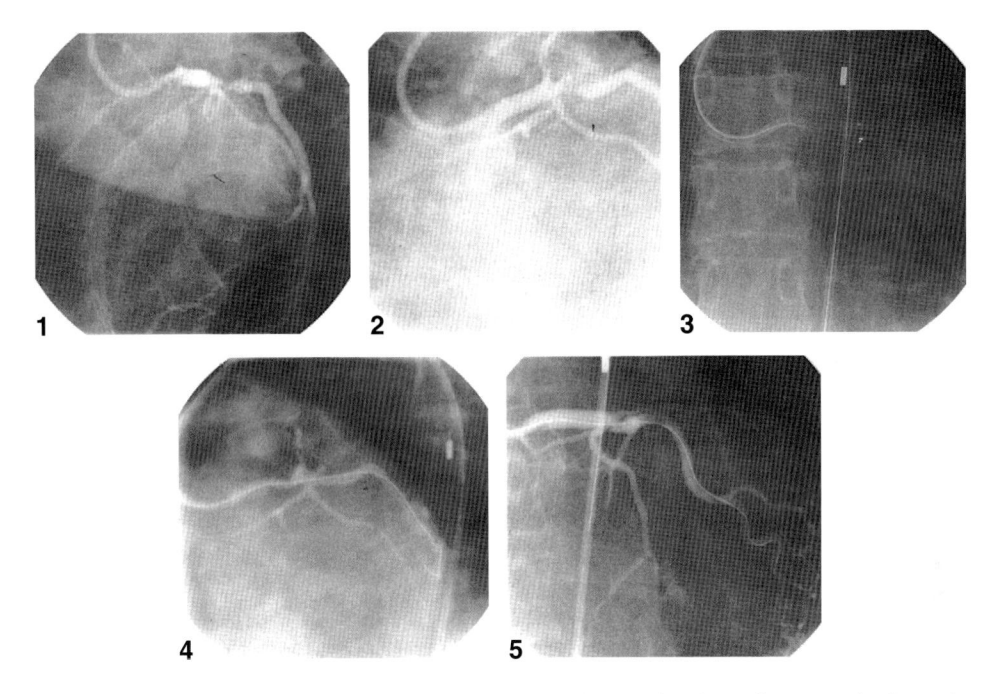

Angiogram 6.1. *PTCA of last remaining artery.* The lesion on the circumflex artery is shown in LAO 70° (1) and LAO caudal view (2). The LAD is small and diseased and the RCA was occluded. An intra-aortic balloon pump was inserted to cover the procedure and the rectangular marker of its balloon is seen (3). The lesion was dilated with a perfusion balloon and the small dot of its central marker is seen in 3. The end results was satisfactory (4 and 5).

Intra Aortic Balloon Pump (IABP)

There are a small number, about 1–2% of PTCA cases, where an IABP can be very helpful to reduce the risks of PTCA (Angiogram 6.1). These include:

1) those with very poor LV function,
2) patients continuing to have angina as they are brought to the catheter room,
3) those with cardiogenic shock.

Usually severe angina at rest will be promptly relieved and hypotension will not occur when an angioplasty balloon is inflated. If the procedure is a high risk case, it may be useful to slip a small 4 or 5F sheath in the contralateral femoral artery, so that an IABP can be promptly inserted if needed.

Percutaneous cardio-pulmonary bypass using the femoral vein and artery in the conscious patient can technically be performed in the catheter room. Large bore cannulae (14F) are required. The role of the technique is uncertain, as in most cases sufficient circulatory support can be achieved more simply using the IABP.

Routine Supportive Management for PTCA

The technical aspects of a PTCA procedure are described in Chapter 7. This section considers the general care of the patients, in order to support them for the PTCA procedure.

The management will be discussed under the time headings of :

a) Before PTCA
b) During PTCA
c) After PTCA — the first 24 hours
d) After PTCA — Prior to discharge and follow-up.

Medical Management before PTCA

1) *Current Drug Therapy*
   Usually no changes are needed to the drugs that the patient was taking before admission. Most patients will already be on aspirin, but if not, this should be given in dose of 150–300 mgm orally per day. With urgent cases, e.g. primary PTCA for acute MI, 1–2 tablets of 300 mgm aspirin can be chewed in the mouth. Alternatively, 100–300 mgm of aspirin can be given intravenously.

   Many patients will already be receiving a beta blocking and/or calcium antagonist and/or oral or i.v. nitrate drug, which are usually all continued. Some operators will start a calcium antagonist to reduce coronary artery spasm, whilst others like a betablocker drug to possibly reduce the size of M.I. should vessel occlusion occur. A slower rather than faster heart rate makes assessment of RCA and LCX lesions easier, as there is less frequent movement of the vessel within the atrio-ventricular groove during cardiac contractions.

   If the patient is on IV heparin for unstable angina, this is usually maintained until the patient goes down to the catheter lab. Some operators will stop the heparin about 6–12 hours before the procedure, to reduce the risk of heparin resistance during the procedure (see page 157).

2) *Nil by Mouth*
   The patient should have nothing to eat or drink for 3–6 hours before procedure, in case he or she needs to go for emergency surgery. A patient scheduled for the afternoon, should receive food in early morning, such as a light breakfast and drinks, in order to avoid hypoglycaemia.

   For an insulin dependent diabetic, it is better for the patient to be scheduled first or early on the list. A light breakfast should be given. The insulin dose will need to be adjusted downwards. Having the patient somewhat 'sugary', is definitely better than hypoglycaemic episodes occurring during the procedure.

3) *IV (Intravenous) Cannula*
   A large 10 or 12 gauge i.v. cannula is placed, preferably in a left arm vein just above the wrist (as opposed to the antecubital fossa). This allows the arms to be folded up over patients head, with the drip set tubing being on the opposite to that of the operator, working on the right side of the patient. To allow a patient a good night's sleep, it is better to insert the cannula on the morning of the procedure, rather than the night before it. However, if several attempts have been needed to get the cannula in, the patient will not come down in a very relaxed state!

4) *Premedication*

Most operators give one to relax the patient. Some use benzodiazepines, such as oral diazepam 10 mgm or lorazepam 2 mgm 1–2 hours before, or opiates such as omnopon 10 mgm with scopolamine 0.6 mgm given i.m., 1–2 hours before the procedure. If the patient is still very anxious when arriving in the catheter lab, 2.5–5 mgm midazolam or 5–10 mgm of diazemuls i.v. can be very effective.

To reverse the effects, e.g. respiratory depression of benzodiazepines, give 100–200 micrograms of *Flumazenil* i.v. The drug may cause convulsions.

5) *Other Drugs*

Aspirin has already been mentioned, to be started if the patient is not currently receiving it. For patients who are to receive an elective stent, or whose vessel anatomy would allow a stent to be inserted if necessary, ticlopidine 250 mgm given the night before and the morning of the procedure may be given (see page 130).

For patients on corticosteroids, a booster dose with the premedication is advisable.

Medical Management during PTCA

1) *Aspirin*

On arrival in the catheter lab, *ask the patient* whether he or she has had their aspirin tablet that morning. Every now and then, the patient will not have had this drug which is proven value to prevent thrombosis and occlusion during PTCA.

2) *IV Fluid*

At the start of the procedure 100–200 ml of dextrose/saline are run in, followed by a slower infusion of 50–100 ml per hour, to help prevent hypotension. It also determines whether the i.v. cannula is still patent. Many operators no longer give i.v. fluids routinely.

3) *Oxygen*

There is merit in having the heart and the body tissues as fully oxygenated as possible, before ischaemia induced by inflation of angioplasty balloons. The patient receives it via an oxygen mask. This is a personal operator preference and is not proven value. It is not given routinely by most operators.

4) *Heparin*

After the control angiograms have confirmed that the vessel(s) and lesion(s) are still suitable for PTCA, heparin is given, usually via the i.v. cannula by the catheter room nurse. The dose is 5–20,000 units, 10,000 units being the average amount. Further top up doses of 1–5,000 units of heparin may be given after about one hour. If ReoPro is to be used electively a reduced dose of heparin is given (see page 162). The heparin requirement may be simply and quickly assessed by measuring the ACT (activated clotting time) in the catheter lab using a Haemochron machine (Technidyne). For PTCA, the ACT should be above 250 seconds and if a stent is to be deployed it should be above 300 seconds. Note that ACT measurements with the less commonly used machine, the HaemoTec (Medtronic), gives values which are about 25–30% lower than with the Haeochron machine (see reference on page 77).

5) *GTN (Glyceryl Trinitrate)*

This drug or isosorbide used to be given liberally during PTCA to prevent coronary artery spasm, until it was realised that spasm was rare and hypotension caused by GTN was a greater problem. GTN is now usually reserved for special procedures such as Rotablator, and for treating spasm appearing with the deployment of stents and the use of stiffer 'extra back-up' guide wires (see page 30 and Angiogram 11.1 on page 122).

Some operators give a dose of an i.v. nitrate at the start of the procedure so as to judge with the maximum vessel dilatation, the appropriate size of balloon and or stent that should be employed.

Medical Management after PTCA — the First 24 Hours

Whilst this care will mainly be carried out by nurses and the junior medical staff, operators need to ensure that clear regimes and instructions are given to these staff. As with all post operative care, much of the good of the operation can easily be undone by errors and complications at this stage. It is a *good rule*, that before leaving the hospital, you should always go and see every patient on whom you have performed an interventional procedure that day. You and your patients will not regret it.

1) ***Sheath Removal***
   This is the single most important aspect of management after PTCA. If performed badly and the patient becomes hypotensive from bleeding from or into the groin, or from a vasovagal attack associated with the pain from groin pressure, the previously dilated vessel may close down and the patient be in serious trouble. New junior doctors and or nurses, need to be taught the correct procedure. In higher risk cases, especially if the patient is to be maintained on i.v. and oral anticoagulants, the operator or a well experienced junior colleague, should be responsible for 'pulling the sheath'. For sheath removal consider:
   a) *Coagulation Check*
      The sheath may be removed the *same day* as the PTCA, or the *next morning* if i.v. heparin is to be maintained until the next day. The duration of the anticoagulant activity of heparin is very variable, so that before the sheath is removed *it is essential to check that the coagulation has returned to normal or near normal*. This is done by confirming that the PTTK or APTT (Partail Thromboplastin Time with Kaolin or Activated Partial Thromboplastin Time) is 1.5:1 or less, or that the ACT is 150 seconds or less. It is very desirable to have 'near bed side testing' of the coagulation tests, i.e. on the ward to give instant results of the tests repeated as necessary by nursing or medical staff. The CoaguChek Plus (Boehringer-Mannheim) can be used for PTTK/APTT tests and the Haemochron or HaemoTec machines (see page 73) for the ACT readings.
   b) *ECG Monitor*
      The patient should be connected to one so as to easily assess any arrhythmia, especially bradycardia.
   c) *Fluids IV*
      A bolus of 100–200 ml of fluid (dextrose/saline or saline) just before sheath removal, will reduce the risk of hypotension. Should fluids be needed or an i.v. drug be required, there will be no delay, as an infusion is already running and the cannula is known to still be patent.

d) *Analgesics and Atropine*
   These are not needed routinely, but should be available at the bedside and include pethidine 25–50 mgm i.v. or i.m. for pain and atropine 0.6–1.2 mgm i.v., for sinus bradycardia.
   If the patient is rather anxious, or if during PTCA seemed to have a low pain threshold, anticipate the analgesic need and give the pethidine i.m. 30 minutes before sheath removal.
e) *Foot pulses*
   Before sheath removal check the foot pulses and ideally record their position by marking the skin with a cross in biro, unless this has already been done.
f) *Firm Pressure with Fingers Laid Flat*
   The exact method of pressing on the groin after sheath removal varies from one doctor to another. It is better to press with fingers *flat* on the skin, rather than *pressing in* (or down) into the patients groin. It is of less importance whether the pressure is applied at, or above, the puncture site.
g) *Pressure Duration*
   For most patients 30 minutes is sufficient. Towards the end, the pressure on the groin can be slowly reduced. Chat to the patient and if he or she suddenly goes quiet, be concerned! At the end, check the foot pulses to confirm that they are present.
h) *Dressing*
   A simple piece of gauze or small plaster is usually all that is needed. Some operators use a pressure bandage for a few hours.
i) *Fem Stop*
   (Radi Medical Systems)
   This is an effective simple device, which is more comfortable to the patient than manual pressure. It saves valuable medical or nursing time pressing on groins. It is less reliable in very obese patients.
   A sand bag or a clamp are simpler aids for groin pressure to assist haemostasis. Neither is very comfortable nor effective.
j) *Later Review of Groin*
   Check later, especially prior to discharge, that there has not been any late bleeding and bruising at the groin on mobilization.

Medical Management after PTCA — the First 24 Hours Continued

2) *I.V. Fluids*
   Prior to PTCA the patient is routinely starved ('Nil by Mouth'). If little or no i.v. fluid was given during PTCA and especially if nitrates were administered too, then there is a risk of hypotension during the recovery period. A liberal i.v. fluid regime is recommended to avoid this, i.e. 0.5 litres of dextrose/saline in 2, 4, 8 and then 12 hours. Usually, during the final bag, the drip can come down. Oral fluids should be encouraged too. On return to the ward, the patient can eat food from the routine menu.
3) *Heparin*
   Usually heparin is routinely stopped when the patient leaves the Catheter Room, i.e. there is no post-op heparin. This allows sheath removal later that day, with full mobilization and discharge the next day.

Some operators continue i.v. heparin until the morning of the next day. This is done for patients with some degree of dissection, after primary PTCA, or after an indifferent stent result. The value of heparin in these situations is unproven. Some operators who continue to use oral anticoagulants after stent insertion, will maintain i.v. heparin for 3–5 days until the anticoagulant control (INR) is in the therapeutic range. If i.v. heparin is given, its correct dose should be regularly monitored about every 3–12 hours. An ACT of 200–250 seconds, or the PTTK of 2–2.5:1, are the readings to achieve a safe therapeutic level. There is some evidence that i.v. nitrates potentiate and prolong the action of heparin.

4) **Routine Drugs**

The drugs prior to PTCA can be continued, but if the patient was on i.v. heparin or i.v. nitrates for unstable angina, these will be stopped.

Medical Management after PTCA — Prior to Discharge

1) **Restenosis and Return of Symptoms**

Remind the patient that there is about a 30% chance of restenosis and recurrent angina. The patient may restart the previous antianginal medical therapy. The family or local doctor and or the PTCA centre should be contacted and the patient be seen for an early reassessment, which will often involve another exercise test. Inform the patient, that should another PTCA be needed, then usually a repeat coronary arteriogram will be followed immediately by the angioplasty at the same procedure (or 'sitting').

2) **Drug or Medical Treatment**

The medical therapy should be reviewed and can usually be reduced. If the patient is on 'triple therapy' i.e. beta-blocker, calcium antagonist and oral nitrate, then usually two of these can be stopped. Usually the patient is left on a beta-blocker or the calcium antagonist. If the patient is hypertensive, one or both of these classes of drugs may still be needed. When having a two-stage procedure and the patient is to return for a later PTCA, all the current drugs will usually be continued.

Aspirin 75–150 mgm per day should be continued, probably indefinitely. If a stent has been inserted, it is essential for aspirin (150–300 mgm per day) to be continued for at least a month. For stent patients, many operators also use ticlopidine 250 mg once or twice per day for two to four weeks (see page 130).

3) **Mobilization**

For the first 2–3 days the patient should take it quietly at home. After this the groin should no longer be tender and the patient should take regular exercise, with walking being one of the simplest and best. Within a week, progress should be made to a brisk walk for 30 minutes before lunch and or supper. Regular active exercise will identify more promptly, if angina is beginning to return.

Driving can be resumed 2–3 days after discharge, when the groin has settled down. Return to work, usually full-time, can be restarted at about one week. Sexual intercourse can be started again at the same time as driving is resumed, but the two activities are best kept separate!

4) *Lipids*
   The importance of successful serum cholesterol reduction to improve long term prognosis, is now better appreciated. A current serum cholesterol should be known or measured and if above 5.0 mmol/Litre, medical treatment should be given, usually in the first instance with a statin drug.
5) *Other Risk Factors*
   Reinforce the importance of these to the patient, who should not smoke, should have a healthy mixed diet, take regular exercise and attempt to reduce stress. If the patient is hypertensive, a diabetic, or overweight, these conditions will require treatment.
6) *Follow-up Appointment*
   A date for 4–8 weeks should be made for assessment by a Cardiologist, either at the PTCA centre, or at the referring hospital. An exercise test may be considered, especially if angina has recurred. Some operators routinely perform an exercise test and the improvement compared to the pre op test is reassuring and often 'therapeutic' to the patient.

   If the PTCA procedure was difficult, or a complicated one, or if a new procedure or equipment was used, an elective repeat coronary angiogram at 2–6 months may be considered. This should be explained and agreed with the patient.
7) *Discharge Booklet or Sheet*
   Patients find these very useful indeed, as it is well known that doctor-patient communication for a variety of reasons, is often poor. Several manufacturers of PTCA equipment have useful instructive booklets for patients. Cardiac units or individual operators should consider producing their own, which can give local contact addresses and telephone numbers and can be updated as necessary.

Conclusion

Whilst it is possible to consider PTCA merely as a technical procedure, attention to the general measures will lead to a happier and more relaxed patient and ensure that all the 'good work' achieved in the Catheter Room is not undone elsewhere.

Reference

Hasdai D, Holmes DR, King SB, Chronos N. Prevention of Groin Vascular Complications Associated with Percutaneous Procedures. *J Invas Cardiol* **9**, 119–125 (1997).

7 Review of the Diagnostic Angiogram

The diagnostic angiogram is the '*gate keeper*' for the subsequent management of patients with coronary artery disease. After an angiogram a patient will be placed into one of three categories:

1. Continue medical treatment — normal coronary arteries or minor disease only.
2. CABG — extensive, occlusive and usually 3 vessel disease.
3. PTCA — half-way house. Less severe disease, 1 or 2 vessel disease. Rarely, 3 vessel disease, usually not totally occluded.

The *decision* to consider an angioplasty rests on the *diagnostic angiogram*. This angiogram decides the *feasibility* and defines the *angioplasty risks*. The clinical status is reviewed to determine whether a PTCA is *needed* and to asses the *general medical risks*.

Occulo-dilatory Reflex

This somewhat derogatory phrase, has been coined to describe the supposed desire of an angioplasty operator to dilate any lesion that he or she ever sees! However, it is true that the *presence* of a lesion which is suitable for PTCA does not indicate the *need* for an angioplasty.

At one end of the spectrum is a patient with single vessel disease and good LV function, who is asymptomatic, or nearly so. Angioplasty may not be needed. An abnormal exercise test will support a decision for PTCA. The technical ease of the procedure will also be relevant — if it looks straight forward the threshold to consider PTCA will be lower, than if the procedure looks as it would be difficult (e.g. a long chronic occlusion), or risky (e.g. a complex lesion on a tight bend of the RCA).

Another patient may have a single remaining coronary artery, with poor LV function, have had previous CABG and have a poor general medical status. The ease that PTCA can be performed, together with the clinical features, will govern whether the patient is offered a high risk PTCA, elective CABG, or continued medical treatment.

80 Guide to Coronary Angioplasty and Stenting

This chapter will discuss assessment and decisions that are arrived at by reviewing the diagnostic angiogram. Assessment of the clinical status and explanation of the procedure and its risks to the patient are covered in Chapter 5.

Reviewing the Previous Diagnostic Angiogram:

The angiogram review simultaneously considers:

a) feasibility and cardiac risks of PTCA and
b) technical equipment to be used, or that might be needed.

During the diagnostic angiogram review consider:

1) **The Feasibility for PTCA of the Lesion**
   (See also page 83)
   a) is the lesion a stenosis, subtotal occlusion, or a total occlusion?
   b) type and length of the lesion.
   c) is the lesion on a bend?
   d) is there thrombus or calcification present?
2) **Left Main Stem (LMS)**
   a) *Is there a lesion present?*
      When reviewing the angiogram prior to PTCA take care to check the state of the left main stem to ensure that there is not a lesion. This is particularly true in older patients, i.e. over 70 years old and for angiograms of patients referred from other hospitals.

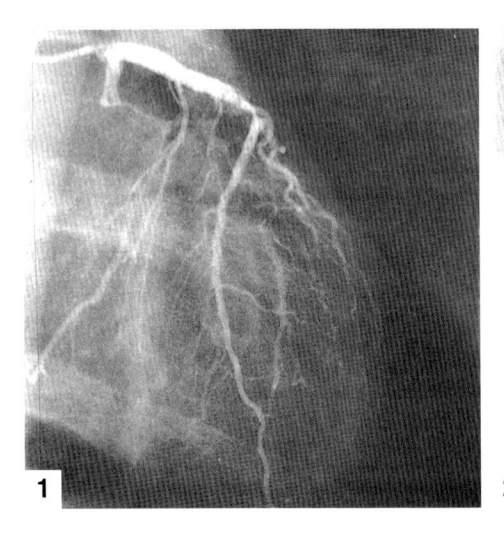

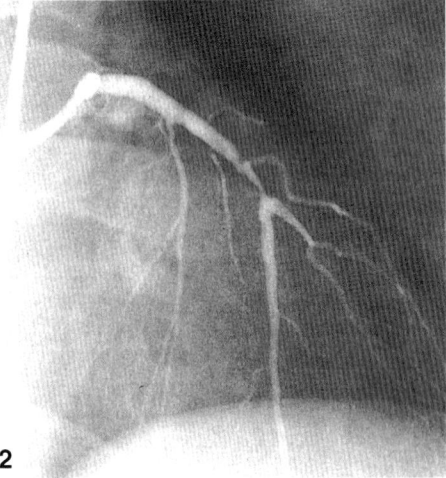

Angiogram 7.1. *RAO cranial projection to show mid-LAD lesion.* The AP projection (1) shows a lesion on the LAD. There is a short left main stem and then the LAD passes downwards. A left Judkins 4 cm (JL4) catheter would be suitable to enter LCA. Note that the circumflex artery is occluded. A shallow RAO cranial (RAO 6°, cranial 28°) shows the lesion well which is at a bifurcation (2). The diagonal artery is relatively small, and the lesion does not involve the origin of the branches. PTCA with a single wire down the LAD was successful, and flow to the side branch (diagonal artery) was not compromised.

b) *The form of left main stem and choice of suitable guide catheter.*
This is best assessed on the A P projection. (See Figure 1.4 page 8).
If the LMS is flat or downward pointing, Judkins JL4 or Voda 3.5 catheter (Angiogram 7.1 and 7.2 on pages 80 and 82).
If the LMS is upward pointing, use JL 3.5, or JL3, or Voda 3.0 guide catheter.
3) **Type of Origin and Initial Course of the Vessel**
   1. RCA — is there an angulated U-shaped course (shepherd's crook) to initial third of vessel? If this is present cannulation of the RCA and tracking a stent around this initial section will be more difficult (Angiogram 22.2 on page 233).
   2. LCX — type of origin of the LCX from the Left Main Stem (Figure 7.1). When assessing a circumflex artery lesion, carefully check the length of LMS and the type of origin of the LCX from the LMS. Two extreme types are:-

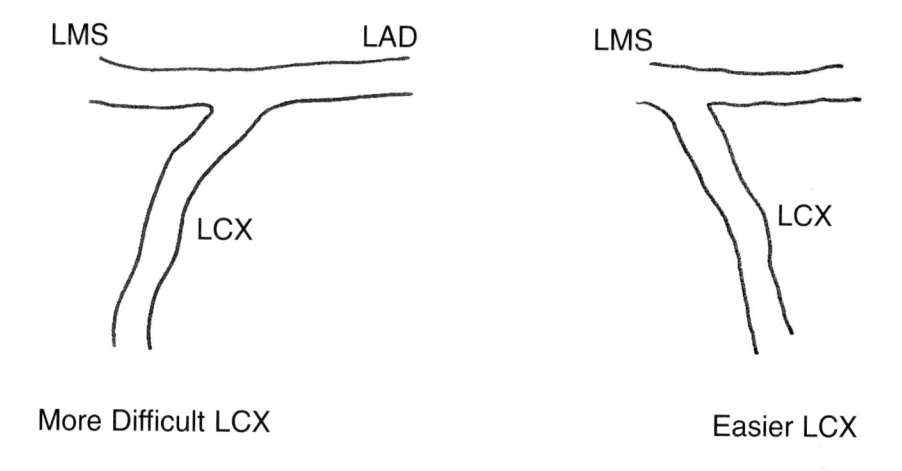

Figure 7.1. Types of Circumflex artery and left main stem.

The More Difficult LCX (Angiogram 8.2 on page 94)
a) Long left main stem.
b) Right angle bend (or less than 90°) present at the origin of LCX.
c) Passage of wire and balloon into and along the LCX will be more difficult.
d) Need good back-up from guide catheter, as may be obtained by an Amplatz or Voda guide catheters.
e) The left Judkins shape guide catheter will often provide insufficient back-up.

The Easier LCX (Angiogram 7.2)
a) Short left main stem.
b) LCX comes off at an obtuse angle from LMS.
c) Passage of guide wire and tracking of balloon are usually easy.
d) Less back-up needed from guide catheter.
e) Left Judkins shaped guide catheter is often adequate.

4) **Is There Proximal Disease?**
This may impede passage of a stent. Is there ostial disease, especially in a saphenous vein graft?

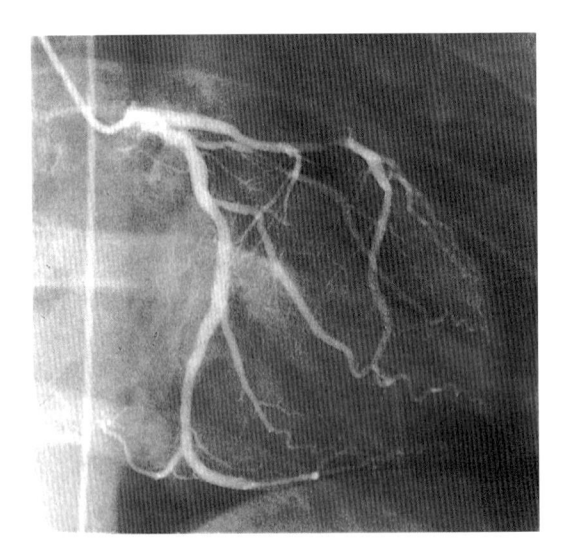

Angiogram 7.2. *'Easier' left circumflex artery.* The LAD in middle third has a lesion on the bend as the artery turns round into the inter ventricular groove. The left main stem is short and the circumflex artery comes off at an obtuse angle. This is an 'easier' circumflex artery, as a guide wire will pass easily into the circumflex, and there will be good backup available from a left Judkins guide catheter for PTCA, if a lesion was present in the circumflex artery.

5) **Collateral Vessels**
   Are they present to the artery beyond to the lesion?
6) **Severity of other CAD**
   Is the case 1, 2, or 3 vessel disease?
7) **Assess LV function**
   It is not essential to have a measured ejection fraction (EF). If the EF is available, Dr G. Hartzler of Kansas City USA divides patients into those with an EF of above or below 40%, i.e. of lower and higher risk.

   Is there angiographic evidence of previous MI in the territory of the vessel to be dilated? This will not preclude PTCA but if angina is mild or absent, medical treatment may be more appropriate. In unstable angina post MI and primary PTCA for MI, angiographic evidence of an infarct will routinely be expected.
8) **Assess Overall Risk**
   From reviewing features 1–7, an idea of the overall *complexity* and *risk* for the PTCA will be gained. Patients may be placed into one of three rough categories, low, medium, or high complexity and risk for PTCA. These categories may influence the order on the catheter list schedule, degree of surgical cover and when discussing PTCA with the patient.
9) **Consider Procedure Details**
   a) Which vessel first, if the case is one for multivessel PTCA? (See page 86 below).
   b) What equipment to use? Guide catheter, balloon size, guide wire and alternative shapes and sizes.

Review of the Diagnostic Angiogram   83

Previous RCA   PTCA + Stent   3 Vessel D.   LV > 40%

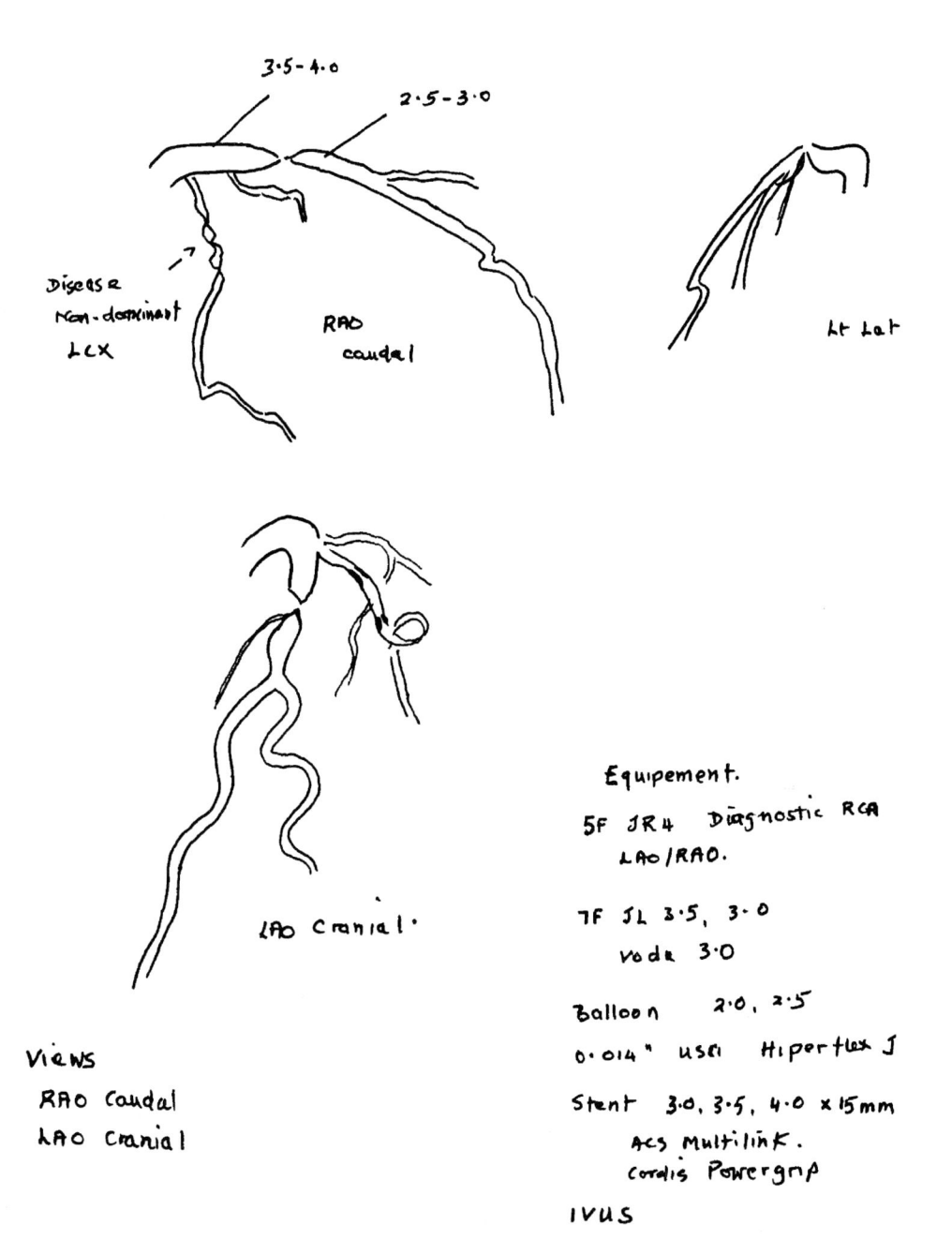

3.5-4.0
2.5-3.0

Disease
Non-dominant
LCX

RAO caudal

Lt Lat

LAO Cranial

Views
RAO Caudal
LAO Cranial

Equipement.
5F JR4   Diagnostic RCA
LAO/RAO.

7F JL 3.5, 3.0
vode 3.0

Balloon   2.0, 2.5

0.014" usci Hiperflex J

Stent 3.0, 3.5, 4.0 x 15mm
   Acs Multilink.
   cordis Powergrip

IVUS

Figure 7.2. Menu sheet.

c) What possible alternative equipment might be needed? e.g. stent, IABP, pacing wire, IVUS, or rotablator.
d) Radiographic views to use.
e) Approach if vessel occludes during PTCA.

10) **Vessel Anatomy**
Review carefully and try to remember the vessel's anatomy as much as possible. Look at the small side branches, especially those near the lesion. These may 'get in the way' by allowing the GW to enter them rather the main channel. On the other hand they can be a 'sign post' or 'land mark' to define a point in the vessel and can be very helpful for accurate stent placement.

As a personal practice a *"menu sheet"* is prepared and given to the catheter room nurse before the start of the procedure (Figure 7.2). It is later stuck up on a nearby wall or screen. On a single sheet of A4 paper the following are recorded:-

1. A sketch of the coronary artery and lesion in the two radiographic planes to be used.
2. The radiographic views that are to be used and other possible views to consider.
3. The equipment to be used, or possibly needed: i.e. guide catheters, balloons and their sizes, guide wire, stents, pacing catheter (see Angiogram 11.1 on page 122) and intra aortic balloon pump etc.

This 'menu sheet' is helpful to the nurses who can inform you if an item of equipment that you are considering using, is not available. Besides its use during the procedure, the sheet can be referred to later if a repeat angioplasty is being considered.

Assessment of Lesion Types and the Risk of Vessel Occlusion at PTCA
(See also page 155)

The Joint Task force of the American College of Cardiology and the American Heart Association, has classified lesions and risks of PTCA into three categories, A, B & C.

<u>**Lesion Specific Characteristics**</u>
Type A Lesions (high success, >85%; low risk)

Discrete (<10 mm length)	Little or no calcification
Concentric	Less than totally occlusive
Readily accessible	Not ostial in location
Nonangulated segment <45°	No major branch involvement
Smooth contour	Absence of thrombus

Type B lesions (moderate success, 60 to 85%; moderate risk*)

Tubular (10 to 20 mm length)	Moderate to heavy calcification
Eccentric	Total occlusions <3 months old
Moderate tortuosity of proximal segment	Ostial in location
Moderately angulated segment, >45°, <90°	Bifurcation lesions requiring double guide wires
Irregular contour	Some thrombus present

Type C lesions (low success, <60%; high risk)

Diffuse (>2 cm length)
Excessive tortuosity of proximal segment
Extremely angulated segments >90°

Total occlusion >3 months old
Inability to protect major side branches
Degenerated vein grafts with friable lesions

*Although the risk of abrupt vessel closure in Type B Lesions is moderate, in certain instances the likelihood of a major complication may be low, as in the dilatation of total occlusions <3 months old, or when abundant collateral channels supply the distal vessel. Reference: Ryan TJ, Faxon DP, Gunnar RM, *et al*. Guidelines for percutaneous transluminal coronary angioplasty. *J Am Coll Cardiol* **12**, 529–545 (1988).

The ACC/AHA classification is valuable to provide a descriptive record in medical literature of the type of cases being attempted by a given method, or with a new item of equipment.

Perhaps of greater practical help is to consider features which are associated with lower or higher risk of acute closure or dissection (see also page 155).

Abrupt Closure

Lower Risk	*Higher Risk*
1. Smooth concentric lesion.	Eccentric, or ulcerated, or cul-de-sac lesion.
2. Short lesion <1cm	Longer lesion >1cm, especially 2–3cm or diffuse disease.
3. Lesion on a straight segment of the artery.	Lesion on an acute bend, especially RCA.
4. Stable angina.	Unstable angina.
5. Absence of thrombus.	Presence of thrombus; often difficult to detect by angiography; a feature of unstable angina or acute M.I.
6. Restenosis	De novo lesion
7. Medium and larger calibre artery.	Small calibre vessel — 2 mm or less.
8. Male patient.	Female patient: usually related to small vessel size.
9. Non-diabetic.	Diabetic patient: usually related to more diffuse disease.

(*Features 1–4 are the more important ones*).

Other Features to Consider

1. **Can the vessel lesion be stented?**
   If the vessel occludes, or for de novo stenting.
   Three important aspects to consider are:-
   a) *Vessel calibre* — when 3 mm or more, there is a lower risk of stent thrombosis and restenosis. Vessels of 2.5 mm calibre are still potentially suitable for a stent.
   b) *Lesion accessibility* — amount of vessel tortuosity and proximal disease which may impede a stent reaching the lesion.
   c) *Lesion visibility* — this needs to be good for accurate placement of a stent to cover the lesion (see also page 147).

2. **Which Vessel First?**
   For cases needing more than one vessel to be dilated, the *first* artery to be dilated will usually:-
   a) *Have the culprit lesion* — e.g. in unstable angina, a critical lesion in a large significant artery supplying the territory where there has been ECG changes.
   b) *Be the more important artery* — i.e. supplying a larger area or territory of myocardium.
   c) *Be the more difficult artery to dilate* — There is usually no point in dilating an easier or smaller artery, if later a more important but more difficult vessel cannot also be dilated.

3. **Attempt to Reopen a Chronically Occluded Artery to Support Dilating the Target Vessel?**
   If dilating for example a severe LAD stenosis and if there is a chronically occluded RCA responsible for an inferior M.I. a few years earlier, some operators will attempt to reopen the RCA to provide collateral support during PTCA especially if the LAD occludes. Unless the RCA has only a very short and favourable occlusion (see page 202), PTCA time and finances are not usually well spent in trying to reopen the chronically occluded vessel. Instead it is better to have a well prepared strategy for the PTCA dilatation and possible occlusion. This might include PTCA with a perfusion balloon, or elective stenting.

4. **LV Function**
   If this is severely impaired an intra aortic balloon pump (IABP) may be considered. The pump should be in the catheter room. A small 5F sheath may be popped into the contralateral femoral artery to allow ready access. Rarely, an IABP may be used from the start of the procedure.

5. **Surgical Cover**
   If the case is of higher risk, such as from very poor LV function, or because PTCA is to be attempted on the last or nearly last remaining artery, or the lesion is on a very dominant LAD or RCA, it is wise to discuss the case with the surgeon before undertaking the procedure. The PTCA can be 'scheduled' to suit the surgeon. At the very least, the surgeon can't complain (or explode) that PTCA should have never been attempted in the first place!

6. **Form of Aortic Arch and Distal Aorta**
   If the LV angiogram shows that the aorta is very dilated and tortuous, guide catheter manipulation may be more difficult. Often this can be improved by using a long

femoral sheath, extending to the lower abdominal aorta. Some interventionists electively use a long sheath in elderly patients, e.g. over the age of 70 where tortuosity of iliac vessels is commoner.

Conclusion

With experience, much of the considerations and thought processes discussed in this chapter will occur automatically. However, time spent in reviewing the angiogram and planning the procedure may reap dividends during the 'heat' of the PTCA itself. *To be prepared is to be forearmed!*

8 Routine PTCA Case

No two operators work in entirely the same manner and even the same case approached on another occasion might be managed in a different way. After all 'variety is the spice of life'.

This chapter discusses the operative procedures in the catheter laboratory during a routine angioplasty (Angiograms 8.1 and 8.2 on pages 90 and 94). The ancillary medical treatment and ward care, are discussed in Chapter 6.

Using standard angiographic techniques, a 6–8F sheath is inserted into the femoral artery. If the iliac vessels are very tortuous, as may occur in elderly patients, consider a long 20–30 cm sheath extending to the abdominal aorta which will facilitate manipulation and rotation of the guide catheter. Through the sheath, the guide catheter is advanced to the ascending aorta. With a 6 or 7F guide catheter this can be done over a guide wire protruding out of the proximal end of the guide catheter. With 8F and 9F guides, there is a liberal back flow of blood. This can be prevented by first connecting the Y connector to both the guide catheter and pressure manifold and having the guide wire protruding through the screwed down 'o'-ring.

The guide catheter is passed into the vessel and control angiograms taken. Sometimes these angios will be done with a diagnostic catheter (which is cheaper and easier to use), if there is doubt whether a PTCA will be needed (e.g. for a restenosis lesion), or be feasible.

It is *important that the tip of the guide catheter sits nicely and is stable* in the coronary artery. If the guide catheter tip easily falls out, or points in the wrong direction, there will be poor support from the guide catheter. Time is much better spent sorting out the guide catheter at this stage, rather than regretting not having done so at a later stage when the balloon or stent won't cross the lesion.

If the arterial pressure recorded at the tip of the guide catheter falls significantly, the guide catheter is too large for the vessel, or there is mild spasm of the artery, or there is an osteal stenosis. This situation is described as 'the pressures damping off'. The problem is relatively common with the RCA. The guide catheter is changed for one with side holes, or downsized in calibre, i.e. from an 8F to a 7F or 6F guide (see p. 6). The practice of drilling sideholes into the guide catheter is best avoided as there is a significant risk of damaging the catheter which will then give less support.

90 *Guide to Coronary Angioplasty and Stenting*

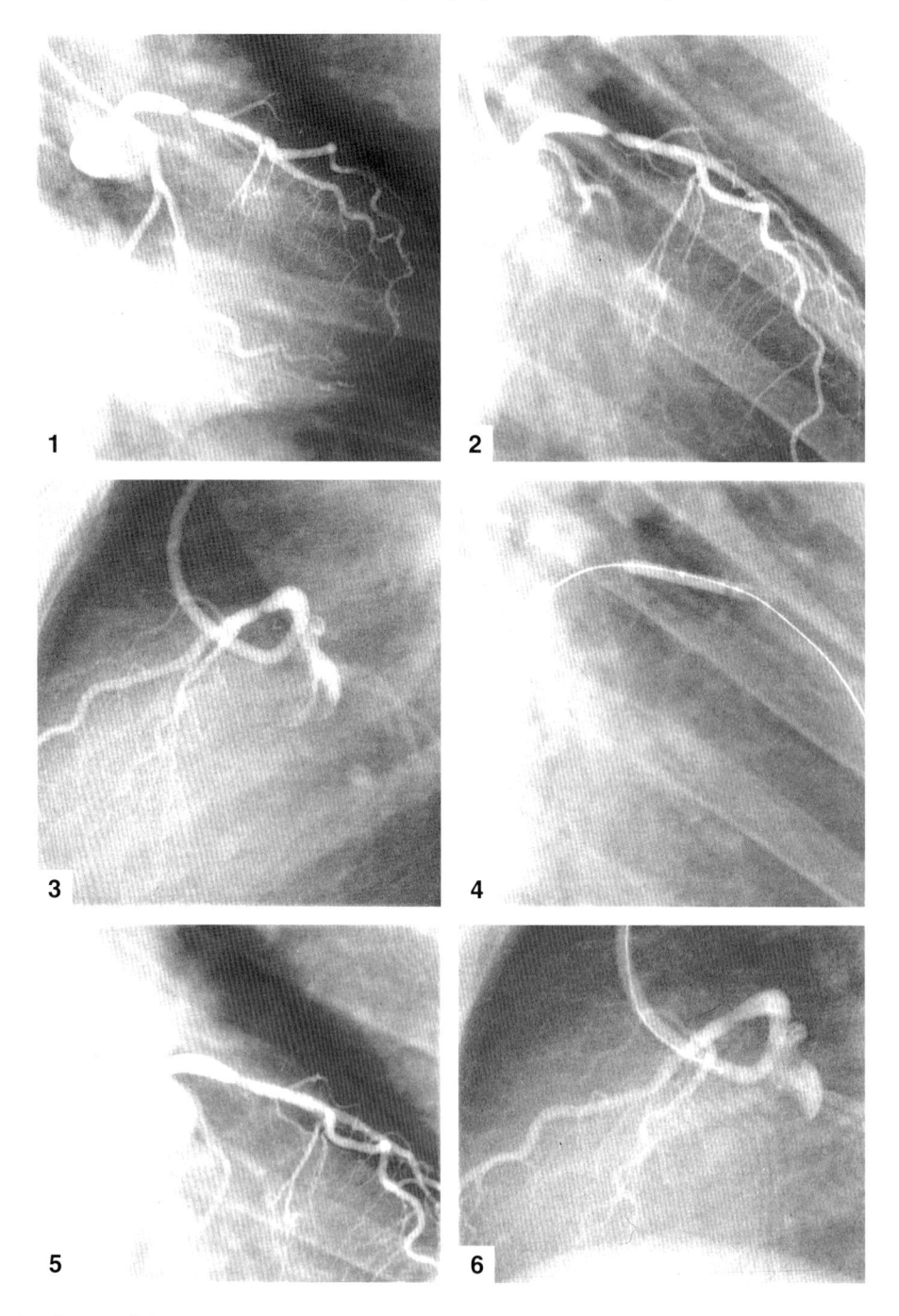

Angiogram 8.1. *Routine PTCA of an LAD lesion.* The diagnostic angiogram shows a very short left main stem with an upward pointing LAD (1). An 8F JL 3.5 guide catheter was used to point to and selectively catheterize the LAD (2) RAO caudal, and (3) left lateral with 5° caudal. The lesion on the LAD was dilated with 2.5 then 3 mm balloons (4). The end result was satisfactory (5) and (6), with approximately a 20–30% residual lesion. There is mild haziness at the site of the dilated lesion. There was no clinical restenosis (i.e. no recurrence of angina).

Once the control angios have been taken there is a short pause, whilst these are reviewed and the balloon catheter is prepared. One or two views are "frozen" on digital or video to be used as 'road maps' to show vessel anatomy. If quantitative analysis (QCA, quantitative coronary angiography) is available the vessel size and lesion severity and length are measured.

Heparin 10,000 units IV is given. If not already done so, the patient is asked to confirm that he or she has taken aspirin that morning.

The balloon catheter is prepared (or "prepped") by aspirating on the balloon port with a 10 ml syringe containing 2–3 ml of dilute contrast at full negative pressure. Most use a 50–50 contrast/dextrose or saline, whilst some use neat contrast. The hub of the balloon catheter (or the syringe) is tapped several times with the fingers, to remove as much air as possible from the catheter. The syringe plunger is released to allow a small amount of contrast to flow into the balloon catheter. A small meniscus of contrast is left just above the rim of the catheter hub. The indeflator (or balloon inflation device) is filled with dilute contrast up to 4–5 ml of a 10 ml syringe, or to about 10–12 ml if the indeflator has a 20 ml syringe. It is connected to the balloon catheter and full negative pressure applied by withdrawing the plunger to the maximum extent and locking it at this position.

The balloon catheter and guide wire are taken to the patient and the guide wire fed retrogradely back along the balloon catheter to either the hub (Over the wire [OTW] balloon), or until it emerges a short distance back from the balloon (monorail/rapid exchange balloon).

With the tip of the guide wire just inside the balloon, the combined balloon and guide wire are passed through the 'o'-ring of the Y-connector and into the guide catheter. The ascending aorta is then screened and the guide wire passed up until it appears in the guide catheter at this level. The balloon catheter is then advanced at first without screening until the markers on the distal section of the shaft reach the Y-connector. The aorta is then again screened until the marker(s) of the balloon itself come into view. A check is made to ensure that the balloon marker is on the wire and not beside it, indicating that the balloon has come off the wire which is relatively easily done with rapid exchange balloons.

The guide wire is then advanced into the coronary artery and across the lesion and as distally as can be reached. Time will be well spent achieving this to reduce the risk of the guide wire coming back across the lesion in error and to have a firmer section of the guide wire approaching and passing across the lesion (see pages 27–29).

The guide wire is checked in more than one plane to ensure that it is in the correct artery. This is especially true for the LAD to ensure that it is not in a diagonal or septal perforating branch (see page 52). It is so embarrassing explaining why the wrong artery was dilated!

The balloon catheter is then advanced along the guide wire and across the lesion. With the modern low profile balloons there is often little or no resistance for the balloon to cross.

The first dilatation is done by slowly increasing the inflation pressure (on the indeflator) to a low pressure of about 3–4 atmospheres. The balloon will often have a clear dumb bell appearance, confirming that the balloon is on the lesion (Angiogram 8.2). The patient is informed that anginal pain may occur and the ECG is observed for changes of ischaemia. After about 1 minute the balloon is deflated. Sometimes even during this initial 'low pressure inflation', the balloon may suddenly be seen to fully expand indicating that the lesion has been dilated (or 'cracked').

Usually some part of the balloon inflation(s) are recorded on fluoroscopy and the inflation pressure and duration documented.

The duration of the initial inflation which can be tolerated may be quite short, of the order of 20–45 seconds. With subsequent ones, more prolonged inflations may be possible with less angina or ECG changes. This phenomenon of *preconditioning*, where after one episode of ischaemia the myocardium can better tolerate a further one, is commonly seen at angioplasty.

With the second (and subsequent) dilatations, the inflation pressure is increased to at least the "nominal pressure" i.e. the pressure at which the balloon reaches its specified size. This is usually about 6 or 7 atmospheres. Sometimes it is necessary to increase to high pressures (10–14 atmospheres), to achieve full balloon expansion, i.e. to 'crack' the lesion. The number and length of inflations used by an operator is very variable. Most use at least one dilatation for one minute.

A small contrast injection is made after a dilatation to assess progress. The balloon is left at the lesion, or with a rapid exchange balloon which is very easy to move along the guide wire, the balloon catheter is withdrawn some distance out of the coronary artery to allow improved visualisation of the vessel with contrast injections. Angios are recorded sometimes in two projections. They are carefully reviewed by playing back the video recording, including on magnified or zoom mode, to inspect the dilated lesion. The amount of residual stenosis and the presence of minor or major dissection are assessed. The proximal and distal vessel are checked too. A decision is taken that the result is satisfactory, or that more dilatation is needed with the same or a larger balloon, or that a stent is needed.

If the result is satisfactory the guide wire is withdrawn across the lesion to outside the artery, or if vessel access has been difficult, to just proximal to the lesion. Further angios are recorded and analysed. If at any stage there is doubt as to how satisfactory the PTCA result is, *"catheter dawdle"* for 5 minutes can be very worthwhile. An angiogram is repeated after about 5 minutes, sometimes with a '5 min' X-ray label. The lesion may be unchanged, or be seen to be deteriorating when alternative strategies such as a stent may be needed. It is much better to detect in the catheter room that the lesion has got worse, than have the patient deteriorate (or "go off") after returning to the ward.

If the procedure lasts longer than 1 hour, or if a stent is to be employed, a blood sample is taken from the side-arm of the sheath or the guide catheter, to check the activated clotting time (ACT). If the value is less than 250 seconds for PTCA, or 300 seconds for a stent procedure, a top up bolus of 2–5,000 units of heparin is given. If the patient is to receive ReoPro, the ACT is maintained at 200–250 seconds (see page 162). For a stent patient, the test may be repeated after about 5 minutes to confirm that the desired ACT level has been reached.

If the lesion is satisfactory on the post dilatation angiograms, the guide catheter is withdrawn carefully and under X-ray screening, especially if removing it from the RCA, or if an Amplatz guide catheter was used in the left coronary artery (see Angiograms 6.1 and 8.2 on pages 71 and 94). If the guide catheter is well 'locked' into the artery, there is a risk that damage to the vessel may occur on withdrawing the catheter. This can be avoided by passing the guide wire and balloon back into the first part of the artery and then withdrawing the guide catheter over the balloon catheter (see page 9).

The femoral sheath is secured with a skin suture, a bung is placed on the side arm and a dressing positioned on top of the sheath.

A record in the notes of the procedure is made. A set of clear instructions is written on the charts for the post operative nursing care. These include the IV fluid regime, post operative heparin (to be given or not to be given and amounts), medical drugs and when the patient can resume eating and drinking (usually immediately). A comment is made as to when the sheath is to be removed (usually the same evening, or next morning).

There is much to recommend a formal typewritten record of the procedure, as is usually done after surgical operations. Reviewing a previous PTCA procedure is greatly simplified if a type written report is available.

Variations on the Technique of the Routine PTCA Case

There are many possible variations to the case described.

(1) **Passing a Bare Guide Wire**

Passing a GW without a balloon catheter, down a coronary artery, allows excellent visualization of the vessel during contrast injections. This makes it easier to pass the GW down to the lesion, especially if the vessel anatomy is complex from overlying branches. The clear visualization may facilitate the crossing of the lesion with the GW. However sometimes a bare GW may be more difficult to cross a lesion, especially a complex cul-de-sac lesion. If the balloon is advanced on the GW into the coronary artery to a short distance (1–3 cm) back from the tip, the GW is stiffened and supported. Often it is then easier to manipulate the GW across the lesion.

With modern large lumen guide catheters and low profile balloon and shaft size to PTCA catheters, coronary visualization is usually perfectly adequate with the balloon already on the GW when using 7F or 8F guides catheters. The bare wire technique is more useful with small sized guide catheters (5F or 6F), or if a diagnostic catheter is used instead of a PTCA guide catheter, as their lumen size is also smaller.

Sometimes after manipulation of a GW across a severe stenosis, ischaemia develops and it is very helpful to be able to promptly advance the balloon already on the GW across the lesion to dilate it.

(2) **Balloon Inflation**

Operator practice varies but as a general rule fewer rather than more dilatations and lower rather than very high pressures (more than 10 atmospheres), are preferable. Most PTCA balloons are made of compliant or semi compliant material. By increasing the inflation pressure to 10–12 atmospheres, approximately an extra 1/4 size can be obtained, e.g. a 3 mm balloon will 'grow' to 3.25 mm. This feature can be used to save the time and expense of going up to the next larger sized balloon.

An angioplasty balloon is usually inflated for about one minute. Using a perfusion balloon (see page 20), a single inflation for 5–10 minutes often produces a very favourable result with minimal dissection (see Angiogram 2.1, page 22). There is less screening and fewer angiograms are recorded; hence the radiation exposure is reduced and less contrast is used.

Some patients can tolerate a prolonged inflation of up to 7 minutes with a standard balloon to achieve a similar result to the perfusion balloon. This is particularly true for PTCA in acute M.I.

The main snag of using a perfusion balloon, is the tedium of a prolonged inflation. Most angioplasty operators have Type A personalities and patience is not one of their virtues!

94   *Guide to Coronary Angioplasty and Stenting*

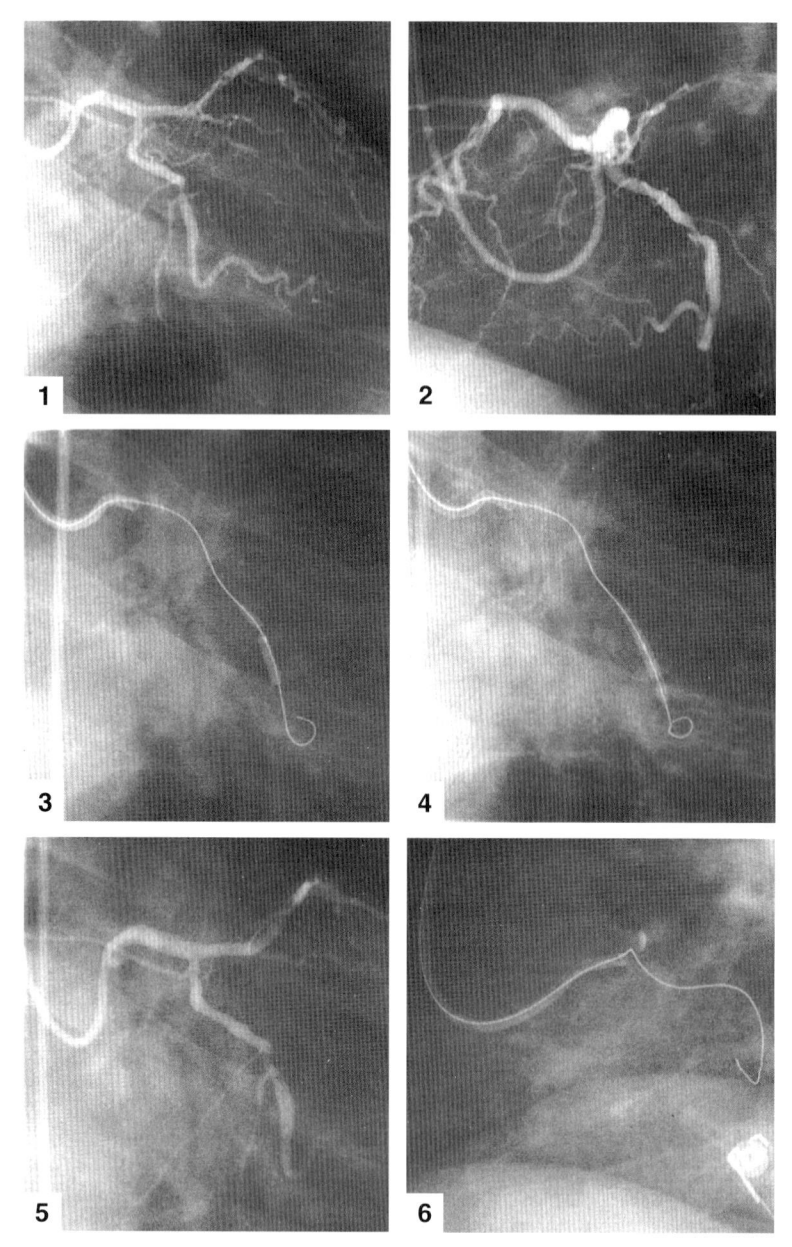

Angiogram 8.2. *Angioplasty of left circumflex artery.* In shallow RAO Caudal (RAO 20°, Caudal 20°) and LAO 80° the lesion is well seen (1 and 2). The RAO Caudal view shows that the circumflex artery is a 'difficult' one for backup. There is a long left main stem, and the circumflex artery arises at nearly a right angle. Later there is another right angle bend before the lesion is reached. Good guide catheter support or back-up is achieved with a left Amplatz II (AL2) catheter (1 and 2). The lesion was crossed without difficulty with a 2.5 mm Europass balloon on a 0.014" guide wire. A waist or nip or hour-glass indentation on the balloon is seen at the lesion site (3). On increasing the inflation pressure from 5 to 7 atmospheres full expansion of the balloon is achieved, and the lesion dilated or 'cracked' (4). The lesion is relieved but there is a haziness at the lesion site (5). The LAO view also shows D-shaped staining of the left main stem (6), from damage by the left Amplatz guide catheter. The contrast cleared quickly and no progression of the damage to the left main stem occurred.

(3) **Predilatation**
   Some operators, especially if the lesion is very tight, will predilate with a smaller catheter and then up-size to the correct balloon size for the artery. This may reduce the risk of dissection. Certainly if there is doubt over the vessel size, it is always better to start with a smaller balloon and go up a size. One can always go *up* a size of balloon, but one can't go *down* a size if the balloon causes dissection! (Note that it was the balloon, not the doctor's choice, that caused the dissection!).

(4) **Recording Angiograms**
   Some operators only record the final result, whilst others like to "tell a story" of the PTCA procedure. For the final PTCA result, most operators will remove the GW from the artery, whilst others will accept an angio with the GW still across the lesion.

(5) **Contrast in the Balloon**
   Neat rather than diluted contrast is used by some operators to show more clearly the inflated balloon. Any dumb bell narrowing or section of incomplete expansion of the balloon, will be seen more easily especially with a small sized balloon such as a 2 mm or 1.5 mm size. A balloon with neat contrast is slightly slower to deflate. These operators 'like their contrast as they like their whisky — neat' !

Failure to Cross the Lesion

If the balloon will not cross the lesion, the tip of the guide catheter will be seen to back out of the coronary artery, while attempting to advance (or 'push') the balloon across the lesion. This problem is now relatively rare with low profile balloons, perhaps less than 10% of cases of PTCA for stenosis (as opposed to chronic total occlusion). It is more difficult for a balloon to cross a lesion, if it has to first pass down a tortuous and or long coronary artery. Hence crossing distal lesions, especially in a tortuous RCA, or where there is a right angled bend to the LCX as it comes of the left main stem, may be difficult. Similarly, a lesion at the anastomosis site of a very tortuous LIMA can be quite a challenge!

Methods to Consider when the Balloon will not Cross the Lesion

(1) **Deeply Engage the Guide Catheter**
   This is especially effective for LAD lesions as it is relatively easy to advance a left Judkins catheter along the left main stem towards or even into the proximal LAD. The balloon catheter is gently withdrawn as the guide catheter is advanced, which eases the process. The balloon catheter is then given excellent support to cross the lesion. Once the balloon has crossed, the guide catheter is promptly withdrawn back to the start of the left main stem; as this is done the balloon catheter is gently advanced to stop it being "sucked back" with the guide catheter.
   There is always a small risk of damaging and even dissecting the left main stem with this manoeuvre. Deep engagement can be used for lesions on other vessels. It is sometimes called "deep throating" the guide catheter.

(2) **Tapping the Balloon**
   With this method, which was greatly favoured by Dr. Geoffrey Hartzler of Kansas City, USA, the balloon is passed to the mouth of the lesion. The catheter balloon shaft held between thumb and index finger is given a series of rapid sharp tapping move-

ments. With these the balloon may slowly advance across the lesion.

(3) **Using a Very Small Balloon Catheter**

Using the smallest size available, i.e. a 1.5 mm balloon, to cross and predilate the lesion and then followed by the balloon catheter originally used. In the past this was quite often necessary and manufacturers would claim that their 1.5 mm balloon 'had such a low profile that where a guide wire would go, so would their 1.5 mm balloon'. They would be prepared to reimburse the cost if one of their 1.5 mm balloons did not live up to expectations.

(4) **Using a Stiffer Guide Wire**

If the problem is believed to be mainly a tracking one, then changing to a stiffer guide wire may allow the balloon to move more easily towards and across the lesion. With an OTW balloon the guide wire is quite easily removed and changed for a stiffer one. This is not possible with a rapid exchange balloon, where the old guide wire has to be withdrawn and the lesion re-crossed with the new stiffer wire.

(5) **Replacement of the Guide Catheter**

This may be essential if the original guide catheter is not in a stable and satisfactory position. Even if the guide catheter position was fine, a guide catheter with more support may be needed such as an Amplatz catheter.

This option is only taken with reluctance and regret, as usually the whole system has to be removed, i.e. the guide catheter and the guide wire with balloon; the procedure is then started anew. There is usually concern that the vessel may close at the lesion site. It is feasible, but difficult and fiddly to extend the GW, leave it in place, remove the original guide catheter and replace with another. If at all possible try to prevent this problem by ensuring good guide catheter support is achieved at the start of the procedure.

(6) **Pass a Fixed Guide Wire Balloon Catheter**

These balloon catheters have a very low profile and some operators such as Dr Tony Rickards of the Royal Brompton Hospital in London, UK, are able to slide one along side the guide wire and across the lesion. When this balloon is inflated, the initial guide wire is still in place and tends to act as a 'cheese cutter' along the artery in contact with the balloon. Usually this doesn't seem to matter (see page 25, Cutting Balloon).

(7) **Inflating the Balloon in the Mouth of the Lesion**

The balloon is advanced as far into the lesion as it will go and then inflated. The aim is to open up the start (or mouth) of the lesion and then advance fully across it after the initial or next dilatation. *This method is mentioned to be* **condemned**. Whilst tempting to try and sometimes it may succeed, more usually it will fail and often lead to a worse situation of vessel closure. The lesion has then become occluded and it is not possible to get that balloon (nor perhaps any other) across it. The surgeon beckons!

Undilatable Lesion

On rare occasions, a lesion cannot be dilated despite the use of high inflation pressures. This problem is discussed on page 235.

Devices to Aid Femoral Haemostasis

The routine patient has the femoral sheath removed about 4–6 hours after stopping Heparin, following confirmation that the PTTK is <1.5:1 or the ACT <150 seconds. There are a number of devices deployed in the catheter room which can achieve prompt haemostasis and early mobilisation, *even if the patient is fully anticoagulated.*

A plug of collagen is passed down the tract to the artery with *Vasoseal* (Datascope) and pressure maintained on the site for about 15 minutes.

With *Angio-Seal* (Sherwood Medical), a small anchor is deployed inside the femoral artery with 2 sutures emerging, which are tied down on to an absorbable plug of collagen. Pressure is maintained on the site for about 20 minutes.

Perclose (Perclose) was invented by Prof. John Simpson of California (who also designed the first 'over-the-wire' balloon for ACS/Guidant), and is a more complicated device. It has 2 needles (4 needles after use of larger sheaths 9 or 10 F) which allow sutures to be passed across the puncture site in the femoral artery and then tied. Usually haemostasis is complete immediately, but sometimes a gentle ooze may require a short period of groin compression. The skin access down to the artery needs to be enlarged, but despite this, later scarring does not occur to any extent. Repuncture within 24 hours (for a PTCA complication), or at a later date, occurs without difficulty. With both Angioseal and Vasoseal the thrombin plug can lead to fibrosis making later puncture of the artery difficult. Rarely, occlusion of the femoral artery by the plug may occur.

Femstop (Radi Medical) is a device with a pressure ring that can be applied instead of manual compression to the groin. It is more comfortable than a sand bag. Its success is variable and usually poor with obese patients.

All these devices add to the *cost* of PTCA. As an aggressive anticoagulant regime is no longer routinely used after deployment of a coronary artery stent, the main requirement for these devices has disappeared. On the other hand, patient comfort is improved and valuable medical or nursing time is not wasted pressing on groins. Complications such as pseudoaneurysm may also be reduced.

Conclusion

There are many ways to cook an egg, and likewise with PTCA many variations on a basic theme are used. Ensuring good guide catheter back-up pays dividends later in the procedure, especially for LCX lesions and when deploying stents. Closure devices for the femoral artery are becoming more successful and popular.

9 PTCA from the Arm

The femoral artery is the usual route for coronary angioplasty. The X-ray intensifier and tube can be rotated and angulated as needed. The foot of the table and the space between the legs provide a stable platform for the PTCA equipment. Repeated catheterizations using the right or left femoral artery is possible. Ready access to a venous route via the femoral vein is available. If an IABP is needed, this may be passed up the contralateral femoral artery.

Angioplasty from the arm may be considered for:

(1) **Difficult femoral access**
   This may occur with:
   a) Peripheral vascular disease, inhibiting cannulation of the femoral artery.
   b) Very tortuous iliac artery and or abdominal aorta.
   c) Abdominal aneurysm.
   It is only rarely that conditions b) and c) give a problem with catheterization from the femoral route.

(2) **Early secure haemostasis**
   The need for this has receded as oral anticoagulants are no longer used routinely after placement of a coronary artery stent. The more secure haemostasis may make the arm approach safer for day-case angioplasty i.e. where the patient is discharged on the same day as the PTCA.

(3) **Operator choice**
   For those who routinely perform diagnostic angiography using the Sones technique.

The main disadvantage when using the arm, is the reduced range of radiographic screening available. This is because the arm often gets in the way of the image intensifier and the X-ray tube, when attempting steep and angulated views.

From the arm there are two access sites available for PTCA:-

a) Brachial artery.
b) Radial artery.

The axillary artery may also potentially be used, and diagnostic catheterization of this vessel via a percutaneous technique is occasionally employed.

Brachial Artery

Catheterisation is usually by an arteriotomy, though some operators use a percutaneous technique and a 6–8F sheath. An arteriotomy repair will give the more secure haemostasis.

Using the *left* brachial artery all the regular catheters of the femoral route will function quite satisfactorily. It is a minor inconvenience to have the patient turned through 180° on the table, or to work from the left side of the X-ray table.

Using the *right* brachial artery the femoral catheters do not need to pass round the aortic arch and some shapes function less well. Usually R. Judkins, Amplatz, and Multipurpose catheters are still satisfactory, but the L. Judkins catheter is not adequate. There are specifically designed *brachial* catheters, including a modified Left Judkins catheter.

The right coronary artery and coronary grafts (especially RCA graft) can usually be cannulated with ease, using a Sones or a Multipurpose catheter. The Sones catheter may give poor backup for angioplasty of the LCA branches, as it may not sit well in the Left Main Stem of the LCA. However, regular operators can often manipulate a Sones catheter into the start of the LAD or LCX artery, which then provides a very good platform for PTCA.

Radial Artery Puncture

This is a relatively recent technique introduced by Dr. Ferdinand Kiemeneij of Amsterdam in Holland. The adequacy of collateral supply of the hand from the ulnar artery is first assessed using the *Allen test*. Both the radial and ulnar arteries are compressed for half a minute, whilst the hand is opened and closed by the patient about 15 times. After release of pressure on the ulnar artery, the pink colour of the hand should return within 10 seconds. Following this there should be no reactive hyperaemia on release of radial compression.

Either radial artery can be used, but usually it is more convenient to use the right, and work from the right side of the X-ray table.

The arm is abducted to 70° and the wrist hyperextended. Five ml of 1% lignocaine are injected subcutaneously over the radial artery. The vessel is punctured at an angle of 45° to the skin, 1 cm proximal from the styloid process, using a 22 gauge needle from an *Arrow Radial Artery Catheterization Set* (Arrow International). Once arterial blood appears from the needle, the small short guide wire that comes with the set is advanced into the artery. The needle itself is then gently advanced over the guide wire into the radial artery. The very short guide wire is removed and replaced by an 0.025 inch 135 cm J-shaped guide wire which is advanced up into the ascending aorta. A small incision is made over the puncture site to enlarge it. The needle is removed and a 6F long (30 cm) sheath and introducer are passed along the 0.025 inch guide wire into the artery.

When the sheath is in position, a 'heparin cocktail' is injected via the side arm of the sheath. The 'heparin cocktail' contains:

10,000 units of heparin
200 micrograms of glyceryl trinitrate (GTN)
1/2 ml of 1% lignocaine.

The GTN and lignocaine are given to reduce the risk of spasm developing in the radial or brachial artery system.

Over the guide wire, 6F catheters can be passed into the sheath and advanced to the ascending aorta. The guide wire is removed and the vessel to be dilated cannulated. As explained above, adequate stability is difficult with Judkins catheters. For guide catheters passed up from the right radial artery consider using:

a) For RCA   Multipurpose catheter
                       Amplatz right catheter
                       Judkins right catheter
b) For LCA   Amplatz left catheter
                       Voda or extra back-up catheter
                       Multipurpose catheter

Kiemeneij has designed a '*Kimmy Radial Catheter*' (Schneider, 6F), which can be slipped into either RCA or LCA.

A modern wide lumen 6F guide is of sufficient calibre to allow virtually any of the current stents available to be passed down it and deployed at a lesion. With care, a multipurpose catheter can be advanced well down into the RCA to near the lesion; this gives excellent support or back-up to cross the lesion with a balloon, or to pass a stent.

With the left radial artery, routine 6F femoral guide (or diagnostic) catheters such as the Judkins versions, can be used.

Sheath Removal

Particular attention is needed with the technique of sheath removal and the method to achieve haemostasis. The sheath is removed slowly, and a small amount of blood is allowed to flow out from the puncture site. Three gauze swabs are laid on top of each other and then folded over double, or even triple. This gauze wedge is placed over the radial artery puncture site. The wedge is secured with a venepuncture tourniquet, trying to avoid compression of the ulnar artery.

A second wedge of gauze swabs is placed about one inch (2–3 cm) higher up the arm and again secured with a tourniquet. The hand is carefully observed at 5–10 minute intervals. If the hand goes blue, the top tourniquet is released. This tourniquet is routinely removed after about 20–30 minutes. The lower tourniquet over the radial artery puncture site is released after about another hour.

It is helpful for the operator or assistant to look at the hand and assess progress at about the 20–30 minute stage after sheath removal. After removal of the second tourniquet the puncture site is usually dry, or there is a very small ooze of blood. A small piece of gauze is placed over the puncture site, followed by 2–3 turns of a lightly applied crepe bandage.

Mobilization of the patient is virtually immediate, and the patient can return from the catheter room to a chair by the bedside. The arm is kept in a horizontal position on a pillow for 2–3 hours.

There is a small risk of late haemorrhage, and about a 10% chance of loss of the radial artery pulse. Repeat puncture of the same artery at a later date can be done. The patient (and relatives) are informed of the potential late problems, and given a contact telephone number at the hospital. This is particularly important for a patient discharged the same day as the PTCA procedure; with these patients it is helpful for the hospital to *telephone* the patient the *next day* to confirm all is well with the arm and the patient.

Conclusion

The main advantage of the radial artery route is early secure haemostasis, which allows prompt mobilization. In the earlier stages of coronary artery stenting, the anticoagulant regime was leading to frequent groin complications. The radial route offered an attractive alternative. However as soon as the post stent regime no longer required oral anticoagulants, much of the need for the radial route receded. For PTCA, the radial artery is now mainly used as a personal preference of the operator, or where there is severe peripheral vascular disease preventing access from the femoral artery.

Reference

Kiemeneij F, Laarman GJ. Percutaneous transradial artery approach for coronary stent implantation. *Cath Cardiovasc Diagn* **30**, 173–178 (1993).

Kiemeneij F. Transradial artery coronary artery stenting. In 'Endoluminal Stenting', pp. 306–310. Edited by Ulrich Sigwart. WB Saunders Co Ltd, 1996.

Lowe MD, Ludman PF. Cardiac Catheterization via the radial artery. *Brit J Cardiol* **4**, 71–74 (1997).

10 Stents (History and Types)

In 1987 an article was published in the New England Journal of Medicine by Dr. Ulrich Sigwart of Lausanne, Switzerland, describing the use of a stent (the Wallstent) to relieve acute closure at the time of PTCA and to prevent restenosis. The immediate result of the stent, fully restablishing coronary flow after acute closure during PTCA, was so impressive that interventional cardiologists were very keen to use stents for acute bail out. The era of coronary stenting had begun, see reference page 119.

There then followed a phase of disenchantment when the risk of stent thrombosis became all too apparent. At this stage oral anticoagulants were not routinely used after stent insertion. Unlike restenosis which develops slowly as recurrent angina, stent thrombosis led to acute myocardial infarction and death.

The response in the next stage was to give "aggressive anticoagulant" treatment with aspirin, dipyridamole, IV heparin and dextran and oral anticoagulants. Though stent thrombosis was less, it still occurred in about 5% of cases in an unpredictable manner. Furthermore the heavy anticoagulant regime led to groin complications of haemorrhage and pseudo aneurysm in about 10% of cases.

Dr. Richard Schatz of San Diego, USA, using the new Palmaz-Schatz balloon-mounted stent, showed that careful attention to anticoagulation, to sheath removal and to ensure full expansion of the stent, led to a low stent thrombosis and groin complication rates of about 3–4% each. Under the initiative of Dr. Schatz and Prof. Patrick Serruys of Rotterdam the two clinical trials of Stress and Benestent were mounted, which showed that the Palmaz-Schatz stent approximately halved the restenosis rate when used electively for de novo lesions. Here at last, after so many failed medical treatments and unsuccessful laser and atherectomy trials, was a treatment that could reduce the 'Achille's heal' of PTCA, i.e. restenosis.

Dr. Jean Marco of Toulouse in France, found that stent thrombosis (and restenosis) was less common in larger vessels (3 mm or more) and with saphenous vein bypass grafts.

The next critical contribution was made by Dr. Antonio Colombo from Milan. He demonstrated that if a Palmaz-Schatz stent was fully expanded to the vessel wall, as achieved by high pressure balloon inflation of 15–20 atmospheres and this was confirmed by intravascular ultrasound (IVUS), then oral anticoagulants were not needed. At this time (1991–1994), when stent thrombosis was the feared and dreaded complication, this view was greeted with amazement and disbelief. However his approach was fully confirmed and aspirin with perhaps ticlopidine has become the standard post stent medical regime.

The French Stent Registry, as reported by Dr. Marie Claude Morice from Paris, France, showed that a regime using high pressure inflations, aspirin and ticlopidine could achieve a very low stent thrombosis rate of about 1%, without the need for IVUS studies.

With the stent trials showing reduced restenosis and Colombo's simplified and safe post stent regime the stage was set in 1994–1995 for a wide expansion in the use of stents. The era of *'stentomania'* had begun. Many centres now use stents in 50–70% of PTCA cases with a few centres reaching up to 90% of PTCA cases. The manufacturers also got the message and from about 5 coronary stents available in 1993, by 1997 there were 25 and their numbers continue to grow.

Prof. Patrick Serruys summarised the place of stents as the *'second wind of PTCA'* reducing both the acute complication of vessel closure and the late problem of restenosis.

Stent developments continue with new designs to make them easier to deliver and to deploy. Heparin and other coatings may reduce further the risk of stent thrombosis. Different drug coatings for stents and radioactive stents may limit intimal hyperplasia and lower restenosis further.

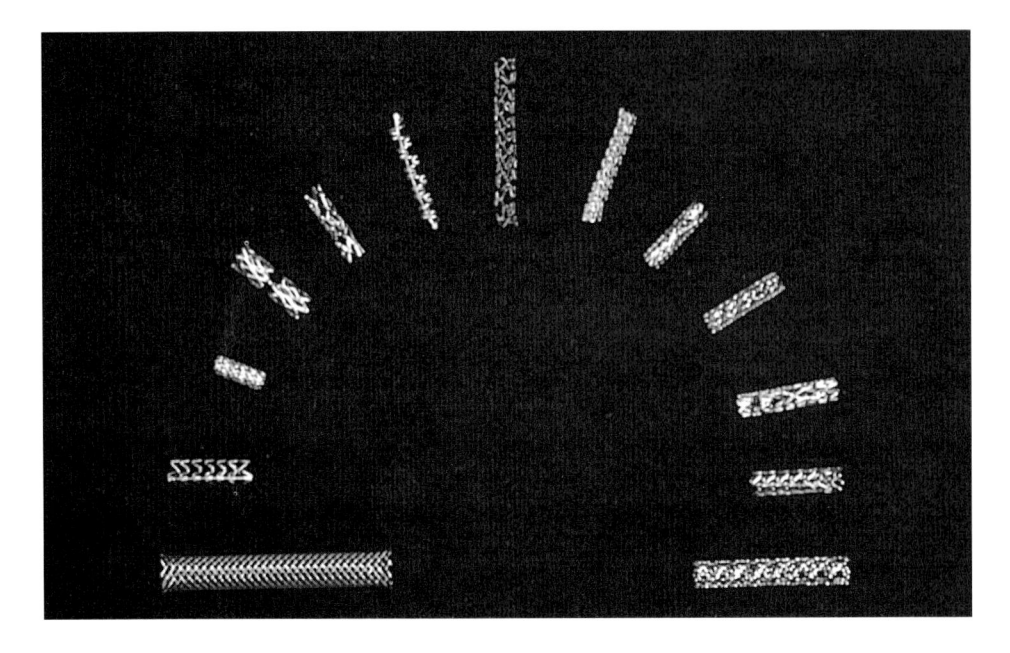

Figure 10.1. The photograph shows examples of thirteen different stents expanded with a 3 mm balloon, or recommended size for a 3 mm vessel (Wallstent). Starting from the left and passing round clockwise the stents are: 1. Wallstent (Schneider). 2. X-T stent (Bard). 3. Jo-Stent (Jomed). 4. Palmaz-Schatz PS153 stent (Cordis, J&J). 5. Modified Spiral Palmaz-Schatz stent (Cordis, J&J). 6. Gianturco-Roubin II stent (Cook). 7. Wiktor-i stent (Medtronic). 8. CrossFlex stent (Cordis, J&J). 9. NIR stent (SciMed). 10. Multilink stent (ACS/Guidant). 11. Micro stent (AVE). 12. BeStent (Medtronic/Instent). 13. Palmaz-Schatz Crown stent (Cordis, J&J).

Types of Stents

A stent is a tubular scaffold within a vessel at a lesion site to enlarge the lumen and support the vessel wall (Figure 10.1). All the ones in current clinical use are metal. Though there were two early forms of temporary stents which could be withdrawn from the vessel, they are no longer used. Now all stents once they have been deployed are permanently positioned in the vessel.

'Stentomania' has influenced the manufacturers so that a plethora of new stents are becoming available. Their design and characteristics vary widely (Figure 10.1) so that *not all stents are the same*. Studies on ease of deployment, thrombosis and restenosis are needed for each new variety. The numbers do allow for variations in clinical use, e.g. some with more strength, or more trackability or more radiopacity and competition may lower costs. As with drug treatments such as beta blockers or ACE inhibitors, learn how to use a few and know their limitations.

The stents that will be described are those that have been assessed for longer and about which the author has personal knowledge.

Stents may be classified into:-

(1) Balloon Expandable Stents
   a) Tubular Mesh Design
      1. Palmaz-Schatz stent   (Cordis, Johnson & Johnson)
      2. Multilink stent   (ACS/Guidant)
      3. NIR stent   (SciMed)
      4. Jo stent   (Jo-Med)
      5. BeStent   (Medtronic/Instent)
      6. ACT-One stent   (Progressive Angioplasty Systems)
   b) Z Loops
      1. Micro stent   (AVE)
      2. XT stent   (Bard)
   c) Coil Construction (usually from a single wire)
      1. Wiktor stent   (Medtronic)
      2. Gianturco-Roubin stent   (Cook)
      3. Cordis stent   (Cordis)
      4. AngioStent   (AngioDynamics)
(2) Self Expanding Stent
      1. Wallstent   (Schneider)

Balloon expandable stents are mounted on a deflated angioplasty balloon which is inflated to deploy the stent. The balloon is then deflated and withdrawn.

A stent can be supplied as the stent alone (so-called 'bare' or 'free' stent), which is hand crimped onto a balloon by the operator. Alternatively, the manufacturer premounts the stent onto a balloon. Most premounted stents are uncovered, but some have a protective sheath (described sometimes as a '*stent delivery system*'). The sheath acts as a protective cover whilst the stent is passed to the lesion down the coronary vessel. It prevents the stent coming of the balloon before it is delivered at the lesion. However the sheath also makes the balloon catheter and stent more rigid and less trackable.

106 Guide to Coronary Angioplasty and Stenting

The balloons chosen by manufacturers for premounting stents are often less good than regular angioplasty balloon catheters. They tend to rewrap poorly after inflation and may catch on the proximal vessel or tip of the guide catheter as they are withdrawn. These balloons usually possess a radiopaque marker at each end of the balloon marking the end of the stent, which is very helpful to accurately place the stent.

Bare stents allow the operator to choose any balloon for mounting the stent. Often it will be the balloon used to predilate the lesion. Bare stents are small items which can be used for a variety of sizes of vessels. Hence less stock and space are needed than with premounted stents.

The major advantage of premounted stents is that they are easy and quick to use, as no time is needed on the fiddly procedure of hand crimping a stent. There is virtually no risk of balloon perforation by the stent, as may occur when a stent is hand crimped. The risk of a stent becoming dislodged off a balloon is similar between a premounted and a well hand crimped stent.

Most stents are made of stainless steel, but the Wiktor stent and the Cordis coil stent are of tantalum and the Angiostent is made of platinum. Both these metals are highly radiopaque. The ACT-One stent is made of nitinol.

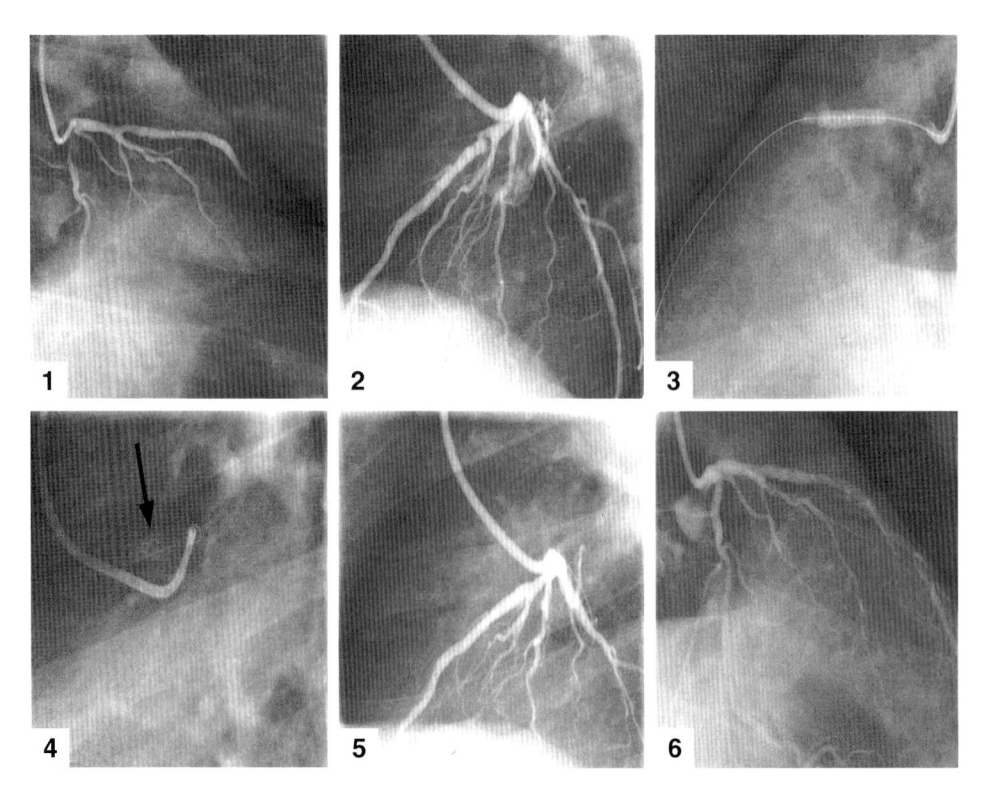

Angiogram 10.1. *PTCA and stent deployment for complex LAD lesion.* A complex LAD lesion, is poorly seen on the RAO projection (1), but shows clearly on the Left Lateral with 10° Cranial projection (2). After predilatation with a 2.5 mm balloon, a 15 mm Palmaz-Schatz (J & J PS153) stent, hand crimped onto a 3 mm Speedy balloon (Schneider) is deployed (3). In the Left Lateral view the stent can be seen on fluoroscopy (4). The final result showing mild over dilatation of the stented region (5 and 6).

Though the Wallstent was the first stent to be used clinically, when the complication of stent thrombosis began to be recorded, this stent was withdrawn and only became easily available again in 1996.

Palmaz-Schatz Stent (Angiograms 10.1, 13.1, 15.1, 16.1 and 20.1 on pages 148, 170, 178 and 212)

A very large number of the original Palmaz-Schatz PS153 stent have been deployed and there have been extensive publications on their use. This stent was used for the two major restenosis trials of Stress and Benestent. It has mainly been implanted as a bare stent, but a version premounted on a balloon with a protective sheath has also been available.

The Palmaz-Schatz stent is constructed from a stainless steel tube from which rectangles have been cut out by laser (Figure 10.2). Hence, the stent is described as having a 'slotted tube' design. When the stent is expanded, the rectangles become diamond shaped (Figure 10.2) and there is 2.5–5% shortening depending on the calibre of the vessel; the larger the vessel the more the shortening. The design produces strong radial strength, so that only minor vessel recoil occurs.

The Palmaz-Schatz stent has two sections joined by a short strip, the central articulation (see Figure 10.2). This arrangement allows some flexing of the stent at its centre to aid trackability. However, the stent has poor trackability and is best used for proximal lesions in straight vessels, free from disease down to the lesion. Tissue from the vessel wall tends to prolapse at the central articulation site. This is rarely a clinical problem but IVUS usually shows the centre of the stent to be the narrowest site.

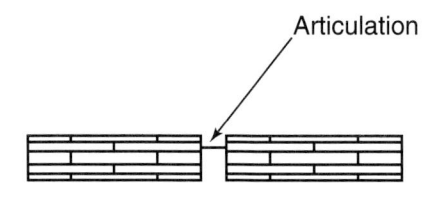

Before expansion

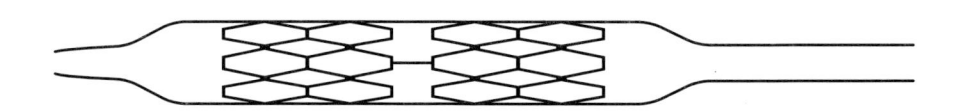

After balloon expansion

Figure 10.2. Palmaz-Schatz stent (PS153).

The struts of the Palmaz-Schatz stent are 0.0025 inches thick and the stent is poorly radiopaque (see below with AVE Micro Stent). With modern radiographic equipment the Palmaz-Schatz stent can just be identified. The poor radiopacity with this and other stents makes it very difficult or impossible to 'find' the stent should it come off the balloon (or be 'dropped').

Relatively high pressures of 12–20 atmospheres are needed to fully expand the stent. This important discovery was made by Dr Antonio Colombo (see above on page 103). With full expansion of the stent out to vessel wall, there is less turbulence with less risk of stent thrombosis and a larger lumen is produced leading to a lower risk of restenosis.

The Palmaz-Schatz PS153 stent has now largely been superseded by newer designs. The *Modified Spiral* Palmaz-Schatz stent is premounted on a monorail balloon ('Powergrip') and has two or more spiral articulations instead of the one central articulation (see Figure 10.1 and Angiogram 18.2). It is relatively rigid and poorly trackable. The *Palmaz-Schatz Crown* stent has a similar design to the Multilink and NIR stents. It is much more trackable yet retains good radial strength. It can be deployed at 8–10 atmospheres. It is supplied in 3–4 mm sizes and in lengths of 15, 22 and 30 mm lengths. It is available as a bare stent or premounted on a balloon.

The Palmaz-Schatz stent has been a pivotal stent in the development and use of coronary stents.

AVE Micro Stent (Applied Vascular Engineering), Figure 10.1 and Angiogram 10.2

This stent is constructed of stainless steel struts in the form of Z-shaped loops which have been joined together. It was one of the first balloon expandable stents to be supplied already premounted on a balloon, but without a cumbersome protective sheath that had been employed with the so-called 'stent delivery system' of one version of the Palmaz-Schatz PS 153 stent. Hence it was quick to use compared with the hand crimping needed for the usual form of the Palmaz-Schatz PS 153 stent. The struts are of thicker stainless steel compared to most stents (0.008 inches as opposed to 0.0025 inches for a Palmaz-Schatz PS 153 stent), so that the stent is relatively radiopaque and is easy to see on screening (see Angiogram 24.1, see page 255). This feature has been particularly useful for osteal lesions of the RCA and saphenous vein grafts (see Angiogram 22.1, see page 230). Finally, from when the stent first became available, short 8 or 9 mm length versions have been supplied, which are very useful to tack up minor dissections at either end of a previously delivered stent, e.g. a Palmaz-Schatz stent (see Angiogram 18.2, see page 197). For all these reasons, this stent rapidly became very popular after its introduction.

The Z loops of the stents form separate segments (almost like railway carriages) and were originally held together by sutures. Later designs have even shorter segments (reduced from 4 mm to 2 mm) and have joints spirally arranged between segments to allow longitudinal flexibility and moderate trackability. The Micro stent is more trackable than the earlier Palmaz-Schatz stent (PS 153), but is less good than 'second generation' stents such as the NIR and Multilink stents.

The Micro stent, as with most premounted stents, is not enclosed within a protective sheath. Though the stent is securely mounted onto the balloon in the factory, it can still

Stents (History and Types) 109

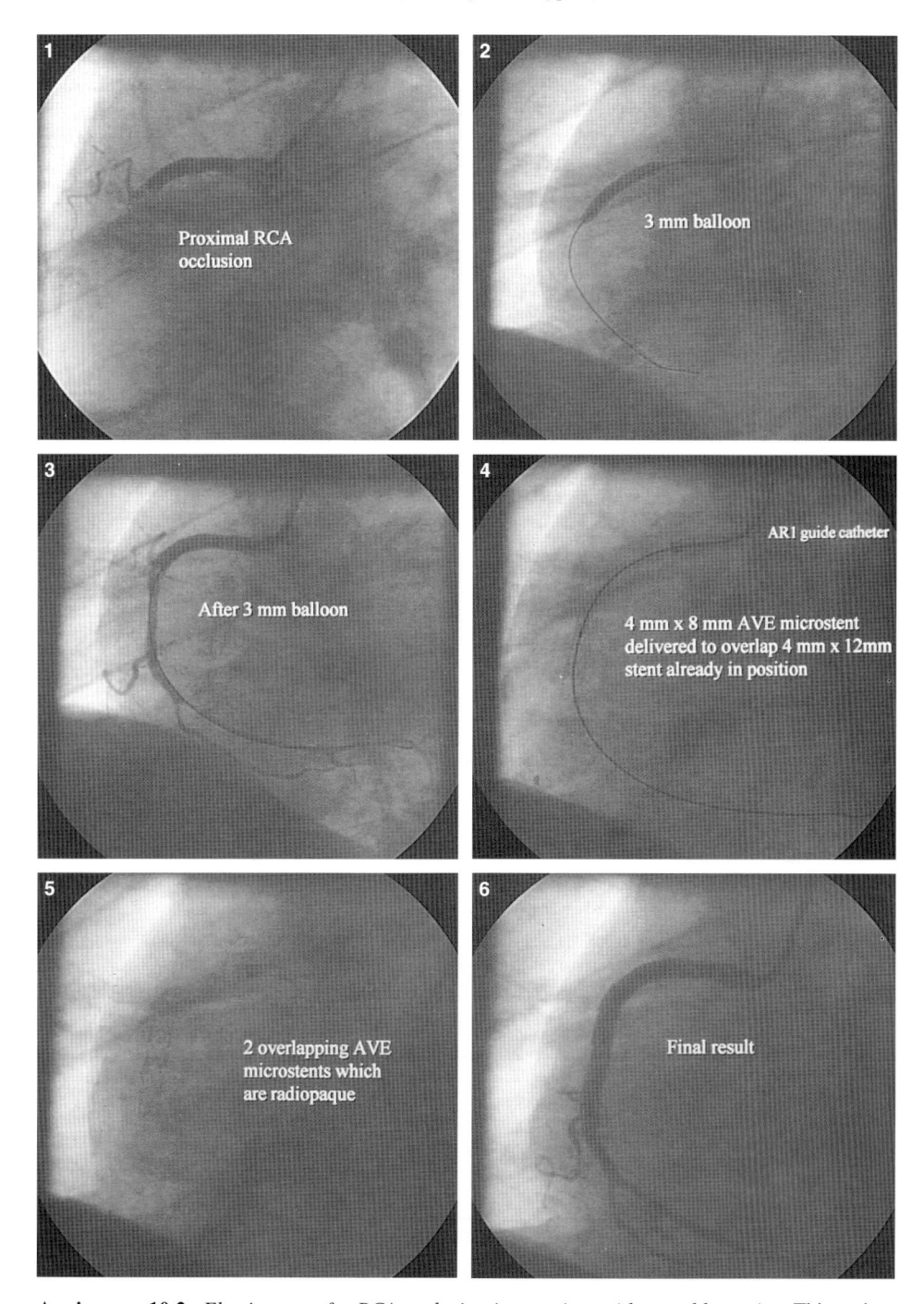

Angiogram 10.2. *Elective stent for RCA occlusion in a patient with unstable angina.* This patient had a previous unsuccessful PTCA when a Wiktor stent could not be delivered to the lesion (see Angiogram 12.2). During the second procedure 24 hours later, the RCA occlusion (1) was crossed with a firm wire (0.014 inch USCI Standard wire), and a 3 mm balloon (2). The reopened vessel has a long lesion (3) and two AVE Microstents were deployed (4 & 5). The end result was good (6).

become dislodged especially when a stent has been passed too distally and when attempting to withdraw the stent back across the lesion it may be left behind, distal to the lesion whilst the balloon comes back.

The Micro stent has radial strength similar to that of a Palmaz-Schatz PS 153 stent, but lower balloon pressures of 9–10 atmospheres are considered adequate to deploy the stent. However, IVUS studies show progressive stent expansion occurs when using higher pressures, i.e. to 14–18 atmospheres.There is some initial stent recoil, so that a stent slightly larger than the vessel should be used.

The Micro stent was one of the first available in 2.5 mm size and the range extends in half mm sizes to 4.5 mm and lengths including 8, 12, 24, 30 and 40 mm. The longer versions are less trackable.

The AVE Micro stent was a major advance when it first appeared, but now has strong competition from a number of 'second generation' stents. The GFX version has improved trackability and remains one of the few stents easily seen on X-ray screening.

Multilink Stent (ACS/Guidant), Figure 10.1

This is described as a '*second generation*' balloon expandable stent. The design gives very much improved flexibility, trackability and lower profile compared to the Palmaz-Schatz PS 153 stent. It comes premounted on a balloon and a sheathed version is also available. Covering the surface of the balloon on which the stent is seated, there is a fine sheet of material. This aids equal and smooth deployment of the stent along the whole of its length as the balloon is inflated. The stent is available in 3.0, 3.5 and 4.0 mm diameter sizes and in 15 and 25 mm lengths. The stent is poorly radiopaque. Balloon inflation to 8–10 atmospheres to deliver the stent, followed by a second inflation to 14–16 atmospheres, is recommended.

NIR Stent (SciMed), Figure 10.1

This is another 'second generation' balloon expandable mounted stent. The stent is cut from a sheet of 316 stainless steel and the sides are spot welded to form a tube. There is a very interesting design to the stent which before expansion has horizontal and vertical U-shaped struts or loops (Figures 10.3 and 10.4). The U of the vertical loops can enlarge

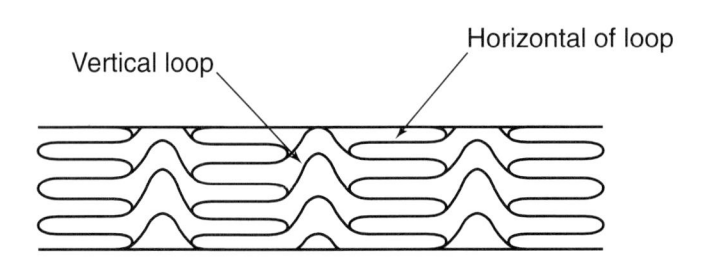

Figure 10.3. NIR stent before expansion.

Stents (History and Types)

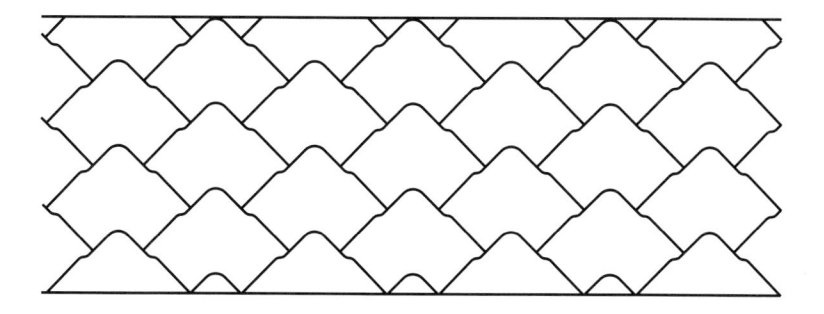

Figure 10.4. NIR stent after expansion.

or contract to allow the stent to flex longitudinally, which with the low profile of the stent makes it very trackable.

With deployment of the stent at the lesion, as it expands, the horizontal loops foreshorten and the vertical loops elongate (Figure 10.5), leaving the total length of the stent unchanged, i.e. there is less than 3% shortening. On deployment the geometry of the cells change to give a regular diamond like pattern (see Figure 10.4), which has good radial strength. For deployment, balloon inflation to 8 atmospheres is recommended and a further balloon inflation to 12 atmospheres may be given.

It is supplied premounted, or as a bare stent which crimps well onto low profile balloons, or comes already premounted on a balloon. The stent is produced in 9, 16, 32 mm lengths and diameters of 2–3.5 mm and 3–5 mm. The smaller stents (2–3.5 mm) have a pattern made up of 7 mm cells. The larger stents (3.5–5 mm) have 9 mm cells. The 7 mm cell

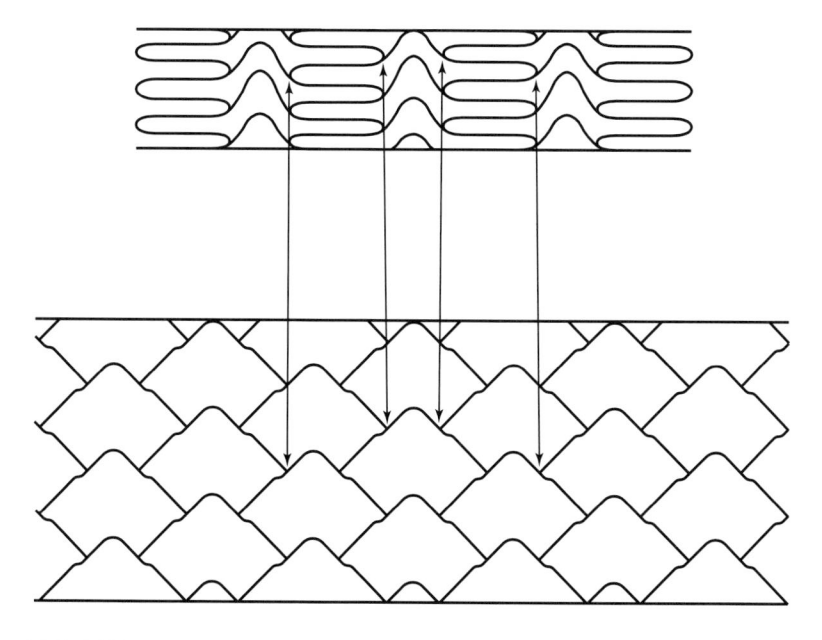

Figure 10.5. Differential expansion of loops, leaving length of stent unchanged (ie. minimal shortening).

design has a slightly larger gap between the struts after stent expansion and is more suitable for bifurcation lesions, as it allows a guide wire to more easily enter a side branch.

The NIR stent, as with most modern stents, can pass down a 6F guide catheter. The stent is poorly radiopaque but a new version, the NIR Royal stent, is gold coated and therefore adequately radiopaque.

Both the ACS Multilink and the NIR stents are now well established and are much improved compared to the Palmaz-Schatz PS 153 stent. Newer stents are mainly compared with these two stents, the Palmaz-Schatz Crown stent and the AVE Micro stent.

Jo Stent (Jo-med), Figure 10.1

The design of this stent is very similar to the NIR stent. It has a 6 mm cell design (for 2.25–3.25 calibre vessels), or a 9 mm cell construction (for 3.0–5 mm vessels). It is poorly radiopaque and is hand crimped onto a balloon. One version has its central struts reduced to a 4 mm cell design over about 0.5 mm. This is for use with a bifurcation lesion to allow easier entrance into a side branch with a guide wire (see page 241). The lengths available include 9, 16, 26, 32 and 38 mm. A heparin coated version is available.

BeStent (Medtronic Instent), Figure 10.1

This is a further 'second generation' balloon expandable stent. The struts have serpentine-like design, which straighten both in longitudinal and radial directions as the stent is expanded. The stent has virtually no shortening on expansion and there are two radiopaque end-markers to assist positioning of the stent. There are two sizes of stent, for 2.5–3 mm and for 3–5.5 mm vessels, supplied in lengths 15, 25 and 35 mm. It is hand crimped onto a balloon and deployment at 8–10 atmospheres, followed by a second inflation at 14–16 atmospheres, is recommended.

XT Stent (Bard), Figure 10.1

This stent consists of a series of Z loops mounted on a central spine. It has good radiopacity as the spine and the struts are made of relatively thick stainless steel (0.006 inches). There are relatively large gaps between the struts, so that side branches are not 'jailed'. It is supplied as a bare stent with a special mounting or loading device to assist transferring the stent onto the balloon, which is then hand crimped. It can pass down a 6F guide catheter and is moderately trackable. It is supplied in sizes of 3, 3.5 and 4 mm and in a variety of lengths from 6 to 37 mm.

ACT-One Stent (Progressive Angioplasty Systems)

This is a slotted tube stent resembling the Palmaz-Schatz PS 153 shape but is made of Nitinol. It is available as bare stent, in 3–4 mm sizes and 8 and 17 mm lengths.

Coil Stents

These stents are constructed from a single wire weaved into a coiled meshwork. This design allows the stent to be very flexible along its length and hence the stents are more able to track down tortuous vessels and to more distal lesions. The design of these stents gives less radial strength and may not prevent a lesion recoiling significantly. Another stent, e.g. a Palmaz-Schatz, may need to be placed across to correct the recoil.

There is usually more space between the struts than with the coiled mesh design and prolapse of the vessel wall is more prone to occur between the struts. The larger gaps do allow easier access to side branches whose origin may be covered by a stent positioned in the main vessel. They are useful in the stent treatment of bifurcation lesions (see Angiogram 23.1 on page 246).

The major disadvantage of a coil stent is the risk that it may uncoil into a single wire. This may occur if an attempt is made to withdraw the stent when it is partially stuck against a lesion or the vessel wall of a coronary artery, or if there is a problem withdrawing the balloon from the stent (see Angiogram 12.2 on page 136). The mark II version of the Gianturco-Roubin stent has a spine to prevent this problem (see below).

Wiktor Stent (Medtronic), Figure 10.1

This stent is made of a single tantalum wire constructed into a meshwork. As a coiled stent it offers good flexibility and conformity with the curvature of the vessel. The stent comes premounted on a balloon (monorail or OTW) which is inflated to 7–9 atmospheres. It is well *radiopaque* and has good flexibility and trackability. The stent is 16mm in length and available in sizes from 3–4.5 mm in diameter.

If there is proximal vessel disease or the lesion has not been adequately predilated, the stent can relatively easily become dislodged off the balloon. If there is a problem with stent deployment (see above), the stent may *unravel or uncoil* (see Angiogram 12.2 on page 136). This can be a great worry, with the stent uncoiled like a piece of spaghetti within, or half in and half out of the coronary artery ... not a pretty sight!

The gaps between the "weave" of the stent are relatively large and vessel wall prolapse through them can occur. The mark II version, the Wiktor-i stent, has smaller gaps between the struts to reduce this problem. The stent is less strong than the Palmaz-Schatz PS 153 stent and lesion recoil may not be prevented by this stent.

The problem of stent uncoiling is a major disadvantage of the Wiktor stent. Its main advantages are good radiopacity and trackability.

Gianturco-Roubin Stent (Cook), Figure 10.1

This stent is made of a coil of interdigitating loops of flat 316 stainless steel wire mounted onto a balloon (OTW or monorail type). At each end of the stent there is a gold marker, which is helpful for accurate positioning of the stent. The model Mark II has a spine running the whole length of the stent to prevent it uncoiling. It is also of lower profile, allowing it to be delivered along a 6F guide catheter. It is relatively flexible and trackable.

The gaps between the struts are relatively large (Figure 10.1), so that prolapse of vessel wall may occur between them. The larger gaps make it easier to pass a guide wire across the stent into a side branch, for example when treating a bifurcation lesion (see Angiogram 23.1, page 246). It is available in 2.5–4 mm sizes and 20–40 mm lengths. See also page 245.

Cordis Stent

This stent is constructed of tantalum wire and is *very radiopaque*, almost excessively so for it tends to obscure assessment of the lumen. Detection of restenosis can be more difficult. The stent comes premounted on an OTW or monorail balloon and is available in diameters of 3, 3.5 and 4 mm and in one length of 15 mm. The *Cordis CrossFlex* stent is a stainless steel version of this stent (see Figure 10.1) and is less radiopaque.

AngioStent (AngioDynamics)

This stent is made of platinum (90%) and iridium (10%) alloy wire, which is connected end-end by a longitudinal wire to prevent uncoiling of the stent. The platinum alloy makes the stent adequately radiopaque and is possibly less thrombogenic than stainless steel. It is available in sizes 3, 3.5 and 4 mm, with lengths of 15 and 25 mm.

Wallstent (Schneider) (Figure 10.1, and Angiograms 11.2 and 20.2 on pages 123 and 217)

Although this stent was the first to be used clinically, the high thrombosis rate led to its withdrawal by the manufacturer. It only became readily available once more in 1996.

The Wallstent is a *self expanding* stent and is more complicated to use than balloon expandable stents.There is a definite learning curve, for the selection of the correct stent size and length and to correctly position the stent allowing for the shortening that occurs when it expands. Furthermore, the stent is ideally used in long diffuse lesions and these are technically difficult cases to treat. For all these reasons, it may be wise to delay the use of the Wallstent until experience has been gained with simpler stents.

The Wallstent has a 16 filament weave of fine wire constructed into a tube (Figure 10.1). Each wire filament is 0.08 mm in diameter and consists of a cobalt based alloy, with a platinum core which makes the stent radiopaque. The Wallstent is self expanding and therefore does not not require a balloon for deployment. It is mounted on a catheter shaft and is constrained or held in a collapsed state by an outer sheath, which can be retracted to release and deliver the stent (see Figure 10.6 and 10.7). Whilst within the sheath, the stent can be safely delivered to the lesion and the whole delivery mechanism is moderately trackable.

The second generation of the Wallstent, the Magic Wallstent, is simpler to use. The mode of deployment is easier and there is less shortening of the stent (20% versus 25%). Potentially, at any stage before complete removal of the enclosing sheath, it is possible to reapply the sheath and abort the deployment of the stent. This is very helpful, for if

Stents (History and Types) 115

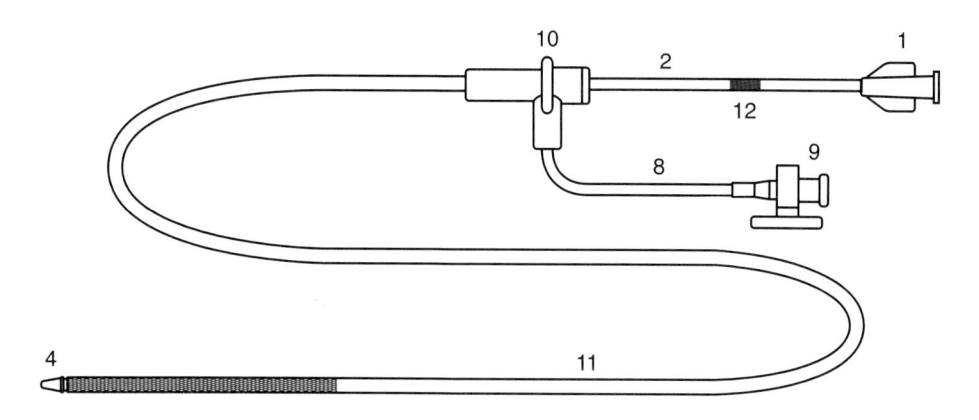

INNER CATHETER (On which the stent is mounted)

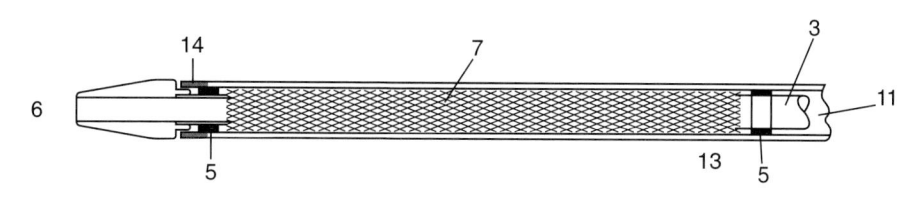

OUTER SHEATH

Inner Catheter

1. Luer lock
3. Shaft
5. X-Ray Marker (Stent End)
7. Wallstent
2. Steel Tube
4. Tip
6. Guide Wire Lumen
12. Repositioning Marker
13. Stent Fixation Area

Outer Sheath

8. Side Arm
9. Stopcock
10. T-connector
11. Outer Sheath
14. X-Ray Marker (end of Outer Sheath)

Figure 10.6. The Magic Wallstent delivery system.

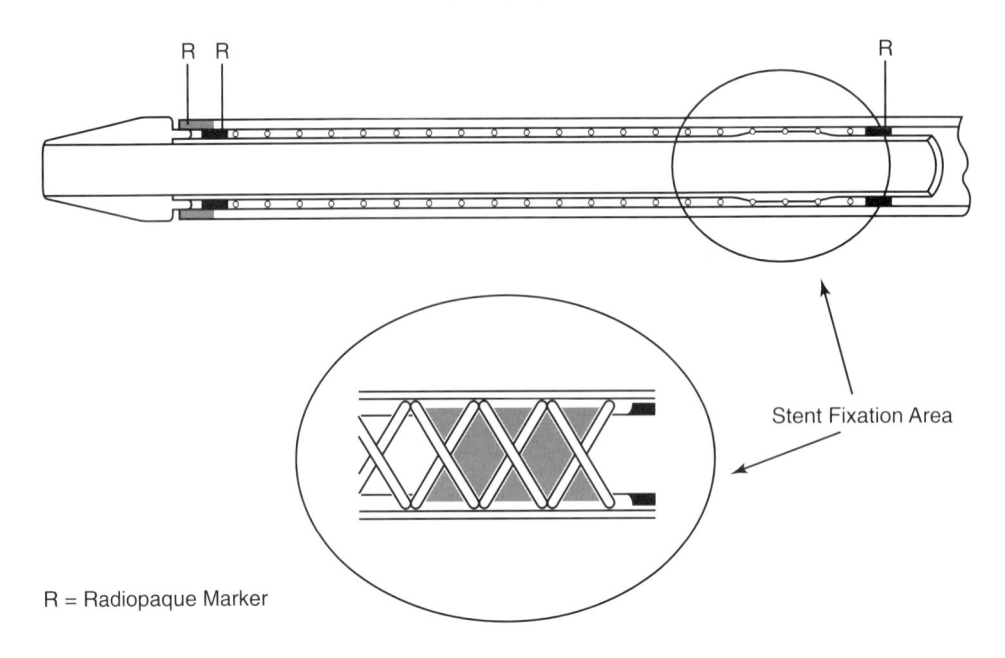

Figure 10.7. Distal end of Magic Wallstent delivery system.

during the deployment of the stent the position is found to be unsatisfactory, the stent can be 'recaptured' and repositioned. The Magic Wallstent can be passed through a wide bore 6F guide catheter. The stent delivery is an 'over-the-wire' (OTW) system and no monorail version is available.

There are three radiopaque markers with the Magic Wallstent delivery system (Figure 10.7):

a) Two markers on the delivery shaft, with one at the level of each end of the constrained stent. These are seen as a round dot on screening.
b) One marker at the distal end of the sheath, seen as a square-shaped dot on screening.

The Magic Wallstent is produced in 4–6 mm sizes and lengths from 15–48 mm. The long lengths available makes the stent particularly useful in *long diffuse disease*, such as in a large calibre RCA or a vein graft, or for long dissections. The stents are moderately radiopaque and so it is relatively easy to ensure that if two or more stents are used, they overlap each other.

The principal disadvantage of the Wallstent is the *shortening* of the stent, by about 20–25%, that occurs as it expands. This makes accurate placement of the stent difficult. The stent tends to 'migrate' proximally from the distal end of the lesion as the outer covering sheath is retracted to progressively release the stent. There is a danger that the full length of the lesion may not be covered by the stent.

A second significant limitation is that it is virtually impossible to cross the close mesh of the Wallstent with a guide wire. If the Wallstent is positioned across a significant sized

Stents (History and Types) 117

side vessel, the branch is 'stent-jailed'. Whilst this problem applies in varying degrees to all stents, it is probably greatest with the Wallstent. It is partly because of this problem that the Wallstent is particularly suited to RCA and saphenous vein graft (SVG) angioplasty, where side branches are usually small or absent (SVGs).

Deployment of the Magic Wallstent (Figure 10.8)

1. *Sizing of the Stent*
   The stent size is chosen both for calibre and length.
   a) Vessel Calibre
      Add 1 mm to the size of the vessel at its widest point to select the stent calibre, e.g. for a 3 mm vessel size, choose a 4 mm size stent. This ensures that the expanded stent will be in close contact with the vessel wall.
   b) Lesion length
      Add 4 mm to each end, i.e. the stent should be 8 mm (or approximately 1 cm) longer than the lesion. The stated length of a stent described on the packaging and in the catalogue, includes or allows for the 20% shortening that occurs, i.e. is the implanted length, not the constrained length when the stent is on the stent shaft enclosed within the sheath. The implanted stent needs to cover a longer length than the lesion, as there are no fixed or welded points at the ends of the stent (Figure 10.1), which therfore have less radial force than the body of the stent.

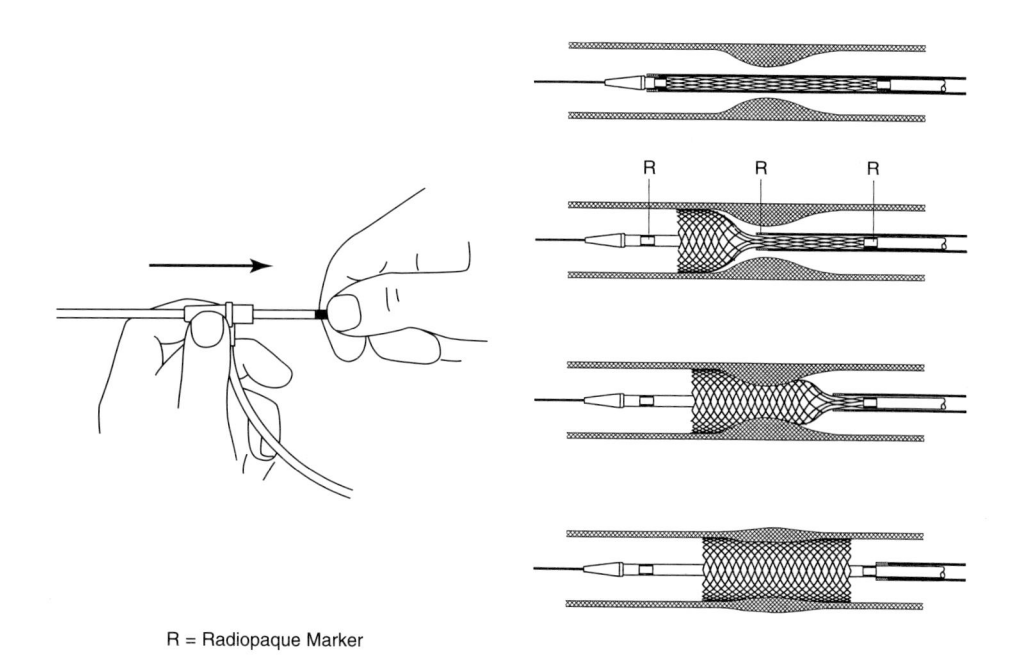

R = Radiopaque Marker

Figure 10.8. Deployment of Magic Wallstent.

2. *Preparation*

   The guide wire lumen and the side arm of the sheath (Figure 10.6), are flushed with 5–10 ml of heparainzed saline. The tap on the side arm can be left open or closed.

3. *Stent Deployment*

   The lesion is predilated with a balloon of the *same* size as the vessel and the balloon is then removed. The guide wire is extended, or a long 260–300 cm guide wire is used from the start of the procedure.

   The stent delivery system is advanced over the guide wire to the lesion. The distal stent radiopaque marker (Figures 10.7 and 10.8) is positioned approximately 1 cm beyond the distal end of the lesion. The steel tube, which is the proximal end of the catheter shaft, is held firmly with the right hand at the level of the *repositioning marker* (Figure 10.6) and remains *fixed*. The T-connector of the sheath is held with the left hand and is *moved slowly backwards towards* the right hand, to uncover and release the distal end of the stent (Figure 10.8). Approximately half of the wallstent is released when the T-connector has reached the repositioning marker. If the position of the stent is satisfactory on screening, the stent is fully released by progressively withdrawing the T-connector towards the luer lock at the end of the steel tube.

4. *Recapturing a Partially Deployed Stent*

   If the stent needs to be repositioned because the distal end retracts too far (see above), it may be recaptured providing the sheath has not been withdrawn beyond the repositioning marker.

   With the T-connector of the sheath held *firmly and stationary* with the left hand, the metal tube is held in the right hand and is *pulled or retracted away* from the T-connector, i.e. the steel tube is moved to the right (see Figure 10.9). The stent is pulled or withdrawn back into the outer sheath. The stent may now be advanced forwards and repositioned. The alternative method is to keep the distal end of the stent in same position and to advance the sheath forwards to cover the stent once more. The stent may not be recaptured more than twice.

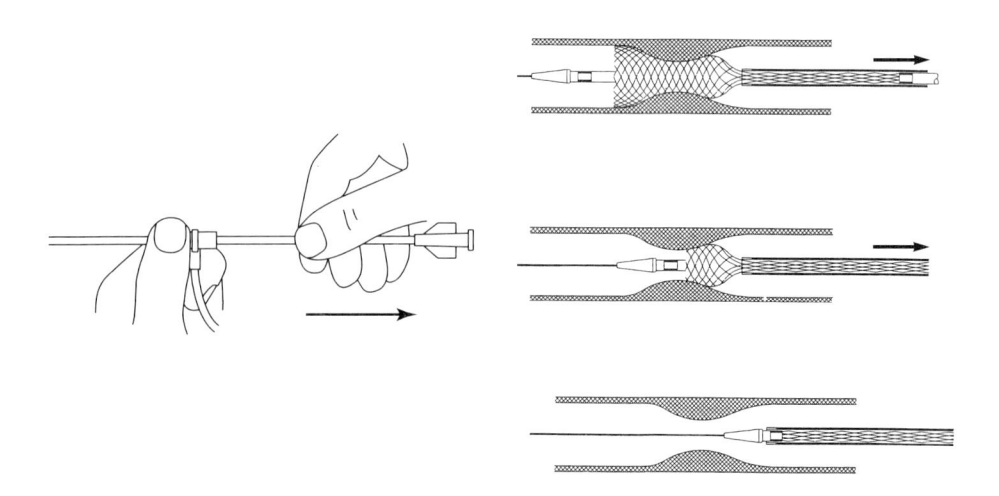

Figure 10.9. Recapture of Magic Wallstent to allow repositioning.

5. *Post Delivery Balloon Dilatation*
   The balloon used to predilate the lesion, may be used again to post dilate the stent to 10–12 atmospheres. This ensures full expansion of the stent to the vessel wall throughout its length. Particularly with long stents, i.e. 30 mm and more, it is desirable to perform an IVUS study to confirm full expansion along the *total* length of the stent.

The Magic Wallstent should end in a straight section of a vessel and not in a curve, where there is a risk of incomplete stent expansion. If two stents in sequence are needed, they should overlap each other by at least 4 mm. It is preferable to implant the *distal* stent and post dilate it to embed the stent firmly in the vessel wall. Then deploy the proximal stent overlapping the start of the first stent. Finally, the second stent is post dilated too.

Other Stents

There are many other types of stents already available and yet others are in development. It is best to use and become experienced with a few types and to assess new ones as they become available. Keeping large stocks of many sizes of different manufacturer's stents takes up valuable storage space and has cost and security implications.

Conclusion

Initially stents were kept in the cupboard to be used for the rare emergencies when angioplasty led to vessel occlusion. The results of stenting were uncertain, particularly with the later risk of stent thrombosis. When Antonio Colombo showed the way to avoid this complication and the Benestent and Stress trials indicated that stents lowered restenosis, the stage was set for a large increase of stenting. The engineers and manufacturers are producing more and more stents. The newer designs have improved trackability and yet have maintained radial strength. The next step requires all the stents to be adequately radiopaque, so that stenting will no longer be done 'in the dark'. Coating of stents with materials to lower intimal hyperplasia is a hope for the future.

It is likely that the large and increasing numbers of stents available, will later diminish into groups of stents for given lesions and vessel types.

References

Colombo, A., Hall, P., Nakamura, S., *et al*. Intracoronary stenting without anticoagulation accomplished with intravascular ultrasound guidance. *Circulation* **91**, 1676–1688 (1995).
Sigwart, U., Puel, J., Mirkovitch, V., *et al*. Intravascular stents to prevent occlusion and restenosis after angioplasty. *N. Eng. J. Med.* **316**, 701–706 (1987).
Endoluminal Stenting. Edited by Ulrich Sigwart. WB Saunders Co Ltd, London, 1996.
Handbook of Coronary Stents. Editor in chief: Patrick W Serruys. Martin Denitz, London, 1977.
These two books give much detailed information on the types, design and use of stents. They are strongly recommended.

11 Indications for the Use of Stents

A stent (or stents) may be used for:-

(A) Unsatisfactory Result from PTCA
   1. Vessel Dissection
   2. Lesion Recoil
(B) Elective
   1. Higher risk lesion for dissection
   2. To reduce restenosis
   3. Vein grafts

Unsatisfactory PTCA Result

1. Vessel Dissection
There are various degrees of the this complication at PTCA and all may be helped by stenting (see page 167).

Stents first showed their value for the treatment of dissection and acute vessel closure (see Angiogram 15.1, page 170). A stent supports the vessel wall and can thereby relieve dissection and improve an unsatisfactory result after PTCA. Furthermore, since the advent of stents, the result of a PTCA procedure is more critically assessed. If there has been a poor angiographic result with moderate dissection, this might have accepted it in the past, albeit with concern for the increased risk of vessel closure over the next 24 hours. Now, if the vessel is suitable for stenting (calibre > or = to 3 mm with relatively straight course to the lesion), a stent should be inserted.

With a poor angioplasty result it is much better to deploy a stent *early*, rather than repeatedly attempting to improve the result by balloon dilatation which may lead to complete vessel closure. The logical extension to this view is to *electively use* a stent for a *higher risk* lesion (see below).

2. **Lesion Recoil**
Sometimes with an eccentric lesion, when the balloon is inflated, full expansion of the balloon is seen. There is no dumb-bell appearance, or narrowed section to the

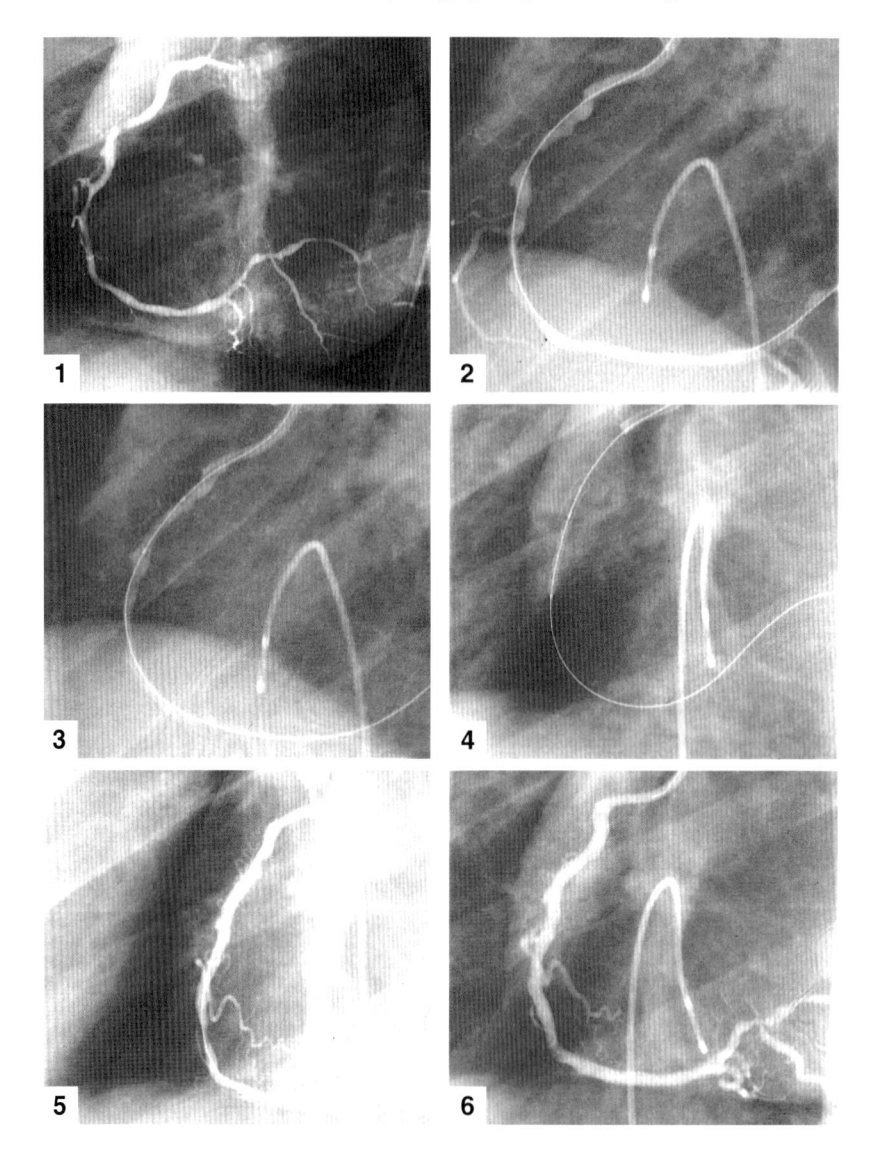

Angiogram 11.1. *PTCA for diffuse RCA disease.* The RCA has diffuse disease with 3 scalloped lesions in the mid-portion shown by angiography using 4F Cordis JR4 diagnostic catheter (1). The patient also had a short concentric LAD lesion which was dilated at a later session (2 – stage procedure).

Electively the decision was taken to use two stents. The Wallstent was not yet available for use. As the case was a higher risk one, a temporary pacing catheter was inserted at the start of the procedure (2). Good back-up for the guide catheter would be needed and was obtained with 7F Cordis right Amplatz I (AR1) guide. The catheter caused some spasm at its tip (2). Pre-dilatation with a 2.5 mm. Europass balloon was followed by deployment of a 3 mm. × 12 mm. AVE Micro stent to the short first lesion (3). A second 3 mm. × 12 mm. AVE Micro stent was passed through the first stent with the two stents overlapping (4). Both stents were inflated to 9 atmospheres.

After deployment of the second stent a new lesion appeared (5). This was due to spasm as it disappeared after 0.3 mgm. of Glyceryl Trinitrate is given into the RCA (6). The final result is satisfactory and no re-stenosis of the RCA had developed when the LAD was dilated one month later.

balloon. However when the balloon is deflated, the lesion is seen to be virtually unchanged. This prominent recoil of the lesion can be abolished by using a stent.

Elective Use of Stent(s)

1. **Higher Risk Lesion**
   If the lesion is ulcerated, irregular, very eccentric (see Angiogram 10.1, page 106), or is on a bend (especially in RCA or LCX), there is an increased risk of dissection (see page 84 and Angiogram 11.1, page 122). Elective stenting can prevent this complication which, if it occurs, may be a long dissection down the vessel, which then requires several stents to relieve as opposed to one used electively.

2. **Vein Grafts**
   Short discrete lesions in vein grafts do well with stenting (Angiogram 20.1, page 212). Vein grafts are usually large calibre, relatively straight vessels which make them very suitable for stenting. Lesions in vein grafts have a *higher risk of restenosis* after PTCA, perhaps as much as 50% and over a longer time period of 9–12 months. The restenosis rate after stenting a localised lesion in a vein graft is about 10%.

   High pressure inflations may not be needed and 8–10 atmospheres with a Palmaz-Schatz stent may be sufficient. The soft friable nature of vein graft atheroma and the relatively bulky size of a stent, increase the risk of atheroma becoming dislodged and embolizing distally. The atheroma of vein grafts is prone to prolapse between struts of wire coil stents, such as the Wiktor and the Gianturco-Roubin stents. Diffuse disease with long lesions in SVGs may be treated with one or more Wallstents (Angiogram 20.2, page 217), but the risk of restenosis is higher than with short discrete lesions.

3. **To Reduce Restenosis**
   Stents are valuable to reduce restenosis with each of the following:
   a) de novo lesion
   b) restenosis lesion
   c) chronic total occlusion
   d) osteal stenosis

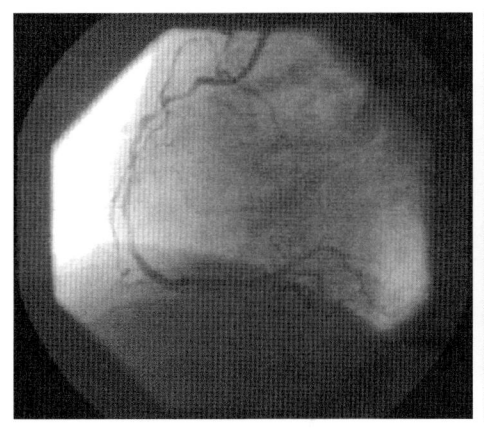

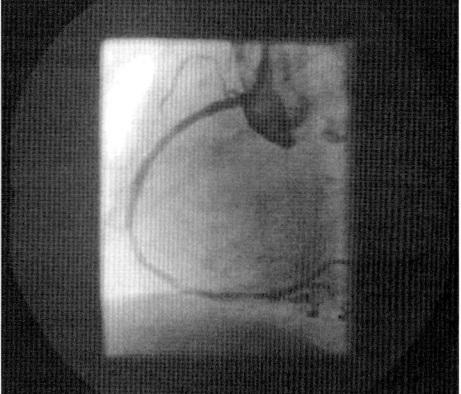

Figure 11.2. *Diffuse RCA disease treated with Wallstent.* (Angiogram kindly supplied by Dr Ulrich Sigwart, Royal Brompton Hospital, London.)

a) De Novo Lesion

After 15 years following the introduction of angioplasty, coronary stenting was the first treatment to reduce the restenosis rate after angioplasty — the so called *'Achilles' heal'* of angioplasty.

For a de novo lesion, in a vessel considered to be of suitable size for stenting i.e. 3 mm or larger in calibre, the two landmark clinical trials were **Stress** and **Benestent.**

The results of these two trials may be summarized:-

	STRESS		BENESTENT	
	Stent	PTCA	Stent	PTCA
Death	1.5%	1.5%	0.8%	0.4%
Emergency CABG	4.9%	8.4%	1.9%	1.6%
Thrombosis	3.5%	1.5%	3.5%	2.7%
Groin Complication	7.4%	5.0%	13.5%	3.1%
Re PTCA	11.2%	12.4%	10%	20.6%
6/12 Event Free Survival	80%	72%	83%	71%
6/12 Angio Restenosis	31%	42%	22%	32%

The reduction in restenosis is the reason for the *huge increase* in stent usage; in some centres 70%, or even more, of PTCA cases will involve the use of stents. Stents have become *"the second wind of PTCA"*. A large (and increasing) number of stents have now become available (see Chapter 10).

Possible Mechanisms for Reduction of Restenosis

After elective stenting a *larger* lumen is obtained than if following routine PTCA (e.g. Angiogram 17.1, page 185). This is achieved by a stent reducing or preventing recoil of the vessel wall at the time of PTCA and over the succeeding weeks and months. The initial recoil may be 'elastic' after deflating a balloon; the later recoil may be due to scar contraction.

After stenting, intimal hyperplasia as a response to vessel wall injury, is actually greater than following routine PTCA. However because the vessel lumen after stenting is so much larger, the final lumen at 6/12 is larger with a stent. See Figure 11.1.

With a Palmaz-Schatz Stent and probably with other stents too, the sequence is:

	Stent	PTCA
Initial gain at time of procedure	Greater	Less

After 6 months there is late loss of lumen size from:

a) 'Elastic' Recoil of wall	± None	Moderate
b) Intimal Hyperplasia	More	Less

The final lumen size of the vessel at the site of the lesion at *6 months* (i.e. "long term" result) is governed by:-

Final Lumen = Initial Gain – Late Loss
= Initial Gain – (Elastic Recoil + Intimal Hyperplasia)

Indications for the Use of Stents

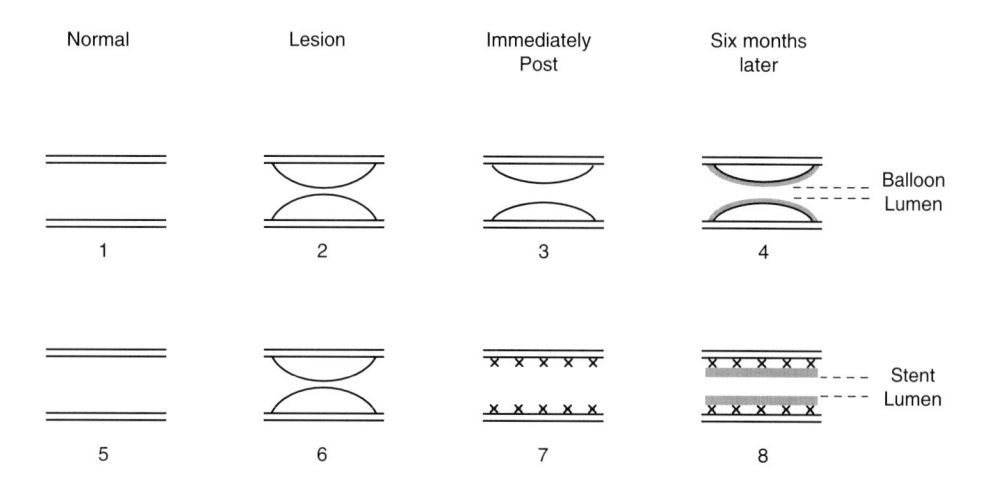

Normal	Lesion	Immediately Post	Six months later	
1	2	3	4	Balloon Lumen
5	6	7	8	Stent Lumen

After balloon dilatation, there is elastic recoil (3), and later intimal hyperplasia (4). After a coronary stent there is virtually no elastic recoil resulting in a larger lumen (7). At six months, there is greater intimal hyperplasia with a stent (8). The lumen after stenting is still larger than after balloon angioplasty (4 and 8).
See text for details.

Figure 11.1. Comparison of balloon angioplasty and stent.

The larger initial lumen after stenting leading to lower restenosis was first proposed, as the theory of *'larger is better'*, by Prof. Don Baim of Boston, USA.

An anti proliferative coating to a stent may reduce intimal hyperplasia and lead to an even lower rate of restenosis. One such coating, heparin, does not seem to have been successful in patients.

b) **Restenosis Lesion**

If a lesion after PTCA restenoses, repeat dilatation is usually a low risk procedure, but is still associated with a 30% restenosis rate. If the vessel is of suitable size 3 mm or more in diameter, then coronary artery stenting can approximately halve the restenosis rate (see Angiogram 24.1, page 254).

c) **Chronic Occlusion**

After PTCA of a chronic occlusion, i.e. one believed or known to have been present for 3 months or more, the restenosis or reocclusion rate is higher than for a stenosis lesion, at about 50%. This is often due to reocclusion which is usually 'silent', i.e. it is not accompanied with acute ischaemia. At the time of reinvestigation for continuing or recurrent angina, the vessel is found to have reoccluded (see Chapter 19).

A stent, by re-establishing and maintaining a large lumen and good flow down the vessel, reduces the risk of reocclusion (by thrombosis) and restenosis. The restenosis rate is about 20% and stenting should be considered for most PTCAs for chronic occlusion of a coronary artery (see Angiogram 19.1, page 207).

d) **Osteal Stenosis**

An osteal stenosis especially of the RCA or of a sasphenous vein graft, has a high restenosis rate of approximately 50% (see page 227). The treatment of choice is to stent the osteum (see Angiogram 22.1, page 230).

Conclusion

The use of stents started slowly but, following their success to reduce restenosis, they are now an essential item of equipment for all angioplasty operators.

References

Benestent Trial

Serruys, P.W., de Jaegere, P., Kiemeneij, F., *et al*. A comparison of balloon expandable stent with balloon angioplasty in patients with coronary artery disease. *N Engl J Med* **331**, 489–95 (1994).

Stress Trial

Fischman, D., Leon, M.B., Baim, D., Schatz, R.A., *et al*. A randomized comparison of coronary stent placement and balloon angioplasty in the treatment of coronary artery disease. *N Engl J Med* **331**, 496–501 (1994).

12 Complications with Stents

There are five main problems with stents:

(1) Stent Thrombosis
(2) Haemorrhage
(3) Problems with placement
(4) 'Stent Jail'
(5) Restenosis

Stent Thrombosis

All the stents currently available are metal and the surface is thrombogenic. The risk of thrombosis (Angiogram 12.1, page 128) is greater in the following situations:-

a) *Small calibre vessels*
   less than 3 mm calibre.
b) *Multiple stents in sequence*
   especially three or more.
c) *Stent used in 'bail out' situation*
   i.e. after total vessel closure.
d) *Inflow or outflow obstruction*
   If blood flow is poor or reduced in the vessel before or after stent; so-called inflow or outflow obstruction. If there is poor flow then the risk of thrombosis is considerable.
e) *Inadequate expansion of the stent*
   This results in a residual stenosis within the stent and a lack of firm contact with the vessel wall by one or more sections of the stent. Both these features lead to turbulence and an increased risk of thrombosis. The importance of this problem was recognized by Dr. Antonio Colombo of Milan who introduced high pressure inflation(s) and confirmation of satisfactory stent deployment by intravascular ultrasound (IVUS).

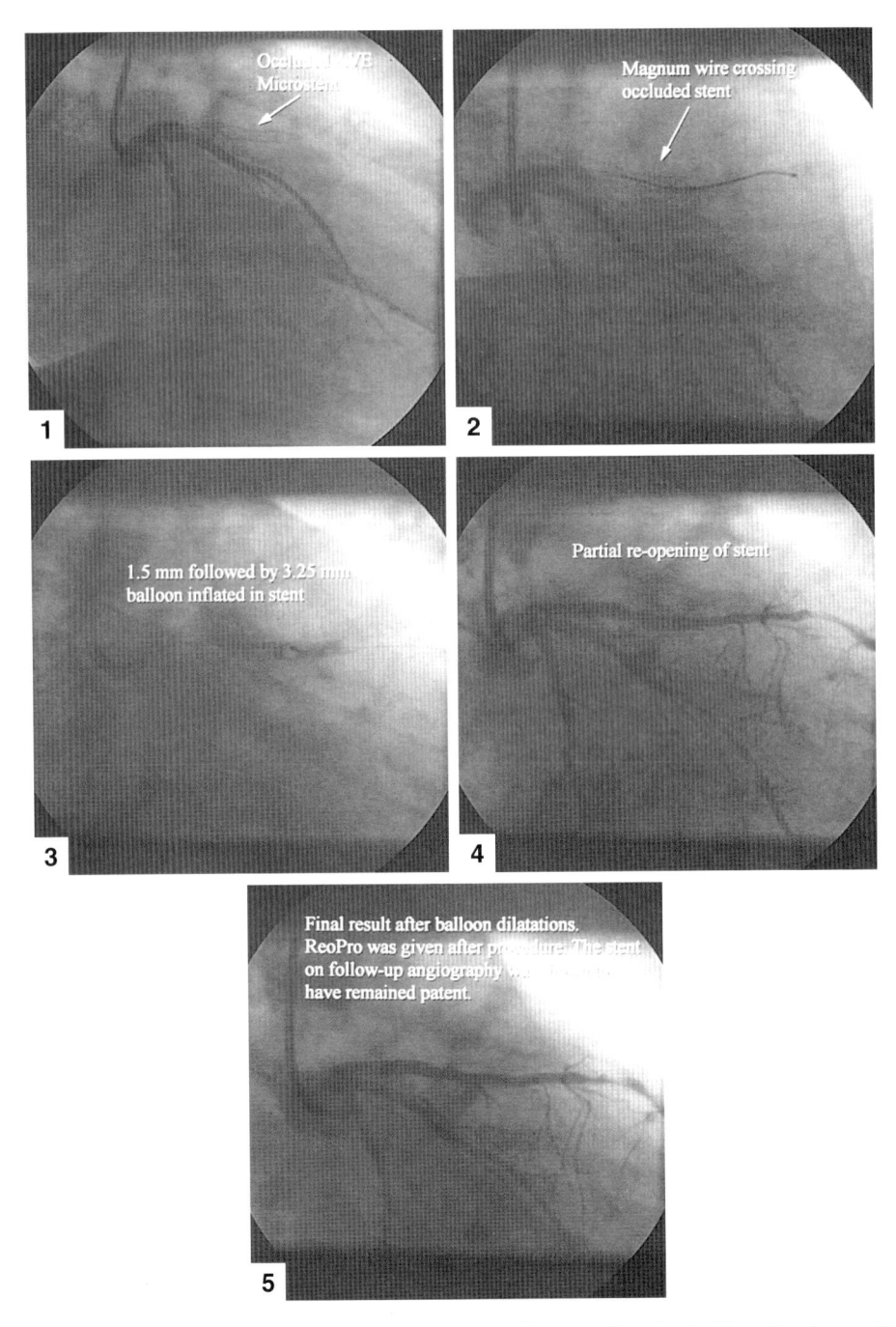

Angiogram 12.1. *Reopening of a stent acutely occluded by stent thrombosis.* Sixty-four hours after stent deployment for an unsatisfactory PTCA result, the patient developed severe chest pain and S-T eleveation on the ECG. Angiography showed that the AVE Microstent had occluded (1). The occluded stent was crossed with a magnum wire (2), followed by redilatation with a balloon (3). Following reopening (4), ReoPro was given, and the final result is shown in (5). The stent did not reocclude, nor restenose (at angiography six months later).

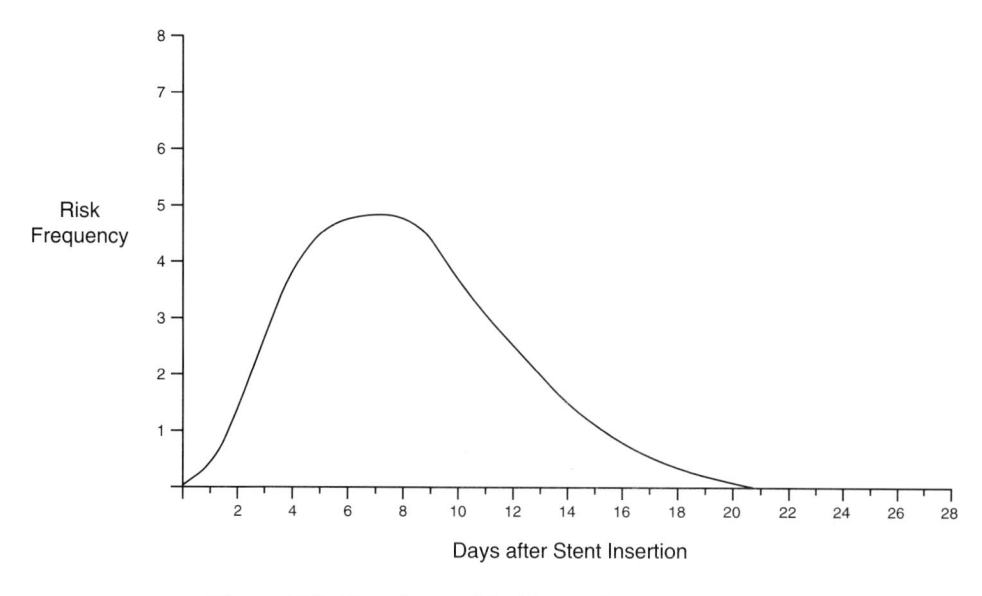

Figure 12.1. Time frame of incidence of stent thrombosis.

f) *Possibly increased in the presence of thrombus*
   However the experience in clinical settings where thrombus may be present, such as acute MI or unstable angina, shows that providing the stent establishes a large lumen and good flow, then stent thrombosis is not increased.
h) *Following a vascular complication in the groin.*
   Previously with aggressive anticoagulant regimes, if the patient had a gastric bleed, or a vascular complication occurred in the groin, the anticoagulants were abruptly stopped. Sometimes vascular surgery might be needed. Over the time frame of 72 hours after stopping anticoagulants there was increased risk of stent thrombosis to add to the previous problem. The increased thrombosis rate may have been due to a 'rebound phenomenon' of hypercoagulation on stopping the anticoagulants.

Time Frame of Stent Thrombosis (see Figure 12.1)

With balloon angioplasty, abrupt vessel closure occurs in the catheter lab or over the next 24 hours. It is then almost unknown. Abrupt stent closure, due to stent thrombosis has a quite different time course. It too can occur in the catheter lab, but is then very rare in the first 24 hours. It may present on the second day and then rises in frequency to reach a peak on day 4–6 and then declines so that it is rare after day 14, but may still occurs up to 4 weeks following stent insertion. After this time, the risk of stent thrombosis is over and the stent has now become covered by a protective endothelial layer.

Effects of Stent Thrombosis

Whereas restenosis is a gradual process over 1–3 months and very rarely complicated by myocardial infarction, the effects of stent thrombosis are very much more serious. The event is usually sudden and presents as total occlusion of the vessel. The patient has severe chest pain and there are prominent changes of acute myocardial infarction on the ECG. Cardiac arrest and sudden death may occur. Ventricular damage from the myocardial infarction may lead to later morbidity and mortality. Stent thrombosis has a mortality rate of about 3–5% and early reports of the use of stents had an overall mortality complication of about 4%, significantly higher than that of routine PTCA (about 0.5–1%). Many of the stents from the early series had been implanted for acute vessel closure at the time of PTCA, when the risk of later stent thrombosis is greater (see page 174). Hence stent thrombosis was and is the feared complication of stenting. Colombo's contribution to reduce this risk has been a major one to allow the increase in the use of stents. Rarely stent occlusion can be less acute, or even silent, as may occur with coronary thrombosis in a coronary artery or a vein graft in the absence of a stent.

Measures to Reduce the Risk of Stent Thrombosis

1. Antiplatelet drugs

   a) *Aspirin*
   In experimental studies and in the clinical setting too, aspirin has been found to be of great value. A number of instances of stent thrombosis have occurred when aspirin has been omitted. If the patient is unable to take aspirin then the use of a stent should be reconsidered. Fortunately, it is rare that a patient cannot take low dose aspirin, i.e. 150 mg per day which is sufficient.

   b) *Ticlopidine*
   This relatively new drug reduces platelet adhesion to fibrinogen. In France, the use of ticlopidine 250 mgs twice a day for one month with aspirin, instead of heparin and warfarin, reduced stent thrombosis from 5–7% to 1–2%. One small controlled trial by Dr Colombo has suggested that aspirin with ticlopidine was superior to aspirin alone, but the evidence of the added value of ticlopidine has yet to be proved by a large controlled trial.

   c) *Dextran and Dipyridamole*
   These were part of the 'cocktail' of drugs used with the initial 'aggressive' anti-coagulant regime for stents. They are not of proven value and are no longer routinely used.

2. Heparin at the Time of Stent Insertion

Heparin is routinely administered for all angioplasty procedures and with stents the aim is to achieve an ACT measurement of 300 seconds or greater, at the time of deployment. If ReoPro is to be used electively a reduced dose of heparin is given (see pages 73 and 163). Often a small increment (2000–5000 Units) of heparin may be needed to achieve this. At the end of the procedure many operators give no further heparin and when the PTTK is less than 1.5:1 or the ACT is less than 150 seconds, remove the femoral sheath. Others leave the patient on a heparin infusion over night and pull the sheath the following day. Dr Colombo has given protamine at the end of the procedure allowing the sheath to be removed there and then.

3. Oral Anticoagulants

Warfarin, together with an IV heparin infusion until anticoagulant control had been achieved, was the mainstay of the post stent treatment to prevent stent thrombosis. However this regime was unsuccessful and lead to an increased risk of groin complications of 5–10%, including haemorrhage, pseudoaneurysm, blood transfusion and groin surgical exploration. Sudden withdrawal of heparin and warfarin to manage a groin complication was associated with stent thrombosis. Oral anticoagulants are not needed if stent deployment has been satisfactory.

4. Meticulous Care with Stent Deployment

The stent needs to be fully expanded out to the vessel wall and high pressure balloon inflations (up to 16–18 atmospheres) may be needed (see Angiograms 19.1, 20.1 and 23.1 on pages 207, 212 and 246). Inflow and outflow obstruction must be avoided (see Angiogram 18.2, page 197).

The use of IVUS may assist in ensuring a good stent deployment. Avoidance of multiple stents (3 or more) and use of stents in a small calibre vessel less than 3 mm, reduces the risk of thrombosis.

Because of the risk of stent thrombosis, the patient should be informed on what action to take in the event and to avoid a vacation during the first month after stent insertion. It is helpful for the patient to be given a named person and telephone number to contact if there is a problem.

Management of Stent Thrombosis

The diagnosis is usually not difficult. The patient presents as an acute myocardial infarction with prolonged and severe chest pain, prominent S-T elevation and sometimes cardiac arrest.

If still an inpatient and the event occurs in routine hours, the patient should be taken immediately to the catheter room, for coronary angiography and an attempt be made to reopen the stent with a guide wire and balloon (see Angiogram 12.1, page 128). This may be followed by Abciximab (ReoPro) given as an IV bolus and then followed by an infusion. This drug can be very effective to clear any residual thrombus and to reduce the risk of its recurrence.

An IVUS study should be considered, which may show that there is a problem with the deployment of the stent. In its absence a further high pressure dilatation of the stent can be given. If there is evidence of inflow or outflow obstruction, this will need attention, perhaps with the insertion of another stent to cover the area.

Having restored flow through the stent a decision should be taken about the future management of the patient. Abciximab (ReoPro) seems to be very effective to prevent rethrombosis. Another option is urgent or semielective surgery.

The use of fibrinolytic therapy such as streptokinase or TPA is usually not successful and complicates haemostasis for emergency coronary artery bypass.

Outside routine hours, a decision is needed whether it is better to call in catheter laboratory staff and attempt reopening, or whether it will be overall quicker to call in the surgical team and perform bypass. If the result of stenting was less than ideal, or if there is proximal or distal disease, or if there is disease involving other coronary arteries, then CABG may be the best treatment.

Haemorrhage after Stent Insertion

This complication was due to the heavy anticoagulation that was used with stents. Groin complications of haemorrhage and pseudoaneurysm were the most frequent, up to 7–10% of cases. Haemorrhage into gastrointestinal tract, the brain and elsewhere occurred too. The complication led to prolonged hospital stays and readmissions. With the aspirin and ticlopidine regime, haemorrhagic complications have fallen to 1–2%, which are no more than after routine PTCA. To reduce access complications the brachial and radial routes were used instead of the femoral approach, but this need has now receded.

Problems with Stent Placement

Stents are relatively "non user friendly". A new learning curve for stents in general and each stent type in particular is needed. Some stents are more difficult to place correctly than others.

The problems in stent placement include:-

A) Problems of Trackability:
  1) Difficulty to reach the lesion.
  2) Difficulty to cross mild proximal disease.
  3) Difficulty to cross the lesion.
  4) Difficulty to enter or cross a stent with a second stent.
  5) Dropped stents.
  6) Damage to proximal vessel.
  7) New lesions appearing.
  8) Distal embolism.
B) Difficulties of Deployment:
  1) Inaccuracy in Positioning the Stent.
  2) Stent migration.
  3) Balloon rupture.
  4) Dissection at either end of the stent.
  5) Inadequate stent expansion.
  6) Persistence of the lesion.
  7) Uncoiling a stent.

Problems of Trackability

(1) Difficulty to Reach the Lesion

Some stents such as the Palmaz-Schatz PS153 stent, are relatively rigid and "do not enjoy going round bends". This type of Palmaz-Schatz stent should be reserved for lesions.

a) in relatively straight vessels without prominent curves or sharp bends.
b) at sites in the proximal to mid portion of a vessel, rather than distal lesions.

If the start of the RCA has even a modest shepherd's crook course, or if the circumflex artery comes off steeply from the left main stem, an alternative stent to the Palmaz-Schatz stent should be considered. There are now many that might be used, such as the Cordis CrossFlex, or Micro stent, or a 'second generation' stent such as the Multilink, Palmaz-Schatz Crown stent, or the NIR stent. These are all more flexible and trackable than the Palmaz-Schatz stent.

(2) Difficulty to Cross Mild Proximal Disease

If the vessel before the lesion has disease, angiographically it may be mild and a balloon may easily pass it. However a stent may be unable to cross and trying to force it across may damage the vessel or strip the stent off the balloon.

(3) Difficulty to Cross the Lesion

If the target lesion has been predilated with a 2.5 mm or larger balloon, there should not be a problem of later crossing it with the stent.

To avoid problems of tracking the proximal vessel and crossing the lesion:

- *Ensure good guide catheter back-up.*
  At the start of an angioplasty procedure, if later a stent might be needed, do not accept an indifferent guide catheter position and back up. Electively change to a better guide catheter if needed, such as from Left Judkins (JL4) to a Voda or Amplatz Catheter for LCA lesions.
- *Increase guide catheter back-up.*
  Just prior to passing a stent up the guide catheter from the groin, check the guide catheter position and consider more deeply engaging it, if necessary.
- *Use of stiffer section of the guide wire.*
  Pass the guide wire as distal as possible so that the stent mounted balloon is travelling on the firmer portion of the guide wire.
- *Use of extra back-up guide wires.*
  These have a firmer core wire extending down the wire with only the final 2–4 cm being soft and flexible. These aid tracking of the stent, by providing a firmer rail for the balloon to ride and also by straightening out the artery, especially the RCA (see page 29).

(4) Difficulty to Enter or Cross a Stent with a Second Stent

Sometimes a second stent is needed to overlap the proximal end of a first stent, or pass through the first stent to be deployed more distally. If there is resistance to enter the first stent, inflate the balloon of the second stent to 0.5 atmospheres. This helps to prevent the balloon tip catching on the proximal end of the first stent and aids passing of the second stent balloon into the first stent.

(5) Dropped Stents

With a bare or free mounted stent (i.e. one on a balloon without a protective sheath), the stent may come off the balloon and be "dropped" and lost.

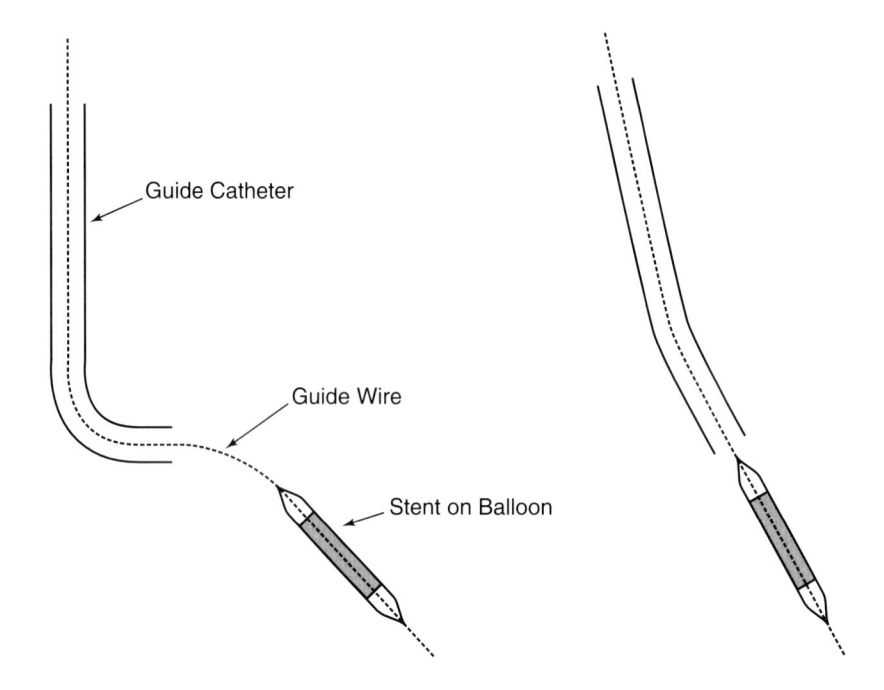

a) Stent may catch on the edge of the mouth of the guide catheter.

b) By withdrawing the guide catheter a short distance from coronary osteum, it is straightened. The end of the guide catheter, and the stent-mounted balloon, are in a straight line, ie. co-axial.

Figure 12.2. Safer withdrawal of a stent on a balloon back into a guide catheter.

This may occur:

a) When trying to advance the stent against resistance from a curve, proximal vessel disease or an inadequately dilated lesion.
b) For a stent that has been passed too distally; when attempting to withdraw the stent back across the lesion, it may be left behind distal to the lesion when the balloon comes back.
c) Withdrawing a stent mounted balloon into the guide catheter. Usually this can be done but there is always a risk of stripping the stent off the balloon. To avoid or reduce this risk, try to straighten out the final section of the guide catheter so that the stented balloon has a straight run into the guide catheter and is less likely to catch on the mouth of the guide catheter. This usually means withdrawing the guide catheter a short distance from the coronary osteum which reduces or removes the final curves of the catheter, e.g. a Judkins JL4 with its L-shape comes to resemble a multipurpose catheter with a smooth straight final section (see Figure 12.2).

Complications with Stents

d) Trying to engage the guide catheter more deeply by 'sucking' it in, whilst withdrawing the balloon catheter. This might be attempted if extra backup is needed to advance the stent. However the manoeuvre which is often used during PTCA, especially of LAD lesions, must not be done with stents as there is a risk that whilst withdrawing the balloon catheter, the stent may be 'sucked' back into the guide catheter and be stripped off the balloon.

e) Ostial lesions of RCA and saphenous vein grafts. Accurate placement can be difficult and the stent may drop off the balloon and out of the ostium.

If a stent comes off the balloon it may either lodge in the coronary artery or be lost outside the coronary in the general circulation. The former is more serious.

1) *Dropped Stent in the Coronary Artery or Saphenous Vein Graft*

   This may lead to partial vessel closure, which may identify the site where the stent has lodged. If the stent is poorly radiopaque it may be difficult to see. Be very careful to maintain the guide wire distally and well beyond the lesion. An attempt can be tried to pass the balloon back into the stent, either progradely or retrogradely, depending where the stent is. However this is usually not possible and it is better to try and recross the stent with a small calibre balloon, e.g. 1.5 mm. Inflate the balloon to widen the channel and return with larger balloon(s) as necessary to expand and deploy the stent where it has lodged i.e. at the proximal "wrong" site.

   Sometimes, inflating a 1.5 mm balloon in the stent may allow it to be trapped and withdrawn out of the coronary artery. Once near the tip of the guide catheter, withdraw the balloon plus stent and the guide catheter as one unit. This prevents the stent being stripped off the balloon when attempting to re-enter the guide catheter and then being dropped near the start of the coronary artery. Once the tip of the guide catheter is round the arch and in the descending aorta, attempt to withdraw the balloon and stent back into the guide catheter. It should be able to re-enter, but if it does not bring the stent down to the ilio-femoral region and retrieve as described below (see section 2).

2) *Dropped Stent Outside the Coronary Artery*

   Usually there has been a problem advancing the stent to the lesion. The stent mounted balloon is withdrawn into the guide catheter but when the balloon catheter is withdrawn from the Y-connector at the proximal end of the guide catheter, the stent is no longer on the balloon "*the stent is not there*". Where is it? It is somewhere in the general circulation and unless the stent is radiopaque it will not be visible. It usually ends up in a leg vessel where it can be detected on an MRI scan. Very fortunately, embolism of a stent to the brain or intestines is extremely rare.

   It is possible to retrieve a stent that is still on the guide wire or is lodged in the iliac or femoral vessel. An *Amplatz 'Goose Neck' Snare* catheter (Microvena), is passed up on a guide wire via the same sheath, or via the contralateral femoral artery (Angiogram 12.2, page 136). If the later route is used, via a 6 or 7F sheath, a pigtail catheter is passed to the lower abdominal aorta and an exchange guide

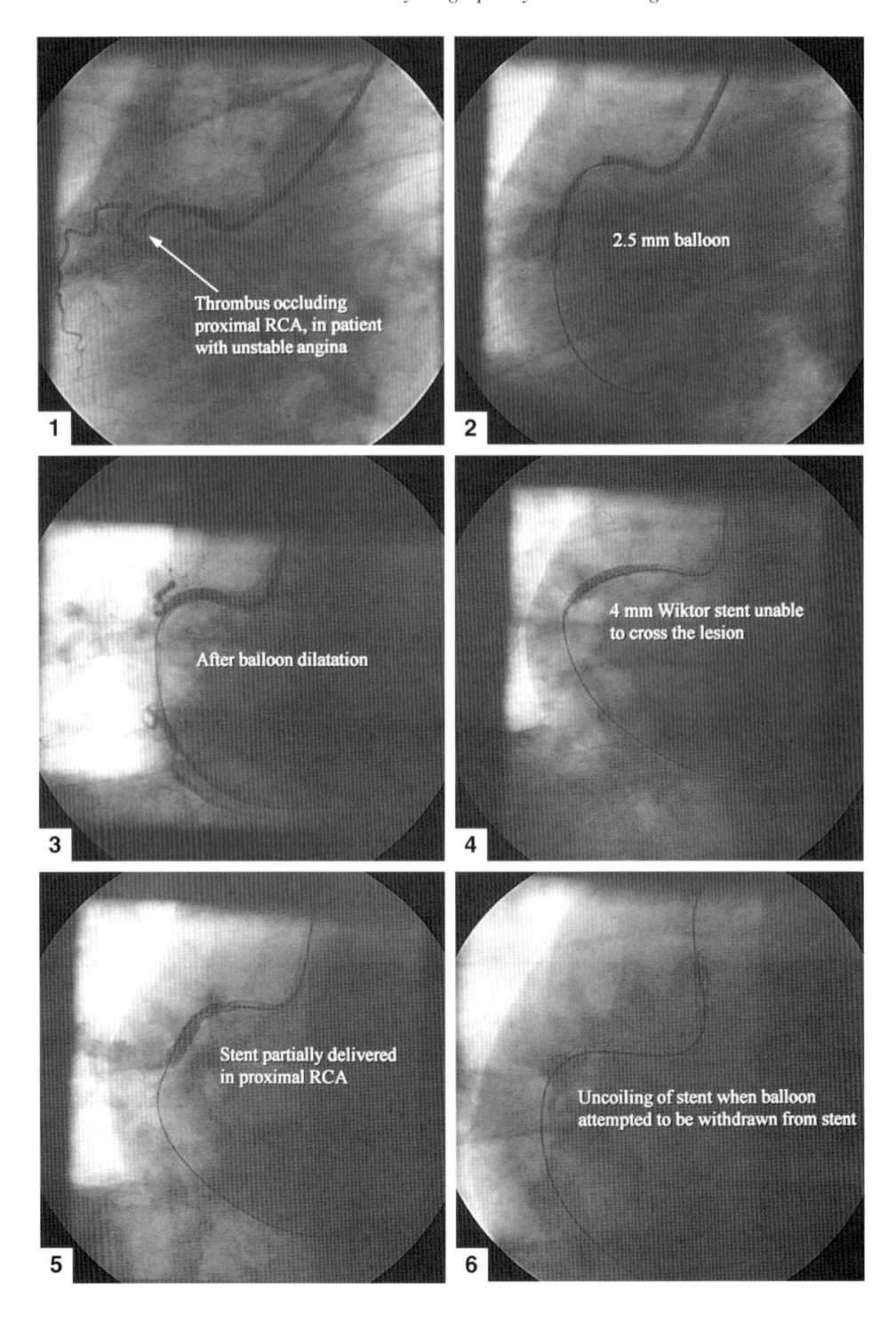

136 *Guide to Coronary Angioplasty and Stenting*

1 Thrombus occluding proximal RCA, in patient with unstable angina

2 2.5 mm balloon

3 After balloon dilatation

4 4 mm Wiktor stent unable to cross the lesion

5 Stent partially delivered in proximal RCA

6 Uncoiling of stent when balloon attempted to be withdrawn from stent

Complications with Stents

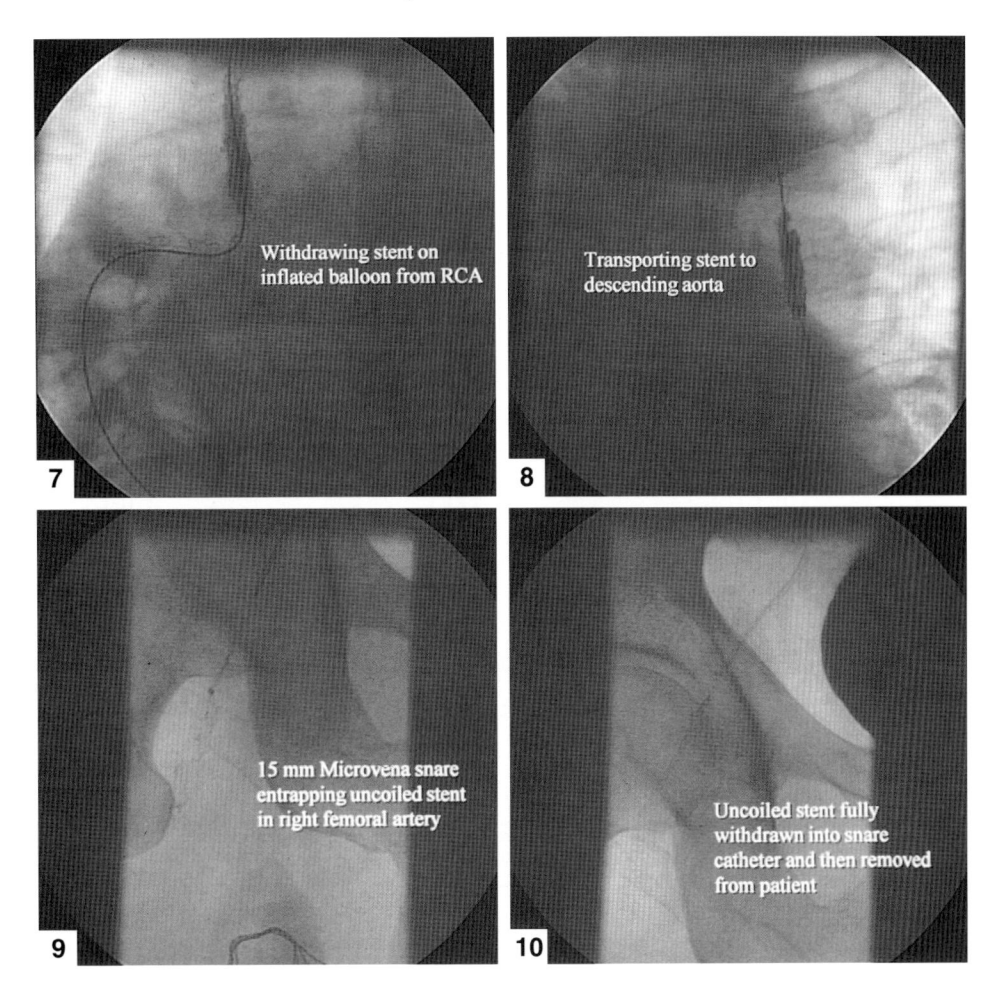

(Image panels 7–10 with labels:)
- **7:** Withdrawing stent on inflated balloon from RCA
- **8:** Transporting stent to descending aorta
- **9:** 15 mm Microvena snare entrapping uncoiled stent in right femoral artery
- **10:** Uncoiled stent fully withdrawn into snare catheter and then removed from patient

Angiogram 12.2. *Retrieving an uncoiled Wiktor stent.* The patient presented with unstable angina, and the RCA had thrombus seen as a filling defect at the start of the vessel, prior to total occlusion of the RCA (1). A soft guide wire would not cross, so that a firm wire (0.014 inch USCI Standard J wire) was used, followed by a 2.5 mm balloon (1). The result showed a long lesion (3), which was not improved with a 3.5 mm balloon. It was not possible to cross the lesion with a Wiktor stent, which became stuck at the start of the lesion (4). The balloon was inflated to deploy the stent at this site (5). On withdrawing the balloon the stent began to uncoil and come out of the RCA too (6). The balloon was then inflated to hold the stent (7), and withdrawn out of the RCA to the descending aorta (8). It was then taken down to the right femoral artery where it was entrapped using an Amplatz snare (9 and 10), introduced via the left femoral artery. The retrieved stent was taken out from the patient via the left femoral artery. The lesion was successfully treated 24 hours later, see Angiogram 10.2.

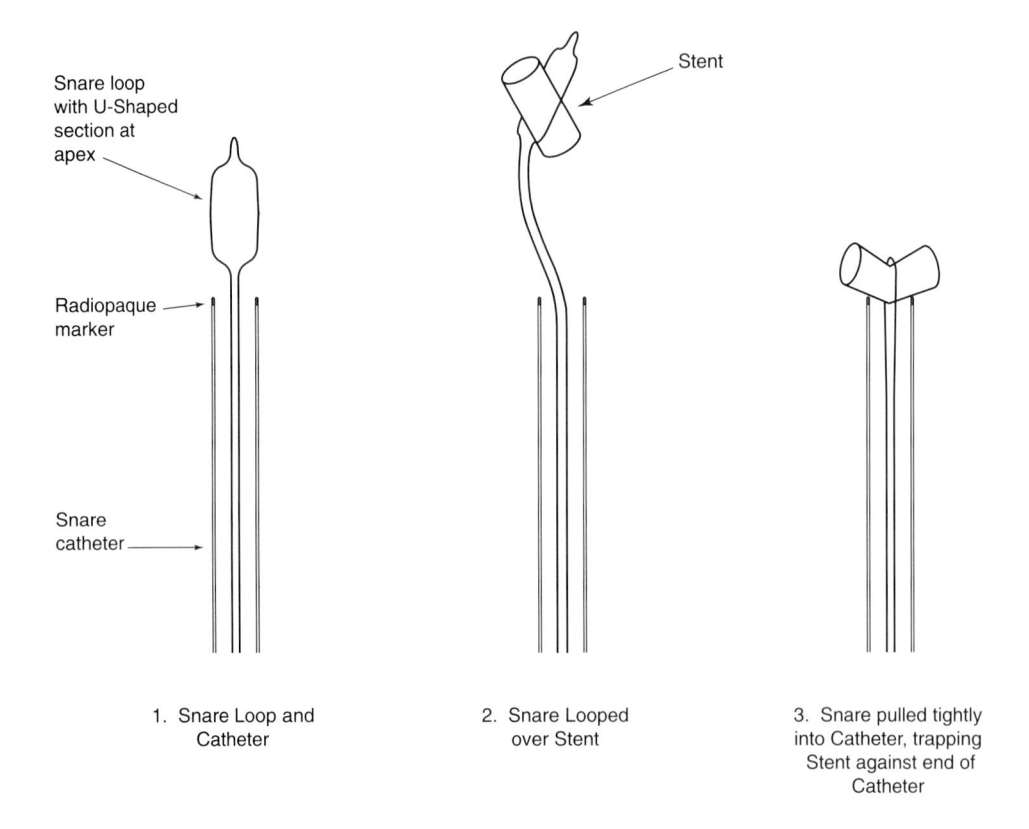

Figure 12.3. Retrieval of dropped stent using Amplatz "Goose Neck" snare.

wire passed through it, which as it emerges faces the other iliac artery. The pigtail catheter is replaced with the special snare catheter. This is 6F in calibre and has a radiopaque ring marker at its tip.

The snare wire has a small fixed U-shaped curve or 'goose neck' at its apex (see Figure 12.3). Through its catheter, the snare loop is advanced over and around the stent. The snare catheter is advanced slowly up to the stent. The snare wire is then withdrawn tightly into its catheter, pulling the stent back and trapping it against the end of the catheter. A Wiktor stent may uncoil and be pulled progressively up into the snare catheter.

The snare catheter and the entrapped stent are withdrawn into the femoral sheath and out of the patient. If the snared stent will not enter the femoral sheath, gentle repeated manipulation may achieve this. If still not successful, the sheath may be changed to a larger one over a guide wire and the snaring process repeated again. Alternatively, the entrapped stent and femoral sheath may be removed by surgical exploration of the artery. A further possibility is to pass another guide wire along the sheath into the abdominal aorta. Next, withdraw the femoral sheath and entrapped stent directly out of the femoral artery. This may damage the femoral artery and with the patient heparinized, significant bleeding may occur. When it is confirmed that the stent is out, another sheath is passed up into the femoral artery which will aid haemostasis.

The Amplatz 'Goose-Neck' snare wire is available with loop sizes of 5,10,15, 25 and 35 mm. The 15 mm size is suitable for stent retrieval. A bent double 300 cm guide wire can also be used to ensnare a dropped stent.

Once the problem with stent has been sorted out, reassess the target lesion to determine whether simple balloon dilatation will suffice. If not reassess whether another stent should be tried. If the first stent was a Palmaz-Schatz 153 stent and the problem was a tortuous vessel then consider using a more flexible stent such as a Micro stent, ACS Multilink, or Wiktor stent.

Sometimes the problem in the coronary artery is more pressing than retrieving the stent. It may be quicker to catheterize the other femoral vessel and proceed with another guide catheter. If the patient is stable and retrieval of the stent has been lengthy, consider to call it a day for that procedure. The patient *and* operator by this time may have had enough! Return to the case 24 hours later refreshed and relaxed after further thoughts on how best to complete the procedure. Share the problem and discuss it with colleagues.

Prevention is better than cure and the risk of dropping a stent is less with:

- Careful patient and stent selection
  Avoiding tortuous proximal vessels, proximal disease and ensuring predilatation of the lesion.
- Ensuring good guide catheter support.
- Using zero or atmospheric pressure for the stent balloon, rather than negative pressure (see page 149).
- Modifying guide wire support.
- Use of a stent protected with a sheath, when there is more complicated proximal anatomy or a difficult lesion.

(6) Damage to the Proximal Vessel

This is usually due to pushing a stent against resistance in the proximal part of the vessel. Even if the stent does not become dislodged from the balloon, the vessel may be damaged, dissected and this section may then need PTCA or stenting.

The risk is greater if there is proximal disease and in saphenous vein grafts. Any inflow obstruction to a stent will increase the risk of thrombosis of the stent at the target lesion site.

(7) New Lesions Appearing

These can be very worrying! At any time during the procedure, but especially after delivering of the stent, a new narrowing either proximal or distal to the target lesion may appear. If you "have not done anything" which might have caused the lesion and if stent passed quite easily, the new lesion may be due to coronary artery spasm. Spontaneous new lesions are more likely when a stiffer 'back-up' guide wire is used. The lesions will disappear or improve after nitrates sublingually or intra coronary are given (see Angiograms 11.1 and 13.2, pages 122 and 152). After removal of the guide wire at end of the procedure such a lesion will usually completely disappear.

(8) Distal Embolism

This is a problem with old vein grafts, that even when the passage of the stent has been without difficulty, a portion of the friable graft atheroma may embolize. Appropriate drugs and an intra aortic balloon pump should be available and the patient warned of this risk (see page 215).

Difficulties of Deployment

(1) Inaccuracy when Positioning the Stent

Many stents are poorly radiopaque or non radiopaque. This is certainly true for the Palmaz-Schatz Stent and makes all aspects of the use of the stent difficult. The Wiktor, Microstent and the Cordis stent have the great advantage of being well visualized on screening, both before and after deployment. Most premounted stents now have a radiopaque marker at *each* end of the balloon. The Gianturco-Roubin stent and the BeStent have a gold radiopaque 'tag' at each end of the stent. With these methods accurate placing of the stent is much easier, but problems can still occur (see Angiogram 11.1, page 122).

The Wallstent on deployment shortens and will contract proximally. It requires particular care to ensure that the distal end of the lesion is covered by the stent (see page 114).

When deploying any stent before the final position is accepted, *don't be in a hurry*. Check and double check the position. Use the greatest magnified field available. Take a short angiogram run. Review under zoom playback. Look in another X-ray view. Check carefully the position of the stent against vessel landmarks, such as nearby branches, or sternal wires for vein grafts.

Unfortunately with the stent in position, vessel visualization on contrast injection may be less good, especially if small calibre guide catheters are used . However this is not usually a major problem. Only when fully satisfied, inflate the balloon and deploy the stent. Sometimes the stent may partially occlude the lumen and cause ischaemia, so that less time will be available — but still avoid a "smash and grab technique". Once the stent is deployed it can't be taken out! Furthermore, its embarrassing and expensive to find that the lesion has not been fully covered and that another stent is needed.

(2) Stent Migration

A very proximal stent, especially at the ostium of the RCA or a vein graft, may be correctly positioned but become dislodged out of the coronary artery as the balloon is withdrawn. With the ACT – One stent, even after high pressure inflations the stent cannot be expanded any further than the preset 'memory' of the nitinol alloy. This may lead to incomplete apposition to the wall, allowing the stent to become dislodged proximally when the balloon is withdrawn. The original form of the Micro stent was in 4 mm sections secured together with a suture. On high pressures the stent segments could separate and migrate apart leaving a gap between them.

(3) Balloon Rupture

This may occur at the start of the balloon inflation, before the stent is expanded or at the end whilst using high pressures (16+ atmospheres). The former is more serious and is virtually confined to stents hand crimped onto a balloon.

a) *Early Balloon Perforation*

When a stent is hand crimped, a strut may pierce the balloon and lead to a small *perforation* (rather than a rupture) of the balloon. Using an indeflator, if negative pressure is applied it will not be possible to maintain it. The problem of balloon perforation can be recognised *before* the stent is inserted into the guide catheter and the patient. However, often the balloon is kept at zero or atmospheric pressure to reduce the risk of the stent becoming dislodged off the balloon. Perforation of the balloon is then not recognised until deploying the stent, when it is not possible to increase the inflation pressure above 3–4 atmospheres. This is **very serious and is an emergency**. A partially deployed stent may occlude the artery. It may become dislodged proximally whilst trying to withdraw the balloon, which is unable to collapse fully.

When inflating a balloon to deploy a stent always have at least 10 ml of fluid in the syringe of the inflation device. If the pressure will not rise when twisting the handle to increase inflation pressure, recognise the problem of balloon perforation. Quickly unclick the ratchet mechanism and manually push down the syringe plunger as hard as possible. Often, even with a perforated balloon (where the hole may only be pin-prick size), a pressure of 8–9 atmospheres can be achieved which is enough to moderately expand the stent. Usually the balloon can then be safely withdrawn and another passed into the stent to fully expand it.

b) *Balloon Rupture During or at the End of High Pressure Inflation*

As the balloon is expanded to 16–18 atmospheres the pressure gauge may suddenly return to zero. Blood is later seen to be tracking backward from the balloon into the inflation syringe. The coronary artery beyond the stent does not "enjoy" contrast being suddenly shot down the vessel at high pressure. The ECG will often show S-T elevation. Sometimes the blood pressure may fall. Often, there is no, or only mild, chest pain. Nitrates administered sublingually or into the coronary artery may be helpful. After 5–15 minutes the S-T segments return to normal.

(4) Dissection at Either End of the Stent (see Angiograms 18.2 and 19.1, pages 197 and 207)

With a 20 mm balloon and a 15 mm stent perhaps reduced to 12 mm after full expansion, about 2.5 mm of the balloon will protrude from each end of the stent. These segments of the balloon outside the stent will expand further after high pressure inflations, so that for example a compliant 3 mm balloon at 18 atmospheres may approximate to 3.4 mm in calibre. The damage to the vessel wall is greater at the distal end of the stent as the vessel tends to taper. Minor damage is often seen by IVUS to the vessel beyond each end of a deployed stent. If angiographically there is a hazy lesion, or undoubted reduced flow, then IVUS will show a severe lesion, usually a dissection. It must not be left as outflow or inflow obstruction leads to stent thrombosis. Balloon dilatation of the area may be successful, but can also make matters worse. It is preferable to deploy a short 6–9 mm stent (such as Micro or NIR stents, or half a Palmaz-Schatz Stent) ensuring that it overlaps the end of the first stent (see Angiogram 19.1, page 207). A second stent will not increase the risk of stent thrombosis, but *leaving a significant lesion at either end of the stent certainly will do so!* This risk of vessel dissection can be reduced by:

a) *Use of non compliant balloon*
   The protruding segment of balloon will not expand to any extent, even with high pressure inflations. Not many truly non compliant balloons are available. A Non Compliant Viva (SciMed) is an example. Most balloons used to deliver stents are at least relatively non compliant.

b) *Short Withdrawal of the Balloon*
   After a first inflation of 8–10 atmospheres, the balloon is withdrawn a very short distance proximally and reinflated to the higher pressures. The aim is to keep the balloon from protruding beyond the distal end of the stent.

c) *Short Balloon*
   A Palmaz-Schatz stent is deployed using 10–12 atmospheres. A second balloon which is short (9 mm) and relatively non-compliant, e.g. a Chubby (Schneider) or a Non Compliant Viva (SciMed), is passed to the stent. It is inflated at high pressures, up to 18–20 atmospheres, trying to keep the balloon within the stent. However to judge this is difficult with poorly radiopaque stents. To ensure each end of the stent is fully expanded it is necessary to have the balloon across the end and just out into the vessel beyond. Using another balloon for high pressure inflations increases the cost and the time of a stent procedure.

d) *Use of a Balloon with Differential Expansion*
   The CAT balloon (see page 23), has a central section which can expand with non compliant sections at each end. If a stent is mounted on such a balloon, as the stent is deployed at high pressures, the end sections of the balloon which extend out of the stent will not enlarge further, thus protecting the vessel. This balloon is useful for hand mounted stents.

e) *Avoiding High Pressures*
   Not all stents require high pressure to give full expansion, e.g. for the Micro stent and most 'second generation' tubular mesh stents such as the Multilink, Crown, NIR and Jo-stent, 8–10 atmospheres is recommended and seems to be sufficient (see page 110). Vein grafts do not always need high pressure injections. It may be better to go back with a larger balloon and to inflate at 8–12 atmospheres, than to persist with high pressure inflations with a balloon which is less than the vessel size at the lesion site.

(5) Inadequate Stent Expansion

Though angiographically the stent may seem satisfactory, IVUS may still show that the lumen size is still too small and or that a portion of the stent has not been fully expanded out to the vessel wall. Either of these problems may predispose to stent thrombosis, see also page 127.

To reduce this risk:

a) *Accept Only a 'Perfect' Stent Result*
After balloon angioplasty a lesion may still have a residual stenosis, but as it is much improved this is acceptable. In fact the maxim 'perfection is the enemy of good' implies that it is possible to make a good or adequate result worse by yet further dilatations or procedures. This approach does not hold true with stents. Time must be given to ensure that the stent result is very good; that the vessel should look entirely normal (see Angiograms 17.1. and 20.1, pages 185 and 212).

b) *Use Intravascular Ultrasound (IVUS)*
This is the 'gold standard' and the best method to ensure that the stent expansion and the vessel beyond the ends of the stent, are satisfactory. However IVUS is not always available and increases the cost and the duration of the procedure.

c) *Routine High Pressures*
The Palmaz-Schatz stent has been the most extensively studied and 16–18 atmospheres has been established for this relatively stiff stent. The information on the required pressure for other stents is much less definite. Figures of 8–12 atmospheres are often recommended, but with the caveat, that higher pressures can be used if wanted. IVUS is really the only method to confirm whether a stent is adequately expanded or not.

d) *Try to Achieve a Step-Up and Step-Down Appearance*
To ensure full dilatation of a Palmaz-Schatz stent, if the stented segment is slightly overdilated compared to the proximal and distal vessel segments, then the stent is very likely to be fully expanded. However to achieve this appearance runs the risk of vessel dissection at either end of the stent.

(6) Persistence of the Lesion after Stent Deployment

This is very annoying, for instead of seeing a wide open channel, there still is a clear indentation and lesion. The problem is rare with tubular mesh stents (see page 105).
This may occur due to:

a) *Prolapse of the Vessel Wall Between Stent Struts*
This may particularly occur with a coil stent. It may also be seen at the articulation site of the Palmaz-Schatz stent. Angiographically a significant lesion at articulation site is rare, but on IVUS a narrowing can be seen routinely.

b) *Vessel Wall Recoil*
If the stent has inadequate radial strength, a very elastic lesion may recoil despite the stent. It can also occur with a stenosis on a bend or a step-like kink in the vessel, especially the circumflex artery. For such a lesion it is best to avoid a coil stent.

c) *Thrombus*
Thrombus may appear within or near the stent. Thrombus is more likely to develop after bail out stenting, or in the setting of unstable angina or acute MI, see page 198.

If a clear stenosis persists in the stented segment, redilatation at higher pressure may be tried but is often ineffective. It is better to place a second stent within the first stent. Consider using a stronger stent, such as Palmaz-Schatz PS153, NIR, or Crown stent, if a coil stent was used originally. The risk of stent thrombosis with these double stents does not seem to be increased.

If thrombus is suspected redilatation may clear it, but it is likely to reappear. Abciximab (ReoPro) may be effective (see page 162).

If the stent was deployed for a lesion on a bend or step like segment of the vessel, the uneven contour may persist after stenting, as this represents the natural course of the vessel.

(7) Uncoiling of the Stent

This can occur with coiled wire stents such as the Wiktor stent (see Angiogram 12.2, page 136) and the first version of the Gianturco-Rubin stent. If there is a problem reaching or crossing a stenosis, or rarely even after routine stent deployment, the balloon may not easily be withdrawn. When this is attempted by forceful pulling, the Wiktor stent which is radiopaque, uncoils *"before your very eyes like a piece of spaghetti"*! The stent may be stuck distally in the coronary artery and methods to retrieve may be to no avail. The patient will probably need to go to surgery, where even opening the vessel a surgeon may not be able to extract the offending stent. If the problem has occurred with stent near the start of the artery, the uncoiled stent may lie half in and half out of the artery. With the original or another shorter balloon such as a Chubby, attempt to pull the stent out of the coronary artery. Once out of the artery, withdraw the guide catheter to give extra support as the stent is retracted along the guide wire down to the femoral artery. The stent is then retrievable (see page 135).

'Stent Jail'

If a stent is positioned across a side branch, it may not be possible to pass a balloon across the struts into the side branch. The side branch is then 'jailed' and if it has a lesion or develops one later, it may be difficult to perform an angioplasty. 'Stent jail' is less of a problem with coiled stents such as the Gianturco-Rubin, Wiktor and the Cordis stent which have a wider gap between the stent wire struts. Even with the tubular mesh stents it is possible, albeit with difficulty to pass a guide wire through the struts followed by progressively larger balloons. It is virtually impossible to cross the close weave of the Wallstent with a guide wire. 'Stent jail' is mainly a problem with the LAD and a large diagonal branch, especially when treating a bifurcation lesion.

Stent Restenosis

Though elective stenting reduces restenosis to about 10%, it still occurs after the use of stents (see Angiogram 24.2, page 257). The *three main risk factors* are:

1. Diabetes mellitus
2. After multiple stents, for long diffuse disease or treatment of dissection.
3. Final lumen of stent less than 3 mm, i.e. stenting small arteries especially 2.5 mm or less.

These three risk factors are cumulative i.e. the more the patient has the greater is the risk.

Complications with Stents

As stent thrombosis has become rare, *instent restenosis* is now one of the most important problems with the use of stents.

If a long stent has been used, there may be stent '*surgical jail*', i.e. it may be difficult or impossible to graft the stented vessel. It is very difficult to pass a needle into a stent segment of artery to apply a graft at that site. The distal artery may be too small to graft. This problem is more a theoretical than a practical one and it is rare for a stented vessel not be graftable.

For stent restenosis an IVUS study is strongly recommended. This may show that the stent was not fully expanded or deployed. The stent needs to be redilated with a size of balloon guided by the IVUS, usually larger than that used at the original stent deployment.

If the restenosis is due to intimal hyperplasia, this may be treated by:

1. *Redilation*
   Though acute result may be successful angiographically, further restenosis is very likely (perhaps as much as 50%) as the hyperplastic intima is constrained within the metal stent and has 'nowhere to go'. Routinely use a balloon size one (half mm) size up from the balloon that was used for the original stent procedure and consider high pressures. The risk of dissection is small provided that the balloon is kept within the stent (see Angiogram 24.2, page 257).
2. *Deployment of a second stent within the first stent*
   This again has a high further restenosis rate as there is little space for the intimal overgrowth to disperse outside the second stent.
3. *Debulking procedure*
   Using a Rotablator or atherectomy the intima may be removed or debulked. Both these techniques have a record of inducing moderate intimal hyperplasia.

The intimal hyperplasia response induced by a stent is greater than that after balloon angioplasty. Hence, whatever the method used to treat stent restenosis, unless the final lumen achieved is large (2–2.5 mm or more) a moderate risk of restenosis will persist.

Heparin and a variety of other stent coatings are being studied to determine if they can reduce intimal hyperplasia and prevent or lower further restenosis after the use of a stent. Irradiation either using a guide wire, or from a stent coating, greatly reduces intimal hyperplasia, but the long term safety will need to be confirmed.

Other Uncommon Stent Problems

False aneurysm and *vessel rupture* are both probably related to the use of high pressures to deploy a stent. False aneurysm can occur with balloon angioplasty. It is usually benign and may sometimes only be detected on a routine 'follow-up angiogram'. Often an aneurysm will disappear without any specific treatment. Occasionally, it may progressively enlarge and can be closed by placement of another stent across the mouth of the aneurysm. One novel way is to sew a segment of a vein harvested from the arm to enclose a stent and to deliver this to the aneurysm site.

Vessel rupture is virtually unknown with balloon angioplasty. Vessel perforation can occur with atherectomy or laser angioplasty. Vessel rupture is potentially serious as it can lead rapidly to cardiac tamponade. For treatment, pass the original balloon used to deploy the stent back to the site of the leak or just proximal to it. Whilst the balloon is left inflated, get ready a further stent and then promptly remove the balloon and pass the new stent to the site. If this approach is not successful, emergency surgery may be needed.

A stent is a 'foreign body' and is at risk for *infection*. A case has been reported where a stent became infected and surgery was required to remove it. The patient died. When a stent is being implanted extra attention should be given to ensure a sterile technique. Try to avoid 'contaminating' the stent with old blood, contrast, or small fibres of gauze. Even if these do not cause infection, they may predispose to thrombosis or restenosis.

Conclusion

Every new solution to a problem produces its own new problem(s). Stents are no exception to this rule. Some of the problems relate to the learning curve of stents, which are more difficult to use than angioplasty balloons. Other problems such as intimal hyperplasia are intrinsic to the stent itself and await further solutions.

References

For a helpful review of problems with stenting, including stent retrieval, see Brecker JD and Rothman MT 'Implant Complications and Management'. Chapter 42, pp. 296–305. Endoluminal Stenting. Edited by U. Sigwart. W.B. Saunders Company Ltd., 1996.

Gunther, H.U., Strupp, G., Volmar, J., *et al*. Coronary stent implantation: Infection and myocardial abscess with lethal outcome. *Zeitschrift für Kardiologie* **82**, 521–525 (1993).

13 Routine Stent Case

Stents are mainly used electively, or semi-electively and it is better to first learn how to use stents in these situations. Avoid the setting of emergency bail out, with "S-T segments nearly hitting the ceiling", to first use a stent or a new form of stent for the initial time.

Stent patients have come to be managed in a simple manner, which is now very similar to that of routine balloon angioplasty.

A stent procedure for the routine (or elective) case may involve the following stages.

(1) Review of Previous Angiogram

  a) *Vessel suitable for a stent*

  - 3 mm or greater in calibre, judged by comparing vessel calibre with that of diagnostic angiogram catheter (see Angiogram 17.1, page 185). A smaller calibre vessel of 2.5–3.0 mm diameter can still be considered, but long term results may be less satisfactory.
  - straight, i.e. not very tortuous proximal vessel.
  - origin of circumflex from left main stem at obtuse angle (see page 81).
  - check for proximal disease.

  b) *Lesion*

  - easily visible and not obscured by overlying vessels, in at least one plane.
  - complex lesion, e.g. on a bend, where PTCA is at increase risk to cause dissection.
  - a 'straight forward' lesion to reduce restenosis.
  - look carefully at the *length* of the lesion, as a *longer* section of vessel may need to be stented, than merely the obvious lesion. Often at one or both ends of a lesion, the vessel is mildly narrowed with disease before normal vessel is reached. The end of the stent should be in normal vessel and beyond even a mildly diseased or narrowed artery.

148   Guide to Coronary Angioplasty and Stenting

If vessel and lesion are appropriate consider either the elective use of a stent, or the semi-elective use, i.e. if result of PTCA is unfavourable.

(2) Discussion with Patient and Relative

Explain that the planned or possible use of a stent(s), may reduce the risks of emergency CABG and restenosis. Explain the risk of stent thrombosis over the first month and describe the post stent medical regime, with the importance of aspirin (and ticlopidine) (see also page 69).

(3) Admission for Procedure

Review angiogram, clinical status and rediscuss with patient and relatives the procedure and risks.

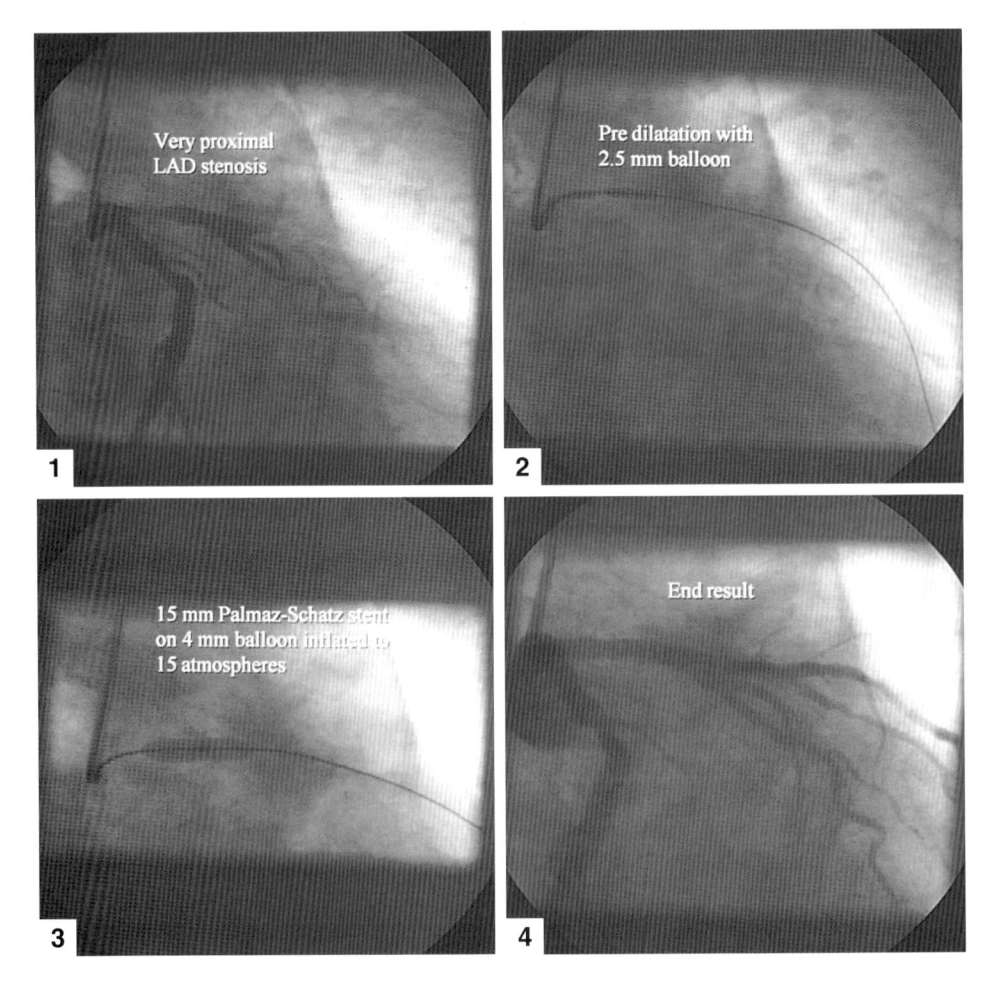

Angiogram 13.1. *Elective stent deployment for very proximal LAD lesion.* The very proximal LAD lesion (1) is at an increased risk for restenosis. The large calibre of the LAD makes the vessel very suitable for stenting. The lesion was predilated with a 2.5 mm balloon (2). A Palmaz-Schatz 153 stent was deployed (3), with a very satisfactory result (4).

(4) Control Angiograms

Confirm that aspirin has been taken that day by asking the patient. Measure the calibre of the vessel by QCA (quantitative coronary angiography). Consider IVUS pre-procedure. Heparin 10,000 units after control angiograms.

(5) Predilatation of the Lesion

A 2.5 mm balloon inflated to 6–7 atmospheres will enlarge the lumen size sufficiently to allow passage of a stent (see Angiogram 13.1, page 148).

Or use the balloon of the 'correct' vessel calibre, e.g. 3.0 or 3.5 mm, which will later carry the hand crimped stent to the lesion. In this case inflate the balloon to low pressures of 3–4 atmospheres, sufficient to remove the lesion dumb-bell.

Try not to cause dissection (does one ever set out to do this ?!).

Before stent insertion check ACT and if less than 300 seconds give further IV dose of 2,000 to 5,0000 units of heparin.

(6) Prepare the Stent

Remember that the stent is a permanent implant. Take care to avoid introducing infection. Try to avoid dried blood from gloves and threads from gauze, collecting on the stent. 'Wash' hands/gloves in a bowl of saline, or change to a new pair of gloves.

Prepare (or "prep") the balloon in the usual way with diluted contrast (see page 91), but use zero or atmospheric pressure rather than negative pressure to provide a more secure platform for the stent.

For a stent supplied premounted on a balloon, there is usually a protective covering tube which is carefully removed. Next, test the stent between thumb and index finger, to ensure that it is securely positioned on the balloon and does not move.

If the Wallstent is being used, follow the instructions described on pages 114–9.

(7) Hand Crimping a Stent onto a Balloon (Figures 13.1–13.7)

If the stent is supplied 'free' or bare, it requires mounting onto a balloon. Any angioplasty balloon can be used for this purpose. Either the balloon previously employed to predilate the lesion, or a new one of appropriate size for the vessel are suitable. If a new balloon is used, it is first inflated to nominal pressure, which slightly reduces its deflated profile. The lubricant coating (see page 15), is wiped off with an alcohol based sterile swab. The balloon is then deflated and left at zero or atmospheric pressure.

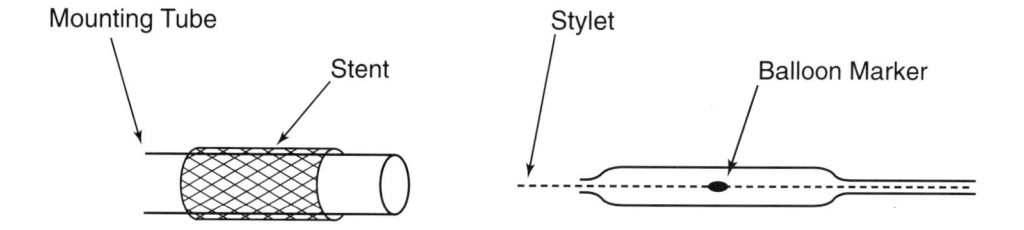

Figure 13.1. Stent on mounting tube. Balloon catheter with stylet emerging from tip.

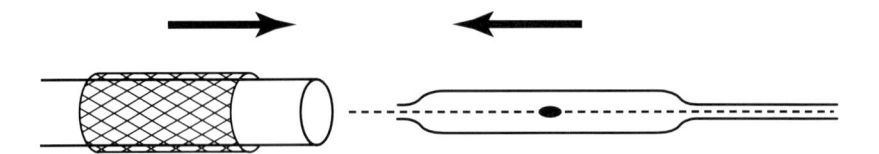

Figure 13.2. Advance stent to balloon.

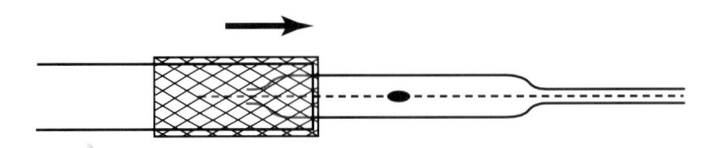

Figure 13.3. Slip mounting tube over balloon.

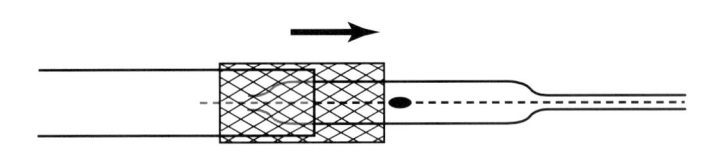

Figure 13.4. Slide stent off mounting tube onto balloon and position in centre of balloon.

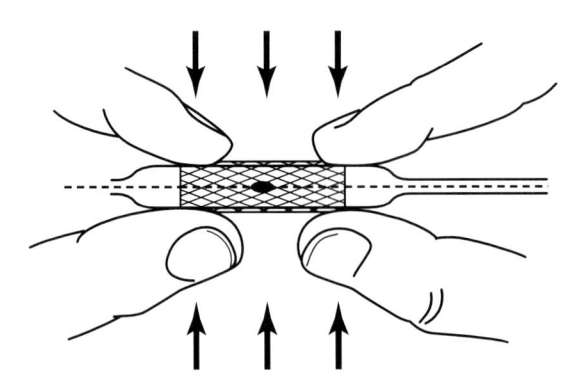

Figure 13.5. Manually finger crimp stent onto balloon.

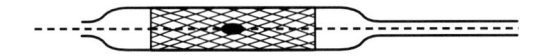

Figure 13.6. Check position of stent, and that it is securely crimped.

Routine Stent Case 151

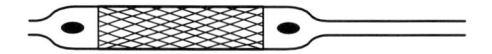

Figure 13.7. Stent mounted onto balloon with end markers.

Many balloons and stents are supplied with a short *stylet or core wire*, which is inserted into the balloon to give it rigidity whilst mounting the stent. Alternatively, the proximal end of the guide wire in the patient can be used, but there is a risk that the position of the guide wire tip may become dislodged.

Most stents are supplied on a short cylinder or *mounting or delivery tube*. There may be a cover to the stent which is removed. With the stylet protruding from the balloon, the mounting tube is slipped over the stylet onto the distal end of the balloon. If feasible, it is preferable to pass the mounting tube over the whole length of the balloon and to turn the tube round a few times. This helps to rewrap and smooth the balloon. (This can even be done on negative pressure, which is released to zero at the end).

The stent is then gently slid off the mounting tube onto the balloon. The mounting tube is removed and the stent is adjusted to lie in the centre of the balloon. This is much easier to assess with a balloon which has a marker at each end, e.g. a Viva Primo (SciMed), rather than a central marker (see Figure 13.7). The stent is then pressed between thumb and index finger of each hand trying not to roll the stent on the balloon, or turn the balloon whilst crimping as these may lead to the stent perforating the balloon. The stent is firmly crimped in one position and then the thumb and fingers are moved through 1/4 of a turn around the stent and the process repeated. Rotating the thumb and fingers through 1/4 turns, the stent is crimped until all the struts have a uniform configuration pressed flat against the balloon. Take particular care to adequately crimp each end of the stent. Remove the stylet and then crimp again to further tighten the stent onto the balloon. Some operators crimp a stent directly onto a balloon without using a central stylet.

Inspect the stent to ensure that it is correctly positioned over the centre of the balloon. Gently tug the stent to check that is secure on the balloon and will not move along it in either direction. If the stent feels loose repeat the crimping process or inflate the balloon to $\frac{1}{2}$–1 atmospheres. If the stent can't be made secure *do not use it in the patient*.

The stent (mounted on the balloon) is now ready to use in the patient.

(8) Deploy the Stent

Carefully pass the stent-mounted balloon onto the proximal end of the guide wire, ensuring that the balloon does not flex whilst trying to pass its tip onto the end of the guide wire. Widely open the 'o' ring of the Y-connector and pass the stent mounted balloon into and along the guide catheter to near its tip. Ensure and or improve guide catheter support. Fix the position of the lesion in your mind, or produce a further 'road map' record.

Pass the stent to the lesion. Take care and be in no hurry, to ensure that the stent is in exactly the correct position. If necessary, use cine or acquisition mode, on the highest field of magnification (see Angiogram 13.1, page 148).

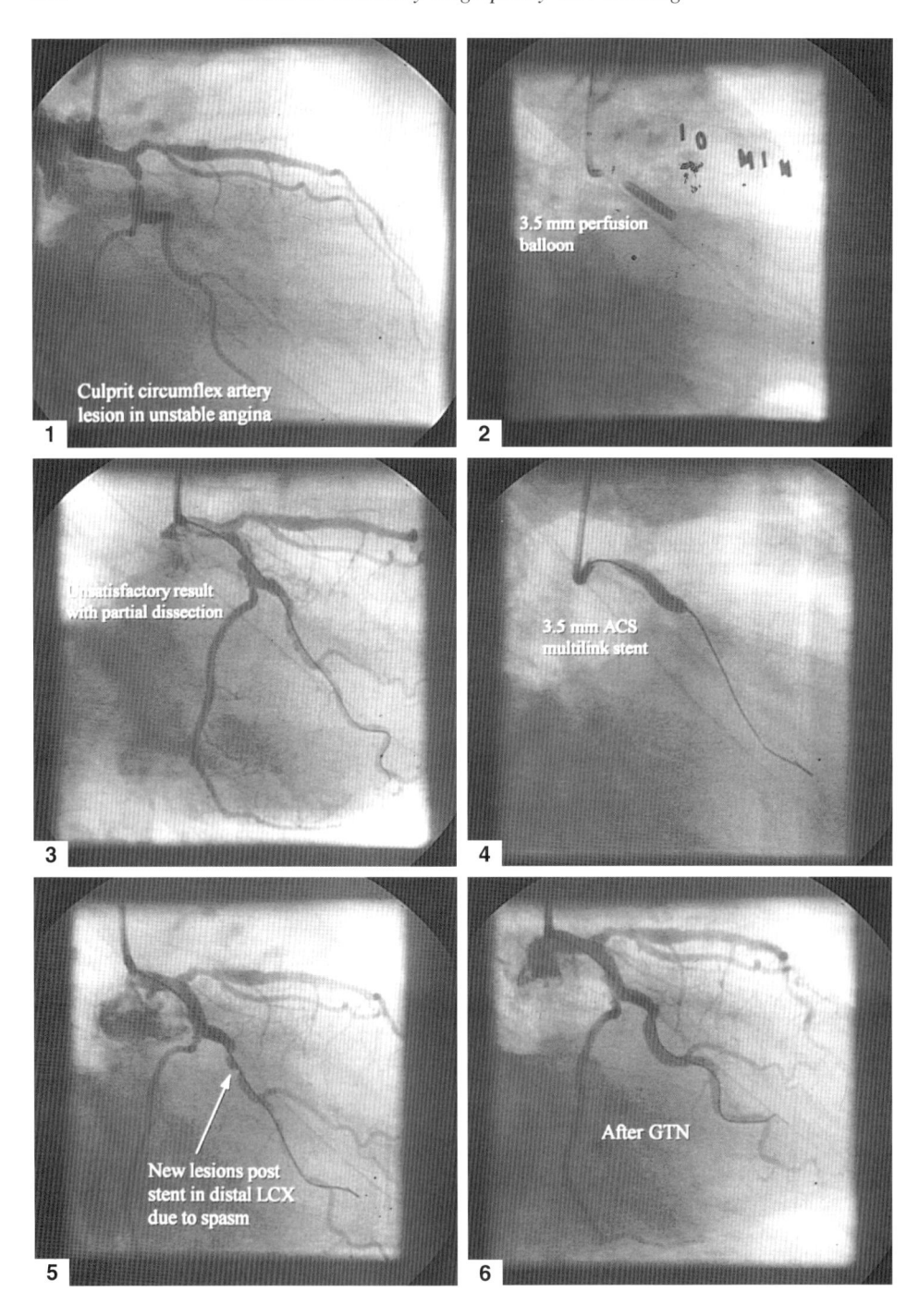

152 Guide to Coronary Angioplasty and Stenting

Angiogram 13.2. *Stent deployment for unsatisfactory result after balloon angioplasty.* There is a severe proximal LCX lesion (1) which is dilated for 10 minutes with a perfusion balloon (2). The result is not satisfactory (3). A 3.5 mm × 15 mm ACS Multilink stent is inserted (4). The lesion is relieved, but a new narrowing has appeared well distal to the end of the stent (5), which is relieved after GTN is given (6). A Judkins JL4 guide catheter was used, but an Amplatz catheter would have given more back-up.

Inflate the balloon to the desired or recommended pressure; 8–12 atmospheres for most stents, but 12–18 atmospheres for the Palmaz-Schatz 153 stent (see Angiograms 13.1 and 13.2 and 17.1 on pages 148, 152 and 185). Hold inflation for 15–60 seconds. Deflate the balloon, allowing sufficient time (perhaps even up to one minute) to allow full deflation under negative pressure. If 8–10 atmospheres is considered adequate to deploy the stent, the balloon is removed. If routinely higher pressures are used withdraw the balloon a short distance, so that its distal end is within the stent and inflate to 12–18 atmospheres.

Advance balloon slightly, to free it from the stent and then withdraw the balloon. Some balloons on which a stent is premounted by the manufacturer, rewrap poorly on deflation. With these there may be resistance to withdrawal of the balloon out of the stent, or along the proximal vessel, or into the guide catheter. *Carefully watch the tip of the guide catheter* to ensure that it is not sucked into the coronary artery whilst trying to withdraw a reluctant balloon. There is a risk that the guide catheter may 'dive in' and damage the proximal end of the stent if it is in the proximal part of the vessel.

Withdraw balloon some distance from the mouth of the guide catheter, perhaps even down to the groin. This allows for optimal contrast injection and vessel visualization.

(9) Repeat Angios

In the primary and backup views (see page 43).

Review angios carefully to ensure that the angiographic result is good, i.e. *near perfect* and considerably better than routinely accepted for a post angioplasty result.

Ideally there should be no residual stenosis; instead aim for a slight "step up and step down" to the stented segment of vessel.

There should be no filling defects in or at either end of the stent. With the Palmaz-Schatz PS153 stent, slight haziness in the centre of the stent may be due to the articulation site and can be acceptable.

(10) Perform IVUS

To confirm that the stent result is satisfactory, i.e. stent struts well expanded out to the vessel wall with a good sized lumen. IVUS is desirable, but not mandatory (see Chapter 5).

(11) Secure Sheath

Review the patient's charts and consider starting ticlopidine if not already being taken. The patient then returns to ward.

(12) Remove Sheath

Remove guide catheter and secure sheath. Some operators will use a closure device e.g. Perclose (page 97). Usually the same day about 4–8 hours later and when PTTK ratio is less than 1.5:1 or the ACT reading is 150 seconds or less. Consider use of Femstop or similar device to assist achieving haemostasis (see page 97).

(13) Next Day

The patient should be able to go home.

Review drug regime; reduce, but not usually stop, all anti-anginal drugs. Prescribe *aspirin* 150–300 mgs per day, with *ticlopidine* 250 mgs twice daily for 2–4 weeks. After 4 weeks stop ticlopidine. It is desirable to give to give a month's supply of tablets, so that the treatment stops when the tablets run out. If on ticlopidine for 4 weeks, arrange for a full blood count to be checked at the end of the second week to ensure that leukopenia has not developed. Inform the patient that a sore throat or fever may be due to leukopenia and to seek medical advice promptly and for a blood count to be checked if there is any doubt.

Give instructions (and preferably written material) of action that patient is to take if chest pain develops which might represent stent thrombosis. Give hospital telephone number and name of doctor and department to contact.

Give an outpatient appointment for 4–8 weeks ... and wish the patient adieu!

Conclusion

In many cardiac units 50–70% of PTCA procedures involve the use of a stent. Hence the routine stent case has virtually become the routine PTCA case. As a result of their use, dissection leading to acute occlusion is now a rare event. Careful assessment of vessel calibre, accurate positioning of a stent and ensuring an excellent 'stent-like' result after deployment without inflow or outflow lesions are all important steps in the stenting procedure. Extra support wires can be helpful for tortuous vessels and IVUS studies, though not essential, can ensure that stent deployment is optimal.

14 Abrupt Closure – 1
(Risks and Causes)

Incidence

Abrupt closure is the feared complication of PTCA and is the cause of death, emergency CABG and myocardial infarction with this procedure. In about 5% of PTCA procedures the result is clearly unsatisfactory with evidence of dissection and or reduced flow. With redilatation about half of these cases can be significantly improved, but there remains a need for emergency CABG in about 2–3% of cases. Since the advent of stents, the role for emergency CABG has fallen to 1–2%, but has not been removed. This complication requires the facility for emergency cardiac surgery preferably on site, or if off site with well prepared and functioning arrangements for speedy transfer of the patient to a surgical centre and operation.

Timing of Acute Closure

With PTCA acute closure or major flow reduction occurs:

a) during the procedure in about 60% of cases,
b) as the patient is leaving the catheter lab and over the next 4–6 hours in about 30% of cases,
c) over the next 24 hours in 10% of cases.

It is very rare after 24 hours and extremely rare after 48 hours following PTCA. This contrasts with stent abrupt closure which is rare during the first 24 hours, rises in frequency on the 2nd and 3rd days and continues out to about 21 days.

Predisposing Factors (See also page 84)

These include:
1) *Lesion morphology.*
   a) complex ulcerated lesions
   b) lesions on a bend

c) lesions with thrombus
   d) long lesions (>2cm)
2) *Smaller calibre vessel.*
   a) less than 2.5 mm in size
   b) hence women have slightly higher risk than men, as their vessels tend to be smaller
3) *Unstable angina and acute M.I.*
   The lesions are often more complex and more often have thrombus present than with stable angina.
4) *Acute M.I.* — where besides proximal vessel damage, embolization to the distal artery or even to another artery (e.g. LAD to LCX) may occur.
5) *Inadequate Antiplatelet or Anticoagulant Treatment.*
   The risk is increased if the patient is not taking aspirin and if the heparin dosage is inadequate, or if there is heparin resistance.

Reduced Risk of Vessel Closure

The risks are lower but not absent:

1) Restenosis cases.
2) Restenosis within a stent.
3) Elective use of stent — for a dissection may occur at the proximal or distal end.
4) Chronic total occlusion — as damage to the proximal vessel may occur.

Results of Vessel Occlusion

The result of vessel occlusion is much more unpredictable than might be expected. Sometimes, with occlusion of the LAD, initially not much happens; there is not much pain, ECG changes or haemodynamic alterations. It may only be the next day that the ECG shows a myocardial infarction. On the other hand a relatively non dominant RCA may sometimes lead to much distress and haemodynamic deterioration. It is for this reason that it is very difficult to predict or pick a " low risk" single vessel disease PTCA case.
   However, there are *higher risk* cases which include:-

1) Last remaining coronary artery — occlusion at the lesion will clearly be very serious.
2) Poor LV function.
3) Post CABG — prompt surgical exposure of the heart is not possible. Revascularization by surgery is relatively slow and a decision may electively be taken not to send the patient to surgery.
4) Poor general medical status — i.e. the elderly, those with poor renal function, chronic airway disease and possibly diabetics, where the risks associated with emergency surgery will be greater.

Discussion with Patients and Relatives

Occlusion of the artery is the principal acute complication of PTCA and its risks and sequelae, of death, M.I., emergency CABG need to be discussed with the patient and relatives. Care needs to be taken especially with ad hoc PTCA procedures in unstable angina, where relatives may not be available and do not know that an operative as opposed to a diagnostic procedure is to be performed. If the relatives are not available to be seen with the patient, consider speaking to them on the telephone.

Discussion with Surgeons

In most cardiac surgical units, PTCA and cardiac surgery proceed daily during routine hours and hopefully *the two don't meet*! Only higher risk cases are discussed and their timing planned to coincide with availability of surgeon and theatre. If a case does go to surgery, before another PTCA patient is brought to the catheter lab(s), the availability of further emergency cover needs to be discussed with the surgical colleagues. Usually an angioplasty emergency causes the cancellation of an elective surgical case and surgeons are naturally sensitive over this matter!

Outside routine hours and even cases to be started later in the day, prior discussion with a surgeon is wise. They and their staff are not enthusiastic to hear at 5 pm, that 'another failed PTCA case' is coming down from the catheter lab. Be considerate to your surgical colleagues and if there is slightest doubt, discuss with them first before rushing into PTCA. This approach is what is meant by 'teamwork' and remember to *promptly* return the compliment when a surgeon asks you to assess a post operative problem in ITU or on the wards.

Causes of Abrupt Closure

These include:

a) Dissection   80–90% of cases (see Angiogram 14.1, page 158)
b) Thrombosis   5–10% of cases
c) Spasm   1–5% of cases
d) Embolism   1–2% of cases.

Thrombosis

Thrombosis is more common with:-

1. *Pre-existing thrombus*
   As occurs in unstable angina or acute myocardial infarction.
2. *Coronary artery stents*
3. *Omission of Aspirin or inadequate Heparin dosage*
   Check with patient at start of procedure that he or she has taken their aspirin that morning.
4. *Heparin resistance*
   This is detected by greater than usual doses of heparin being needed to prolong ACT to therapeutic range of >250 seconds (> 300 seconds for stent placement).

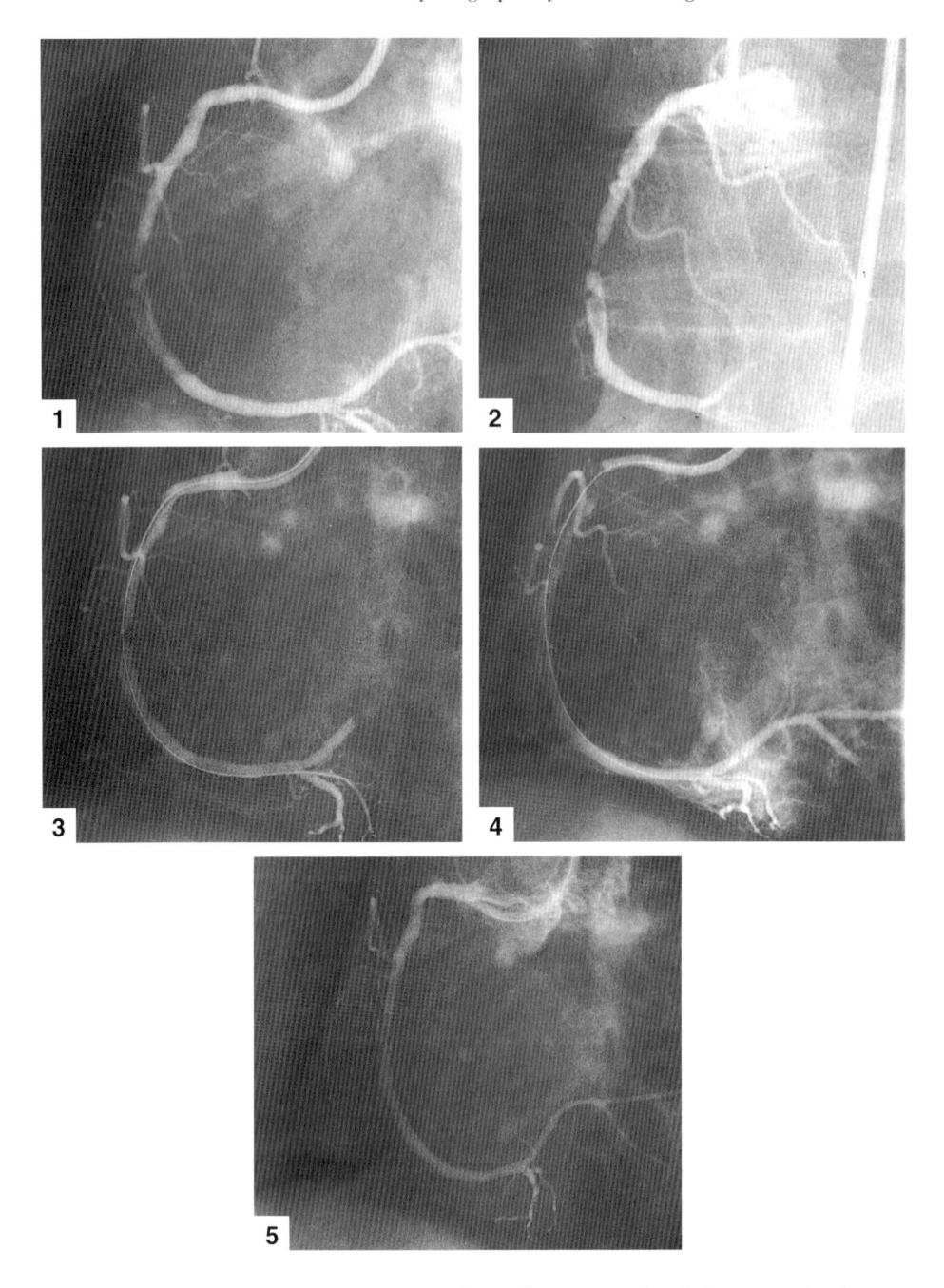

Angiogram 14.1. *Angioplasty of RCA with moderate dissection and embolization to distal artery.* There is a complex stenosis in the mid RCA, and beyond it there is an irregular filling defect suggesting thrombus (1 and 2). After the initial balloon dilatation thrombus has embolised to the atrio-ventricular branch (3). It later moves on (4). The final result shows dissection at the lesion site with a linear streak of contrast outside the main channel (5). The distal artery (A-V branch) is of smaller calibre query due to spasm. The patient later had an uneventful course. This PTCA was performed before the availability of stents. The residual lesion would not now be left, but instead would be stented.

Thrombocytopenia may occur too. Proximal progression of an occlusion up the coronary vessel can be a feature. Sometimes it may develop if a patient has been on IV heparin for treatment of unstable angina.

5. *Haematological Conditions*
   Despite concerns, conditions with a high haemoglobin level and or platelet count such as polycythaemia rubra vera, do not seem to be at increased risk of thrombosis during angioplasty.

Detection of Thrombus

Differentiation from dissection can be difficult and often dissection leads to thrombus formation and extension of an occlusion. Features to diagnose thrombus as the principal problem include:-

1. Irregular filling defect(s) (as in Angiogram 14.2, page 160).
2. Occlusion with a convex upper or proximal end.
3. Progressive proximal progression of an occlusion.
4. Absence of dissection plane(s) outside and parallel to vessel lumen.

The first feature is unreliable and features 2 and 3 are late or advanced features.

Angioscopy is the best current method to detect and assess thrombus. With an acute occlusion during PTCA, the clinical state of the patient may not be stable enough to allow angioscopy studies. IVUS is relatively poor at differentiating soft plaque from thrombus.

Prevention of Thrombosis

1) *Aspirin and Heparin.*
   These are well established to prevent thrombus forming during PTCA.
2) *Glycoprotein IIb-IIIa antagonist (ReoPro).*
   In unstable angina, especially if control angiograms show a complex lesion and perhaps one with identifiable thrombus, giving the IIb/IIIa antagonist, ReoPro (Abciximab), intravenously at the time or just before PTCA reduces the risk of vessel occlusion at PTCA. The need and value of this treatment has to be balanced against the cost (about that of a stent). It does not need to be used routinely for all cases of unstable angina and even in higher risk cases its role needs to be established (see page 162).
3) *Temporary cessation of IV Heparin infusion.*
   Anecdotal evidence suggests that heparin resistance is more frequent after prolonged infusion of the drug. Hence some operators stop the heparin infusion for 2–12 hours before a PTCA procedure.

Treatment of Thrombosis leading to Abrupt or Threatened Vessel Closure

Once the condition is suspected and or diagnosed:

1. *Check Aspirin and Heparin*
   Ensure that these were given. Check the ACT measurement.

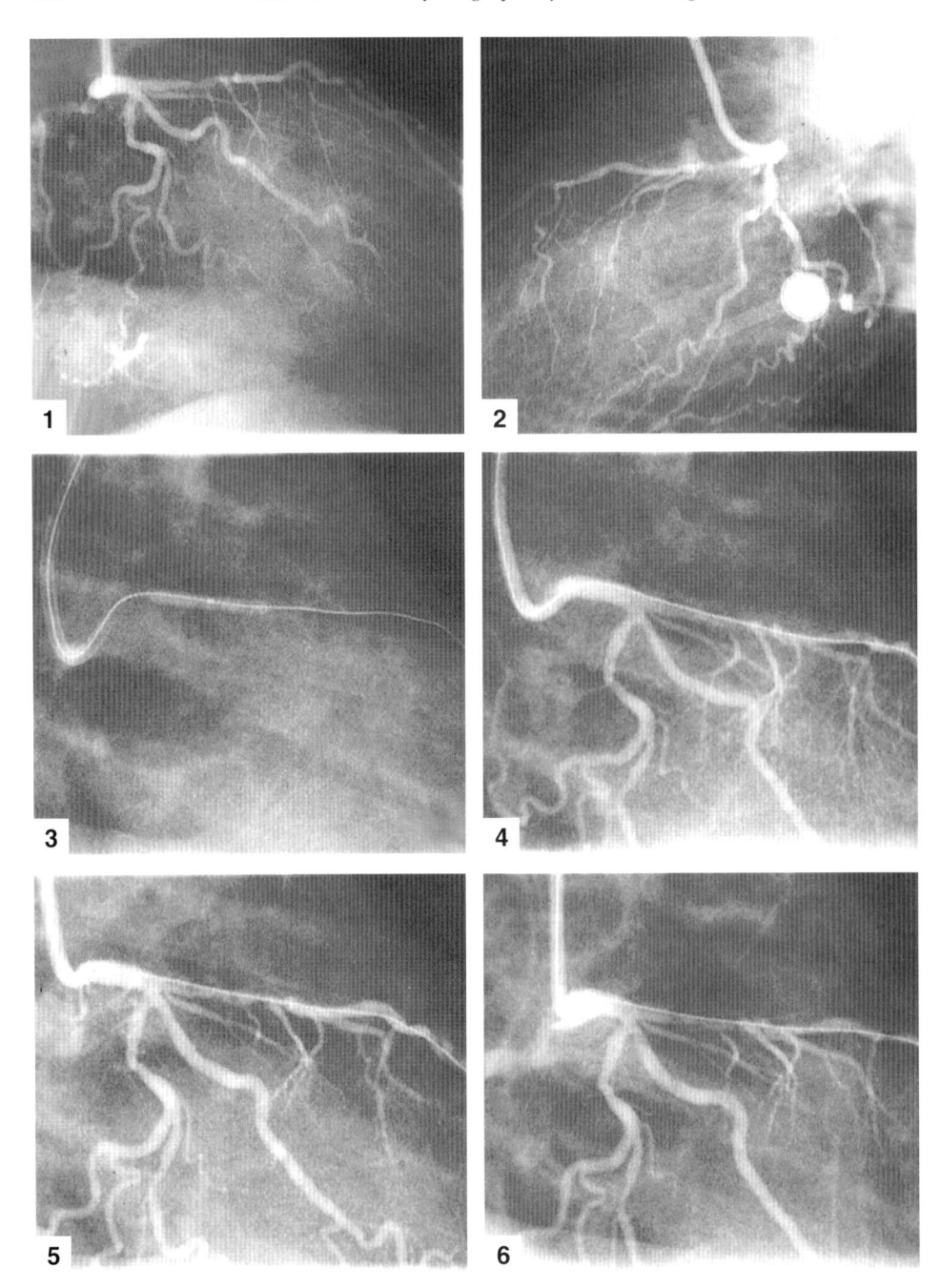

Angiogram 14.2. *Proximal LAD dissection plus thrombus.* The LAD is of small calibre and has a severe stenosis 1.5 cm. after its origin (1 and 2). After PTCA with 2 mm balloon (3) the initial result is satisfactory (4).

The appearance later deteriorates with filling defects suggestive of thrombus at the start of the lesion (5). Despite further dilatations including with 2.5 mm balloon, the flow remained impaired (6). The wire was left across the lesion and the patient referred for emergency CABG. A small anterior M.I. developed.

2. *Glycoprotein IIb-IIIa antagonist (ReoPro)*
   (See below)
3. *Thrombolytic Drugs*
   These drugs have been largely superseded by the Glycoprotein IIb-IIIa antagonist, ReoPro. Thrombolytic drugs are often unreliable and when unsuccessful, there is often doubt whether their lack of success was due failure of the drug, or perhaps that the diagnosis was incorrect and that the problem was dissection rather than thrombosis.

   TPA (Tissue Plasminogen Activator) is the thrombolytic drug mainly used. The dose is 20–40 mgm TPA into the coronary artery followed by a further 20–50 mgs over 3–6 hours IV or slowly down the coronary vessel via an infusion catheter. TPA is probably the best thrombolytic drug, but urokinase (200–500, 000 units intra coronary followed by 20,000 units per hour infusion over 12–24 hours), or streptokinase (100,000 units intra coronary) maybe used as a alternative to TPA.
4. *Heparin IV over 24 hours*
   Having diagnosed and treated intra coronary thrombus it is reasonable to continue with anticoagulant and antiplatelet treatment. For the former this will include IV heparin for 24–48 hours and possibly oral anticoagulants for about one month. For antiplatelet treatment, aspirin and possibly ticlopidine and or glycoprotein IIb-IIIa antagonist may be given. This whole area of post thrombosis treatment is empirical and management regimes vary quite markedly between operators. Intravenous heparin for 24 hours and then continuing with aspirin, is effective in most cases.

Glycoprotein IIb-IIIa Antagonists

IIb-IIIa is a glycoprotein forming a receptor on the surface of the platelet. Each platelet has 50–80,000 such receptors. Fibrinogen, or the Von Willebrand factor, combines with these receptors to achieve platelet aggregation. This mechanism is the *'final common pathway'* involved in platelet aggregation. Hence blocking this receptor will significantly reduce thrombus formation and possibly platelet mediated mechanisms of restenosis..

There are a number of IIb-IIIa antagonists being developed. At present the only preparation readily available for clinical use, is the chimeric fab fragment (c7E3 Fab) of human-murine monoclonal antibody to IIb-IIIa glycoprotein. This chimeric preparation, whereby parts of the rat antibody are replaced by human amino acid sequences, reduces the risk of allergic reactions. The antibody preparation is called *c7E3 or ReoPro or Abciximab.*

Currently ReoPro is only recommended for intravenous use as a bolus and over 12 hours. The duration of treatment is likely to increase and the intracoronary route may also be used.

Oral IIb-IIIa antagonists are being developed and one, xemlofibran (SC 54684), is undergoing clinical trials.

ReoPro (Abciximab) IIb/IIIa Antagonist

As this is a new form of treatment, experience with its use is limited. It is expensive (about the cost of 1–1.5 stents) and is complicated to prepare and administer.

Indications For ReoPro

1. *Electively for a high-risk case.*
   Thrombus within a coronary artery is often present in unstable angina and nearly always present in acute M.I.. These patients and those with more complex coronary artery lesions have a higher risk of acute vessel closure during PTCA, (see page 155). In the two trials EPIC and EPILOG, ReoPro when used electively reduced acute vessel closure and reduced myocardial infarction.
2. *Prevent rethrombosis within a stent.*
   In acute M.I., or after reopening a stent occluded by thrombosis, thrombus may begin to reappear on the stent. This can be very difficult to treat, but responds very well to redilatation (to compress and, or remove the thrombus), followed by ReoPro which inhibits the thrombus reforming.
3. *Established thrombus.*
   ReoPro has poor success at reopening a stent completed occluded by thrombus. Its value to reopen a completely occluded coronary artery, as in acute M.I. is being assessed.

Administration of ReoPro

The drug is given as:
   an initial *bolus* of 0.25 mgm/kgm i.v. as a slow i.v. injection over 5 minutes, followed by an *infusion* of 10 µgm/min i.v. over 12 hours.
   Note that the infusion is not on a weight basis.

Each vial contains 10 mgm of the drug in 5 ml.
Hence for a 70 kgm patient;
   the *initial bolus dose* is 70×0.25 mgm = 17.5 mgm
   $ = 8.75$ ml of ReoPro

This dose = 1 ml of ReoPro per 8 kgm of the patient. Each vial is drawn up via a filter, which takes about 2–5 minutes to accomplish.
The *dose of the i.v. infusion* is 10 µgm/min for 12 hours.

Total amount of ReoPro = $10 \times 60 \times 12$ = 7200 µgm
   $ = 7.2$ mgm
   $ = 3.6$ ml ReoPro

About 3.9 ml of ReoPro is made up with 5% dextrose to fill a 50 ml syringe, and given by an infusion pump at 4 ml per hour for 12 hours. This allows a small amount of leeway and wastage during the preparation of the infusion. With this regimen for patients up to 100 kg, three vials of the drug will be sufficient for the ReoPro treatment. A special filter is needed on the i.v. giving set.

Heparin

Bleeding complications are greatly reduced or avoided altogether if less heparin is used for the PTCA. During the procedure a bolus dose of 50–70 units of heparin per kgm is given to achieve an ACT of 200–250 seconds. There are no follow up doses of heparin, which is not given after the procedure either. If unplanned ReoPro is needed after a PTCA complication, a larger dose of heparin may have already been given. However, if no further heparin is administered, the risks of later bleeding are small.

Sheath Removal

The manufacturers suggest this should be done at about 6 hours after the end of the procedure when the ACT is less than 150 seconds, or PTTK less than 1.5 : 1. However, the ReoPro infusion will still be going through at this time. Alternatively delay sheath removal for 6–12 hours after completion of the ReoPro infusion. When ReoPro has been used for a complication developing during PTCA, re-angiography of the vessel may be considered the next day. For these patients it is not necessary to routinely flush the sheath, but if this is done avoid heparin and only use 5% dextrose. The ACT measurements may be checked from blood taken from the side arm of the sheath. The patient should be encouraged to lie flat, and to move the thigh and hip as little as possible. Removal of the sheath should be by an experienced member of staff, especially if this is done during the ReoPro infusion.

Groin Bleeding and Haematoma

These were a significant problem, but are much less common, as heparin is not used after the procedure and a lower dose is given during the angioplasty (see above). A groin closure device, such as Perclose may be used at the end of the PTCA procedure, and may prevent further bleeding. If oozing and haematoma do develop insert a shortened introducer into the sheath, which may stop the sheath collapsing and reduce bleeding around the side of the sheath. A sandbag over the groin will often supply sufficient local pressure.

Haematological Monitoring

No test is routinely needed but if there is significant bleeding check,

1. *Platelet Count.*
   Despite the platelet count often being reduced by ReoPro, bleeding is uncommon. If the level is less than 60,000 per cubic millimetre, and the patient is bleeding, give 5 units of platelets.
2. *Bleeding Time.*
   This is rarely performed, and management is guided by the platelet count.

Severe Bleeding

If this occurs at the groin or elsewhere, besides local pressure where feasible, also arrange to:

1. Stop the ReoPro infusion.
2. Discuss management with the Haematologist.
3. Give 3-5 units of platelets.
4. Consider giving 1 unit of fresh blood.

Measures to Reduce the Risk of Bleeding with ReoPro

1. Avoid ReoPro for patients with thrombocytopenia. This implies that the platelet count should be checked by the cardiologist before starting *any* angioplasty.
2. Avoid ReoPro in patients after recent surgery, gastrointestinal bleeding or stroke.
3. Avoid its use for patients with a bleeding diasthesis, vasculitis or severe hypertension.
4. Avoid venepuncture, arterial puncture, or i.m. injections during the infusion.

Emergency CABG

If the patient has received ReoPro in the catheter room and needs to go for emergency surgery, stop the infusion and inform the surgeon and anaesthetist that there is an increased risk of bleeding in the post operative period. Five units of platelets should be requested.

Hypersensitivity Reaction

ReoPro is a protein and an anaphylactic reaction may occur.
Intramuscular or subcutaneous adrenaline (0.5–1.0 mgm i.e. 0.5–1.0 ml of aqueous 1:1000 solution), and hydrocortisone 100 mgm i.v. should be available. Hypotension, nausea, vomiting and fever may also occur.

Future of ReoPro

ReoPro is very effective to prevent thrombus reforming on a stent in the hypercoagulable state after acute myocardial infarction, and following reopening of a stent occluded by thrombosis. Whilst it also reduces the risks of PTCA in unstable angina, and with more complex coronary lesions, it is not needed *routinely* for these conditions.

The role, mode and length of administration of ReoPro and other glycoprotein IIb/IIIa antagonists, are under active assessment, and will become clearer in the future.

One aspect currently limiting its use is the cost of ReoPro.

Coronary Artery Spasm

In the early days of PTCA this was considered to be an important cause of vessel occlusion and liberal doses of nitrates were given. This led to hypotension, which can itself predispose to vessel closure. Spasm is a *rare* cause of total occlusion, especially at the lesion site. Spasm more commonly leads to '*new*' lesions proximal or distal to the target lesion. These are more common with stiffer guide wires and after the passage of a stent. They improve and disappear after intra coronary nitrates or removal of guide wire at end of case.

The Rotablator can lead to severe coronary artery spasm, mainly involving the *distal artery*, rather than the treated lesion. Patients should receive intra coronary nitrate and or verapamil prior to its use.

Balloon rupture with high pressure inflation dispatches a bolus of contrast at high pressure down the coronary vessel. There may be vasoconstriction of the distal bed, often with S-T elevation and mild chest pain, which settle after intra coronary nitrates and an interval of 5–15 minutes, (see page 141).

Distal embolism of vein graft atheroma leads to a similar but more severe problem. Pain, S-T elevation and hypotension leading to circulatory collapse can all ensue. Recovery takes longer, often 30 minutes to an hour, or even longer. Treatment involves intra coronary nitrates and circulatory support with IV dopamine, vasoconstrictors such as phenylephrine and sometimes intra aortic balloon pumping, (see page 216).

Vessel Dissection

This important cause of abrupt closure is considered in the next chapter.

Conclusion

Abrupt closure or a serious reduction in coronary flow is now an uncommon event during angioplasty since the elective or early use of stents. The strategy to treat this complication however, still needs to be considered when deciding on the procedure details for an angioplasty. Thrombus formation is usually a secondary event after dissection, whereas spasm usually affects segments of an artery without leading to complete vessel closure. Whilst nitrates easily relieve spasm, clearing thrombus from an artery is a much less certain exercise.

Glycoprotein IIb / IIIa antagonists, such as ReoPro offer a new and exciting approach to the prevention and treatment of thrombosis during angioplasty.

References

The EPIC Investigators: Use of a monoclonal antibody directed against the platelet glycoprotein IIb / IIIa receptor in high risk coronary angioplasty. *N Engl J Med* **330**, 956–61 (1994).

The EPILOG Investigators: Platelet glycoprotein IIb/IIIa receptor blockade and low-dose heparin during percutaneous coronary revascularization. *N Engl J Med* **336**, 1689–1696 (1997).

15 Abrupt Closure – 2 (Vessel Dissection)

This chapter follows on from Chapter 14 and discusses dissection as the cause of vessel closure complicating angioplasty. Dissection may also be accompanied by thrombosis and spasm as secondary events.

Splitting of the Plaque during PTCA

There are various degrees of dissection and the very process of PTCA involves splitting the plaque. Pathological studies show that this is usually at the junction between the plaque and the remainder of the healthy wall, where the vessel is "weakest" to resist balloon dilatation. Varying degrees of splitting of the media and adventitia occur too.

The spectrum of wall damage during PTCA (Figure 15.1) may be divided into:
1. Intraluminal haziness.
2. Minor dissection.
3. Moderate dissection — with or without reduced flow down the vessel.
4. Severe dissection — with or without reduced flow down the vessel.
5. Total vessel closure.

Dissection may pass rapidly from one stage to another and may omit the stage of a severe or long dissection and lead directly to total vessel occlusion.

1. Intraluminal Haziness (see Angiograms 8.1 and 8.2, pages 90 and 94)

After the procedure, in about 50% of PTCA cases the stenosis has been relieved and there is a good lumen with satisfactory flow across the lesion to the distal artery. However at the lesion site there is intraluminal haziness, which some operators call "intimal tearing". This later term is a euphemism, for IVUS studies show that the flow down the coronary vessel is often not along a wide true lumen, but instead to varying degrees along dissection plane(s) between the intima and media. Angiographically the stenosis has been relieved and the flow improved and acutely the patient will usually

1) Prior to PTCA

2) Intraluminal Haziness

3) Mild Dissection
With linear streak of contrast outside vessel lumen

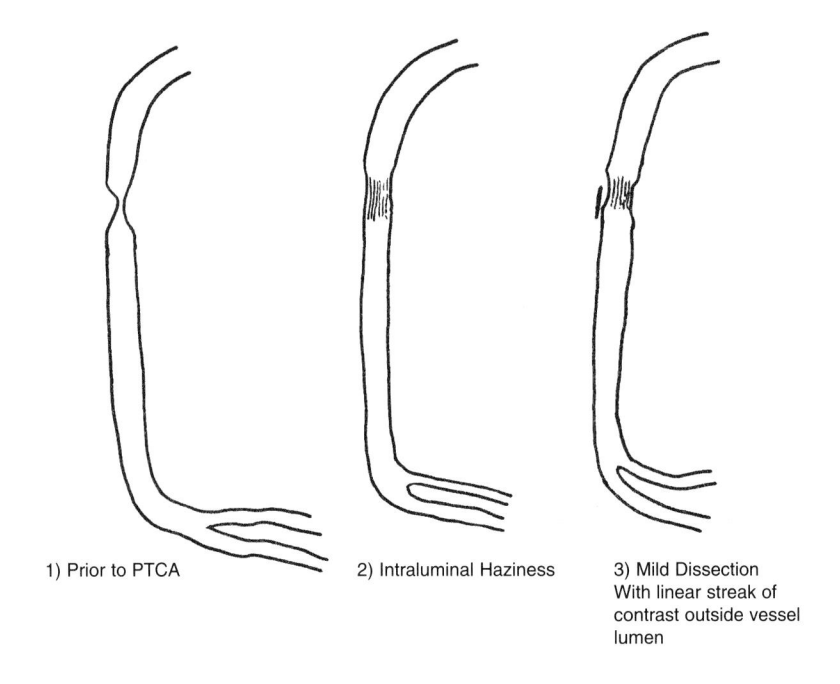

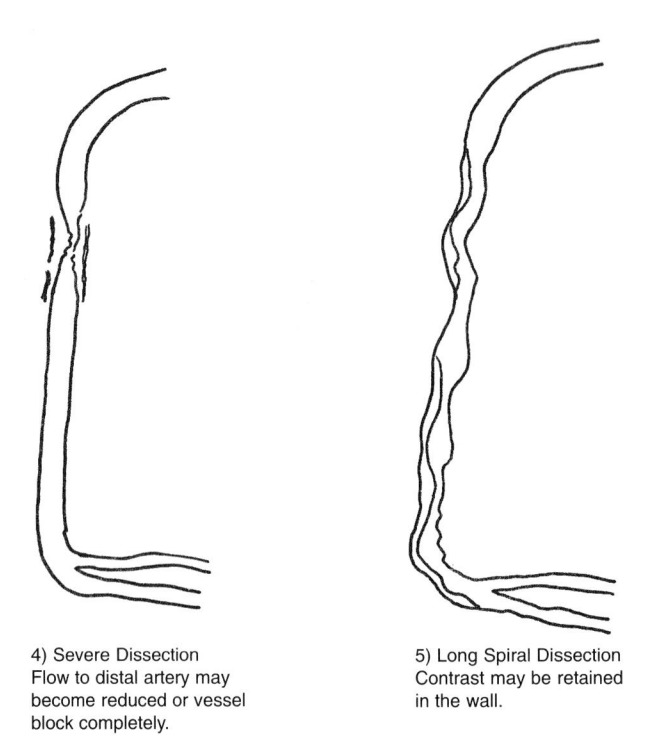

4) Severe Dissection
Flow to distal artery may become reduced or vessel block completely.

5) Long Spiral Dissection
Contrast may be retained in the wall.

Figure 15.1. Degrees of dissection.

progress well. Only time will show if restenosis will develop, perhaps principally because of the residual plaque size and poor true lumen.

2. Minor Dissection

Small fissure(s) are seen as a short narrow linear streak of contrast outside the main vessel lumen and in the wall of the artery. The short line of contrast does not clear, or is slow to do so. It may be seen in one or more radiographic planes. There is good prograde flow of contrast and the stenosis has been well relieved.

3. Moderate Dissection

The splitting is more severe and obvious (see Angiogram 16.1, page 178). The lumen size may be normal, but often will be reduced. The flow down the vessel may still be normal or may clearly be reduced. The dissection may extend for a short distance distally (and proximally) beyond the lesion.

4. Severe Dissection

The flow along the vessel is reduced and within a short time of about 5–10 minutes, may cease altogether (see Angiograms 15.2, and 16.1, on pages 173 and 178). The dissection may be localized to the lesion itself or may propagate down (and up) the artery. The RCA in particular may develop a long dissection with contrast along the vessel wall which clears slowly if at all. A definite double-lumen and spiral dissection may be seen. Sometimes especially with smaller calibre vessels, the severity and length of the dissection is not recognized in one view, but may be more apparent in another radiographic view.

With flow reduction ischaemic pain, ECG changes with arrhythymias and haemodynamic deterioration may develop.

5. Total vessel closure

Blood flow to the distal artery ceases (Angiogram 15.1, page 170) and there is usually chest pain with ECG changes, arrhythymias and haemodynamic changes. Initially, symptoms and changes on the ECG and the blood pressure may be mild or absent. At other times cardiac arrest may occur. Total occlusion requires urgent action to re-establish some flow and then to maintain it by conservative means or by emergency CABG. These procedures are known as 'bail-out' ones to enable the patient to escape from an impending infarction.

Treatment of Dissection

This involves:

A) *Prevention by:*
    1) PTCA strategy – angiogram review.
    2) Prophylactic measures.
    3) Care during PTCA to avoid dissection.
    4) Alternative PTCA techniques.

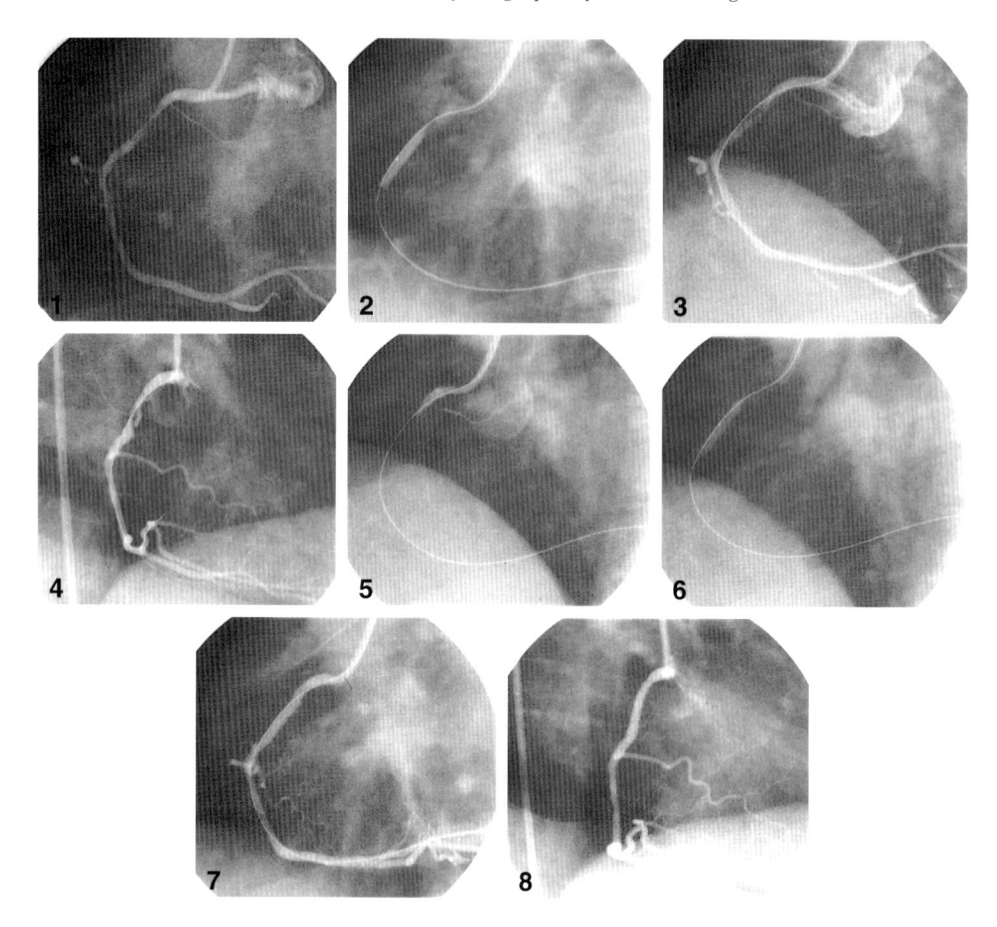

170   *Guide to Coronary Angioplasty and Stenting*

Angiogram 15.1. *Bail out stenting for acute RCA dissection.* The RCA lesion seen in the LAO 30° projection (1) was dilated with a 3 mm balloon (2). The result after PTCA showed a localized dissection, (3) and (4) (RAO 30° projection). Whilst a stent was being prepared, flow ceased altogether — 'bail-out' situation, (5). A 15 mm Palmaz-Schatz PS153 stent was hand crimped onto a 3.5 mm Speedy balloon (Schneider) and deployed at the lesion, (6). Flow was promptly restored, (7), and the end result (8), showed slight over dilatation of the stented region with a step-up to the stent, and a step-down at the distal end of the stent.

B) *Treatment of Established Dissection by:*
   1) Redilatation.
   2) Stenting.
   3) Perfusion balloon.
   4) Atherectomy.
   5) Emergency CABG.
   6) Other measures.

Measures to Prevent or Reduce the Risk of Dissection

1. PTCA Strategy – Angiogram Review

When reviewing the angiogram each lesion and vessel should be assessed as to:

a) Risk of dissection (see pages 84, 155).
b) Suitability to receive a stent.
c) Strategy to use if the vessel dissects.

A lesion may not be at higher risk for occlusion, but in a large calibre vessel consider whether it should be treated by elective stenting.

If the result of treatment by PTCA alone is unsatisfactory, will the lesion and the vessel allow a stent to be used, i.e.

a) vessel at the lesion site of suitable size, 3 mm or more in diameter?
b) proximal vessel, is it straight or tortuous and does it have some disease and narrowing too?
c) which stent and what length might be used?

Is the vessel size and amount of myocardium small, so that if the lesion occludes, will it be better to allow a small infarction, rather than refer the patient for emergency CABG? If this is the decision, it will need to be explained to the patient and relatives. The amount of disease in other vessels will also influence the approach for emergency CABG.

2. Prophylactic Measures

These can include:

a) *Drugs*
   Glycoprotein IIb/IIIa antagonist may be considered in unstable angina, with a complex lesion with thrombus identifiable. The value of this drug to prevent PTCA complications needs further study (see page 162).
b) *Intra Aortic Balloon Pump Stand By*
   If there is poor LV function and/or the vessel to be dilated is the 'last remaining artery', the management of occlusion will involve haemodynamic support. This for most operators will be an intra aortic balloon pump but alternatively percutaneous cardiopulmonary bypass may be used. Rarely, it is necessary to insert the intra aortic balloon at the start of the procedure. However it can be helpful to be "ready and willing to go" by insertion of a small 4 or 5F sheath into the contralateral femoral artery, so that there is prompt arterial access if needed.

3. Care During PTCA to Avoid Dissection

a) *Care with Passage of Guide Wire.*
   Whilst less of a problem with soft flexible tip guide wires, vessel wall damage may occur more easily with stiffer guide wires. *Some dissections first start with the guide wire passing into the wall and lifting a flap* which may not be recognized at that stage. The risks are greater with cul-de-sac lesions, lesions on a bend, very tight lesions and bifurcation lesions. The risks are greater in a recanalised vessel.

The risk of dissection produced by the guide wire is greatest with a chronic occlusion; this will involve the lesion and the vessel beyond it.

Avoid pushing or advancing the guide wire so much, that the tip is seen to buckle. Ensure that after the guide wire crosses the lesion, it can move freely and easily, suggesting that it is in the true lumen. This is especially true after crossing a chronic occlusion.

b) *Care with the Balloon*

Oversizing of the balloon to the vessel size and high pressure inflations, increase the risk of dissection. If in doubt start with a smaller size balloon and progress to a larger one "one can always go *up* with a balloon size, but you can't go *down*, if a dissection occurs!".

If a balloon will not cross a lesion, resist the temptation to inflate the balloon in the mouth of the lesion which can lead to dissection. Instead go down in size or even down to the smallest size balloon and this will almost certainly cross (see page 95).

c) *Care with the Guide Catheter*

The tip of the guide catheter can damage the proximal vessel. Unlike dissection at the site of the lesion, where its occurrence is to some extent "in the lap of the Gods", with catheter induced dissection of the proximal vessel there is no doubt that the *operator* is responsible. Particular care is needed when using an Amplatz catheter within the LCA or RCA (see page 9, and Angiogram 8.2, page 94).

4. Alternative PTCA Techniques

Some measures are claimed to reduce acute dissection and these include.

a) *Prolonged Inflation*

If the balloon can be inflated for 5–7 minutes, a better acute angiographic result may be obtained. A perfusion balloon is usually needed, though sometimes a patient can tolerate this duration of balloon inflation using a routine balloon (see page 93).

b) *Progressive Dilatation*

Some consider that if a smaller balloon is first used, before dilatation with the correct sized balloon for the vessel calibre, dissection is less. The theory, whilst reasonable, has not been proven by clinical trials. The technique seems to be helpful with tight lesions on a bend in the proximal RCA.

c) *Cutting Balloon*

It is claimed that dissection (and perhaps even restenosis) may be less. The cutting balloon may have a role in smaller calibre vessels (see page 25).

d) *Rotablator*

For calcified lesions, the initial use of a Rotablator burr may fracture calcium and reduce the risk of dissection with subsequent balloon inflations.

e) *Predilatation IVUS*

With experience, crossing and inspection of the lesion can be safely performed prior to PTCA in about 80% of lesions. IVUS may help assess the form of lesion, e.g. the amount of calcification and the extent of vessel disease prior to and after the lesion. This information may help in the selection of the best angioplasty equipment and strategy (see page 60).

Treatment of Established Dissection

The results of dissection are quite variable (see page 156) and the management will vary depending on the:-

1) Amount of compromise to blood flow (normal, reduced, total occlusion).
2) Length of dissection.
3) Haemodynamic consequences.

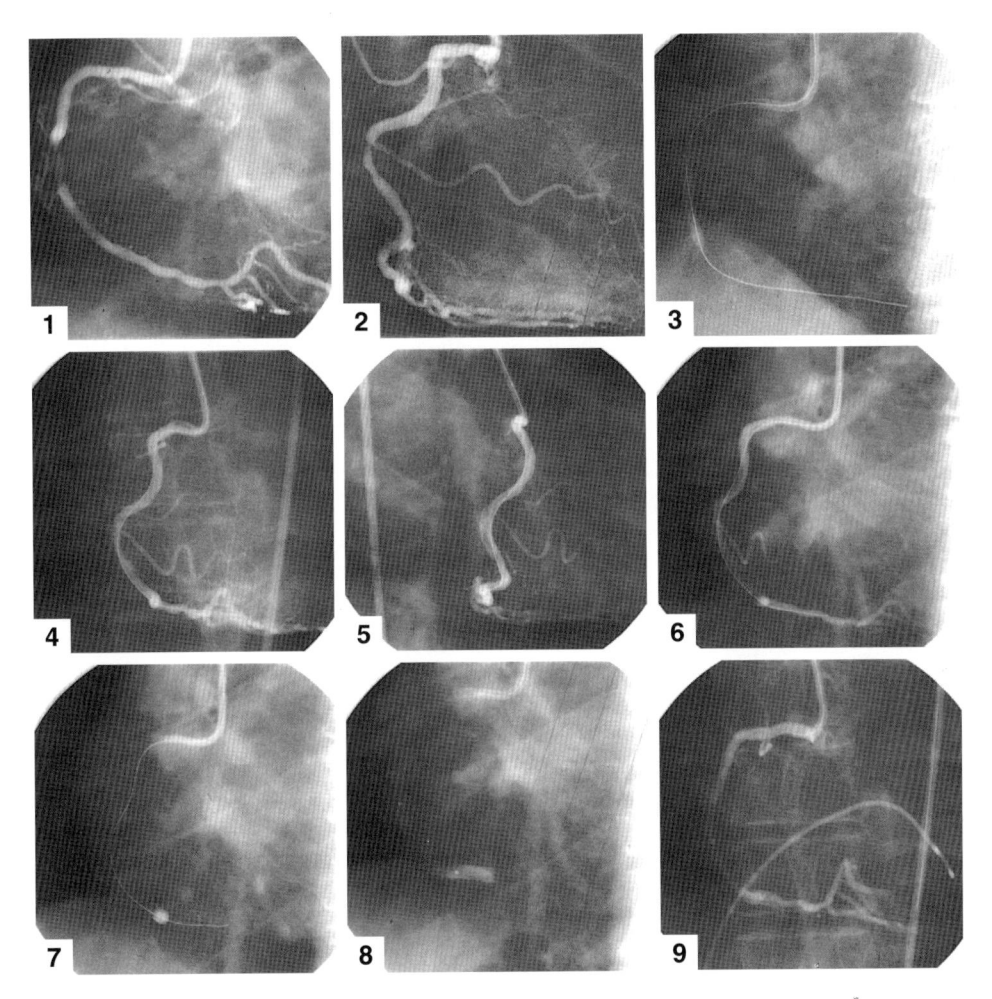

Angiogram 15.2. *Severe dissection of the RCA after PTCA of lesion on a bend.* (1) and (2) show severe stenosis on a bend in a tortuous RCA. Dilatation was with 3.5 mm balloon (3) which produced dissection (4) which is seen more clearly in the RAO projection (5) where a longitudinal dissection is shown. A false lumen with retention of contrast was later seen (6 and 7). Prolonged inflation with a perfusion balloon was unsuccessful (8 and 9). A pacing catheter was inserted and the patient was sent for emergency surgery with a perfusion catheter providing flow to the distal artery (guide wire withdrawn) (9). The PTCA was performed before coronary stents were available.

Measures to relieve a dissection or an unsatisfactory PTCA result include:

1. Redilatation

After the first inflation the appearance may not be satisfactory and redilatation should be performed, ensuring to "catch" or dilate the lesion along its whole length. Consider an attempt at a prolonged inflation of 5–7 minutes, if the patient can tolerate it (see page 94). Consider redilating with a larger balloon if it is clear that the balloon first used was *undersized* for the artery. If the balloon was the appropriate size, redilating with the next size balloon (and some recommend at low pressures of 2–4 atmospheres), rarely helps and more often aggravates the dissection both in its length and further reduction in blood flow.

2. Stent

Placing a stent is by far the most important and successful procedure (see Angiogram 15.1 on page 170). It should be done *earlier rather than later*.

If the result from PTCA is clearly poor, with moderate dissection, don't wait around until the blood flow falls off. Get the stent out and deliver it promptly to the lesion. From the review of the angiogram taken before the procedure, the type, length and size of stent for possible use, should have already been considered.

Stenting works best if the dissection is short and be covered by a single 15–18 mm stent. If the dissection is a *long* one, e.g. down most of the RCA to and even beyond the bifurcation, emergency surgery is a safe and well proven treatment without the risk of early closure or restenosis within a few months.

With a long dissection the Magic Wallstent is the *stent of choice* available in lengths of 15–48 mm. One or two overlapping Wallstents may correct the dissection and "reconstruct" the vessel. With the deep wall injury that has occurred, the risk of stent restenosis, and probably thrombosis may be increased. If the dissection is not too extensive, i.e. about 3–4 cm, a longer version of a Gianturco-Roubin, AVE Micro, CrossFlex, or NIR stent may be able to cover it totally.

An alternative for a long dissection, is to use a small number of shorter balloon mounted stents. Two 15–18 mm length stents, one at either end of the dissection, may be sufficient to seal it. As passing a second stent through the first may be difficult, the distal stent should initially be delivered, followed by the more proximal one. However it may be necessary to implant multiple Palmaz-Schatz Stents to 'cover' the dissection and restore satisfactory flow. Whilst feasible to insert 5–7 stents, this greatly increases the cost of the procedure and the risks of stent thrombosis and restenosis too. For a long dissection it is quicker, safer and cheaper to use a long Wallstent or a long coiled stent, such as a Gianturco-Roubin stent.

3. Perfusion Balloon (see page 20).

This balloon catheter aims to allow a prolonged inflation without causing ischaemia. The design allows blood to perfuse the distal artery beyond the balloon during inflation. The balloon is inflated for 15–30 minutes, with the aim of "sticking back the wallpaper onto the wall". The technique is successful in only about 30–50% of cases. The perfusion balloon may be helpful for short dissections but is rarely successful with long dissections (see Angiogram 15.2 on page 173).

A perfusion balloon, including the more recent versions such as the Lifestream Balloon, is relatively rigid and may be unable to track to the lesion. Flow down a perfusion balloon is dependent upon arterial pressure and if the patient is hypotensive the system is much less effective at perfusing the distal artery. If there is a side branch covered by the balloon, ischaemia in its territory may prevent a long inflation.

To allow maximum blood flow down the shaft of a perfusion catheter, the guide wire should be retracted proximally to before the start of the perfusion holes. This is *very undesirable* when there is a dissection as it may not be possible to return the guide wire along the true lumen to the distal artery. With the guide wire retained distally perfusion to the artery beyond the balloon may be insufficient to allow a prolonged inflation.

Finally, when a perfusion balloon is used there is a lot of "hanging around" (thirty minutes at a time) not knowing whether the balloon will or will not work. The patient's sick, the surgeons are sharpening their knives, whilst the cardiologist is twiddling his thumbs and another operator is trying to get into the catheter lab! Interventionists are men and women of action and hate this uncertainty of hanging around; for many, the perfusion balloon is not for them!

Perfusion balloons were used when there was nothing better. Stents have replaced them, but perfusion balloons may still have a role in smaller calibre vessels and perhaps as the initial PTCA balloon to allow a longer than usual inflation (5–7 minutes) to help prevent dissection (see page 172).

4. Atherectomy

Sometimes a short flap of dissection tissue is obstructing the lumen. This usually will respond to placement of a stent. An alternative strategy is to perform atherectomy. This may require changing the guide catheter from 6 or 7F to an 8F size.

5. Emergency CABG

Cardiac surgery has always been an important 'stand-by' to 'bail-out' a failed PTCA. Inform the surgeons sooner rather than later, when a PTCA problem is not responding to the treatments described in sections 1–4 above. CABG is very effective, but needs to be performed promptly, i.e. avoiding delays in the catheter lab and further delays before an operating theatre becomes available. This is the reason why PTCA is preferably performed 'on-site' to minimize the time for transfer to cardiac surgery.

Emergency CABG is particularly indicated for long dissections, where there is significant disease affecting other coronary arteries (multivessel disease) and when the patient's clinical haemodynamic status has deteriorated.

6. Other Measures

a) *Pain Relief*
   Give diamorphine 2.5 mgs i.v. Consider an anti-emetic such as stemetil (prochlorperazine) 5 mgm i.v. or metoclopramide (maxolon) 10 mgm i.v.

b) *Oxygen*
c) *I.V. Fluids*
   To help maintain the blood pressure. These are needed especially if liberal amounts of nitrates have been given i.v. or into the coronary artery.
d) *Pacing Wire*
   This may be needed for an RCA occlusion (see Angiogram 15.2, and 16.1, on pages 173 and 178). It is preferable to use the contralateral groin to avoid confusion with the guide catheter and to ease groin compression when the sheaths are removed; this may also reduce the risk of groin complications, such as femoral arterio-venous fistula.
e) *Intra Aortic Balloon Pump (IABP)*
   Consider its use, especially if the blood pressure falls and there is haemodynamic instability (see Angiogram 16.1, page 178).

   If the ECG is showing unequivocal ischaemia, such as Q-waves and S-T elevation, the IABP will help maintain circulation and reduce oxygen requirement for the myocardium. This role can be particularly helpful, if there will be a delay before emergency CABG can be mounted.

Accurate Recording of Events

These are very useful when later auditing the outcome. It is best that the technician or nurse does the recording. Though this may be difficult, attempt to document:

1) time that dissection or a problem was first recognised.
2) time that ischaemia was clearly present on ECG.
3) measures taken and at what time, e.g. stent and other balloons that were used.
4) time that theatre and or the surgeon was informed of the problem with the PTCA procedure.

Conclusion

Since the advent of stents, dissection is no longer the major threat of PTCA that it once was. With a high risk case, a stent can be used electively and in other cases, their early use may promptly relieve the situation. However as with all "good news" there is also the downside. Stents don't always work to relieve dissection and sometimes they even cause the dissection. Stents have not removed the need for emergency surgery and the management of the patient going for emergency CABG is described in the following chapter.

16 Emergency Surgery

This chapter follows on from Chapters 14 and 15 on 'Abrupt Closure'. Emergency CABG (emergency coronary artery bypass grafting) is one of the treatments available for abrupt closure.

Whilst both patient and cardiologist dread the need for emergency surgery, from the outset the patient needs to be informed of this possibility and the cardiologist must recognise its value.

The availability of a venous conduit should have already been established, i.e. whether the patient has had previous venous stripping, or whether there are severe varicose veins in the legs (see page 68). Other medical conditions which may affect surgical outcome should also be known, such as diabetes, significant lung, renal or peripheral vascular disease. Left ventricular function and severity of coronary artery disease in other vessels besides that being dilated, should be known by the operator. All this information must be readily available to potentially give to a surgeon, who may be seeing the patient for the first time and who needs to make decisions promptly (see on site or off site surgery, page 155).

The sequence from catheter room to theatre and beyond is variable but often has these identifiable steps.

1) *Inform Surgeon and theatre EARLY.*
   The earlier the surgical staff are informed that there is a problem, the easier it will be to reschedule the operating list. A patient about to be called from the ward, or even anaesthetised can be told of the emergency and that their operation may be delayed. If the problem is 'fixed' in the catheter lab, no tears will be shed in theatre.
2) *Other general measures* (see also page 175).
   Transfer to surgery, of a patient who has arrested and is receiving external cardiac massage, should now be part of history or a very rare event indeed. Give oxygen by face mask and fluids intravenously, especially if nitrates have been used and there is hypotension from vasodilatation. Try to maintain the patient in as fit state as possible. This may mean the insertion of an intra aortic balloon pump as part of supportive measures. However if prompt surgery can be performed, immediate transfer to theatre may be better than further delay inserting the IABP.

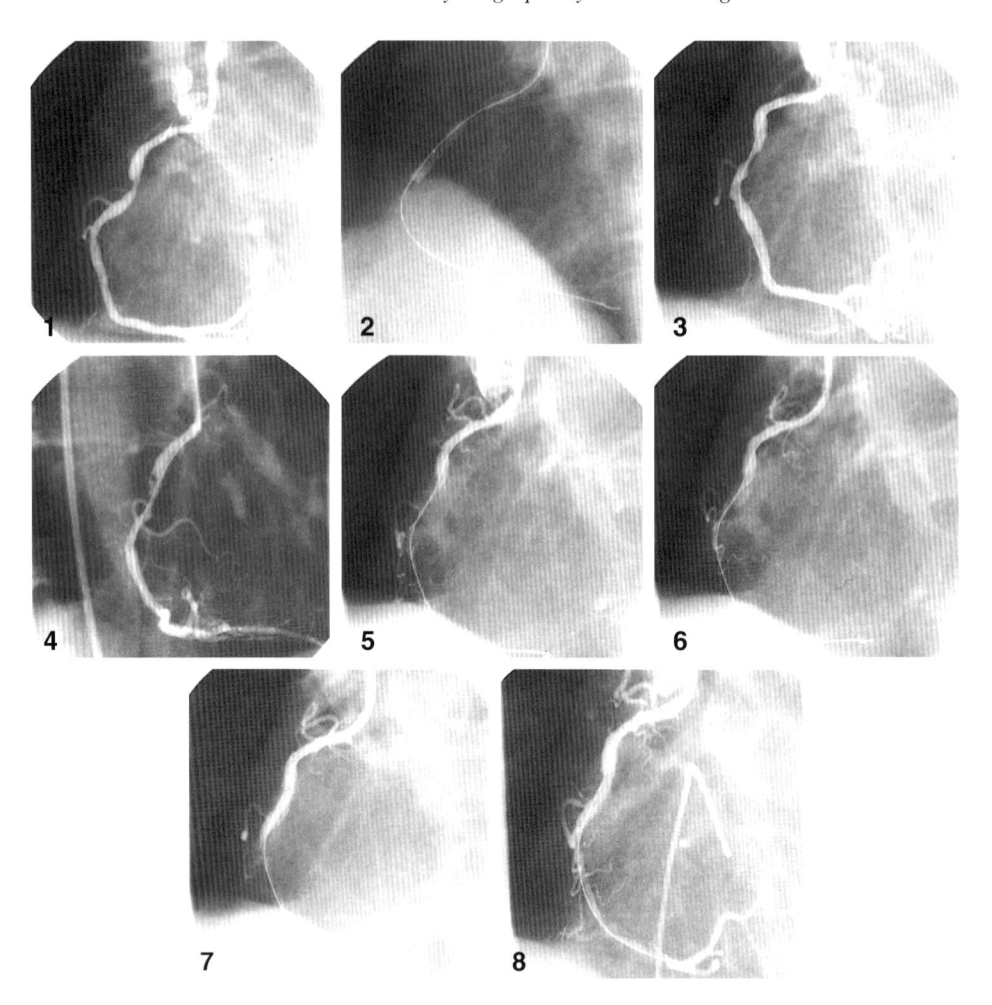

Angiogram 16.1. *RCA dissection requiring emergency CABG.* The moderately severe eccentric stenosis in the proximal RCA (1) was dilated with a 3 mm balloon (2). Initially the lesion was improved (3) but the RAO view was very unsatisfactory suggesting dissection and thrombus (4). The vessel later closed (5). After further balloon dilatation a long dissection is seen (6). A Palmaz-Schatz PS153 stent was deployed at the lesion (7), but the vessel remained closed beyond it, as there was by now a long dissection (7). The guide wire was left insitu allowing some flow to the distal artery. A pacing wire was inserted (7), and also an intra-aortic balloon pump. The patient was referred for emergency CABG, where the dissection was found to stop at the crux of the RCA. Grafts were given to PDA, LAD and the first diagonal artery. The patient made a full recovery without developing infarction.

3) *Refer the patient sooner rather than later.*
   The time clock of ischaemia and infarction commences when the occlusion or dissection first occurs. If measures, such as stenting, to relieve the situation are not successful, resist the urge to go on and on to the bitter end with further attempts to 'fix' the problem. If the patient sustains infarction in the catheter laboratory, it is

unrealistic to expect CABG two or more hours later to reverse or prevent infarction damage. The risk of emergency CABG will be greater if the patient is hypotensive and clearly "well into his or her infarct".

However some patients, despite dissection, seem very stable with little or no ischaemic pain and with a normal ECG or one with only minimal changes. These can be carefully monitored and can perhaps be transferred to surgical ITU to await the next available theatre slot (see page 156).

4) *Maintain the guide wire across the lesion.*

The guide wire acts as a splint and very often will be able to allow sufficient blood flow to the distal vessel to avoid severe ischaemia (see Angiograms 14.2, page 160, and 16.1). A perfusion balloon is now rarely used as a 'bail out catheter', to bridge the time between catheter room and surgery. The small holes often become clotted up and a guide wire alone is usually as effective, if not more so.

Remove the guide catheter from the main left coronary artery (and perhaps from the RCA too), this reduces the risk of any clot forming in the guide catheter ending up in the coronary artery.

Secure the guide catheter, guide wire and sheath at the groin. Allow the hub of the guide catheter and the guide wire to be visible, so that at surgery they can easily be withdrawn.

Connect the guide catheter to a pressure manifold which allows it to be flushed and arterial pressure to be recorded. Alternatively connect the guide catheter to a 10 ml syringe with heparinised saline to allow periodic flushing.

5) *Inform the patient.*

That unfortunately PTCA has not been successful. If true, explain that their cardiac condition is stable. Explain, that as was previously discussed with them, it will be safer and better for them to have prompt surgery. Show your regret, but be optimistic that they will do very well with a bypass.

6) *Inform the relatives.*

Let the nursing staff on the ward know that the patient is going for surgery. The nurses can inform the relatives who may need to come in from home.

7) *Check availability of blood.*

Usually the patient has had the blood group determined and the serum saved. Cross match 4 units of blood or whatever amount is recommended by the surgeon or anaesthetist.

8) *Consider the need for other coagulant products.*

If thrombolytic drugs have been given consider aprotinin (Trasylol) and sometimes also tranexamic acid (Cyklokapron). A test dose of aprotinin of 50,000 units (5 ml) by slow intravenous injection over five minutes, is followed by 2 million units (200 ml) of aprotinin i.v. over 20 minutes. Further aprotinin 200,000–500,000 units i.v. per hour may be given.

The dose of tranexamic acid is 1–5 gm by slow intravenous injection, followed by 1 gm i.v. per hour as needed.

If the glycoprotein IIb/IIIa antagonist, ReoPro has been given, check the platelet level and request 5 units of platelets to be made available (see page 164).

If the patient is on oral anticoagulants, surgical haemostasis will be more difficult if the INR is more than 2.5:1. Order 4 units of fresh frozen plasma.

9) *Promptly record procedure details.*
   In the 'rush' for emergency surgery, documentation of the procedure may be omitted and it will be very difficult to recall later the details. Write in the notes the procedure and the sequence, reasons and results of the measures taken. Ask the physiological measurement technician, nurse or radiographer to record the time that the problem arose, that the surgeon was contacted and that the patient left the catheter room for theatre. Record a 12 lead ECG and document its timings and what it shows.

10) *Review angiograms with the surgeon.*
    Decide whether other vessels besides the dissected one will need bypassing. Discuss the patient's current haemodynamic status. Inform the surgeon if there is an increased risk from bleeding, e.g. if a thrombolytic drug or IIb-IIIa antagonist has been given. Explain any other medical problems or risks, such as diabetes. If the vessel involved is the LAD, discuss whether the LIMA can be taken for the bypass. Whilst a vein graft is quicker to use, a LIMA graft will last longer and is to be preferred if the patient's clinical status is stable.

11) *Try to accompany patient to the anaesthetic room.*
    During induction the patient may deteriorate, especially with arrhythmias. Ensure that the guide catheter and guide wire do not become displaced.

12) *Try to get into theatre.*
    During the operation perhaps with the patient already on bypass, go to theatre. Observe the heart and if feasible the vessel that 'caused' the problem. Sometimes, despite extensive angiographic dissection, the artery appears normal from the outside. Discuss whether the myocardium showed signs of ischaemia. Thank surgical, anaesthetic and nursing colleagues.

13) *See the relatives.*
    Explain that PTCA was not successful and as previously discussed with them, the patient has been referred for bypass surgery. Show your regrets, but explain the benefits of surgery. Describe what is being done and by whom. Inform that the risks are greatest over the first 24 hours. Explain that the initial recovery will be in ITU and then the patient will be transferred to a surgical ward.

14) *Attempt to contact the general practitioner.*
    Try to inform the GP of the complication as the relatives may need support and perhaps a sedative.

15) *Assess patient in ITU.*
    Visit the patient and assess the clinical state, check the ECG to determine if myocardial infarction has developed. Advise on arrhythmia management. Discuss the patient's progress with the relatives.

16) *Subsequent course.*
    Make a special effort to visit the patient and relatives as recovery occurs in the surgical ward. Again express your regrets that PTCA was not successful and that emergency surgery was needed. Explain that the risk of restenosis has been removed and that medical drug treatment will eventually be very small, perhaps just aspirin. Make an effort to see the patient yourself at the first out-patient visit.

17) *Audit meeting.*
    Try to review all cases that require emergency surgery on a regular monthly basis. Review the angiograms, discuss the treatment options, the sequence of events and

the management strategies employed. Try to learn from the complication to assist future cases.

On the otherhand, *don't take complications too personally* — surgery and interventions inevitably involve risks. Remember the saying, 'that failures destroy some people (doctors) ... they make others'. Don't expect any solace and comfort from your surgeon when cases go wrong. Early in their training they learn that some of their operations will go wrong and their patients die. As one surgeon said to me during discussion about a patient who needed emergency surgery, 'If you can't stand the heat — you shouldn't be in the kitchen'!

18) *Thank your colleagues.*

It may not always be possible or appropriate during an emergency to thank those who have *bailed YOU out*. Do ensure that you thank your colleagues and include the anaesthetist, nurses, technicians, your own assistant and catheter room staff. Take the trouble to always see or telephone the surgeon that day. At the very least you have interrupted the surgeon's busy planned schedule and almost certainly caused the surgeon more work and hassle. Attention to and sincerity with your gratitude, will oil the wheels for your next case needing the skills of your surgeon in a hurry.

Conclusion

Though the risk of emergency CABG has fallen to about 2% (and even less for some Units), it is still needed. The surgical mortality has also fallen to about 5%, mainly as the patients are now more often referred in a stable haemodynamic state. Audit of these cases is very important to identify means to reduce the risks of both needing and receiving, emergency CABG for unsuccessful PTCA.

17 Ad Hoc PTCA

This term means, angiography proceeding directly to PTCA in the same procedure. This phrase has been popularised by Professor Bernhard Meier of Bern, Switzerland. Other names used are: 'angiogram? proceed to PTCA' and 'follow-on angioplasty'.

Ad hoc PTCA implies that the diagnostic angiogram is performed by an experienced interventional cardiologist. Perhaps his or her time might be better spent concentrating only on interventions. Many coronary angiograms are made by staff not experienced in performing PTCA and at centres without cardiac surgery on site, or without arrangements for emergency CABG. Ad hoc PTCA may not be an option for these patients.

Advantages of ad hoc PTCA

1. *One procedure* — diagnosis and treatment in the same 'sitting' or procedure.
2. *Avoids a complication occurring between the diagnostic angiogram and PTCA*, such as a stenosed lesion becoming occluded and the patient sustaining a myocardial infarct.
3. *More pleasant for the patient.*
4. *Cheaper.*

Disadvantages of ad hoc PTCA

There are number of disadvantages, none of which are insuperable, especially to experienced operators.

1. *Inadequate Assessment of the Angiogram.*
   Whilst one artery may have a clear lesion, disease elsewhere may be missed, or its severity underestimated.
2. *Inadequate Planning for PTCA.*
   The careful analysis of the angiogram, the consideration of X-ray views to use, the equipment to employ and the strategy if a vessel occludes, all have to be done in a greatly compressed time span.

3. *Inadequate Assessment of the Whole Patient Problem.*
    A very suitable (or 'juicy') PTCA lesion on one or two vessels may stimulate the 'occulo-dilatory reflex' — coronary patient with lesion, cardiologist with balloon catheter, result: PTCA performed, whether needed or not!
    Is the patient still symptomatic and would he or she be content with medical treatment? Would CABG be preferred if a full discussion of both procedures is given.
4. *Inadequate Explanation of the Risks of PTCA.*
    The patient and relatives may have been told that the risks of an angiogram are very low. They may not have been informed that risks of PTCA are of a greater order of magnitude.
    Certainly one can't (or shouldn't) start for the first time, to tell a patient about PTCA whilst he or she is lying on the catheter table. The relatives of a patient transferred for angiography from another hospital may not even be aware that their loved one is going for an operation. If the patient dies, considerable anguish leading to litigation may ensue.
5. *Catheter Room Logistics.*
    It takes 2–3 times longer to perform a PTCA than a diagnostic angiography. It is not known whether a PTCA will or will not follow the angiogram. The PTCA may develop a complication so that the case takes 2–3 hours. All these factors make scheduling in the catheter room difficult.
6. *Inadequate Cardiac Surgical Cover.*
    If a case is scheduled later in the afternoon and a complication ensues, surgical colleagues may not be amused to be referred the case after 6 pm!

Use of ad hoc PTCA

The indications for ad hoc PTCA include:

1. Acute MI ... more or less 100% of primary angioplasties are ad hoc PTCAs.
2. Unstable Angina ... ad hoc PTCA is very desirable.
3. Stable Angina ... it is this indication where there is most difficulty in terms of numbers, to consider ad hoc PTCA (see Angiogram 17.1).
4. Previous PTCA ... if the patient has restenosed, then really the case is a repeat PTCA.
5. Previous Coronary Angio ... if the coronary anatomy is known from an angiogram some months to years earlier, this can be reviewed prior to starting the case (if it can still be found!).

Angiogram and Leave the Sheath In

At the end of the diagnostic angiogram, *the sheath is left in the femoral artery* and secured with a suture. The PTCA is done later that day or the next. This is a 'halfway house' between ad hoc PTCA and returning for a second separate procedure. It saves the patient another femoral artery canulation. It is particularly helpful for patients with unstable angina. After a diagnostic angiogram by a non-interventionist angiographer, if the disease shown is suitable for PTCA, the femoral sheath is left in position and the patient returned to the ward. The angiogram is reviewed by an interventionist and discussion with the

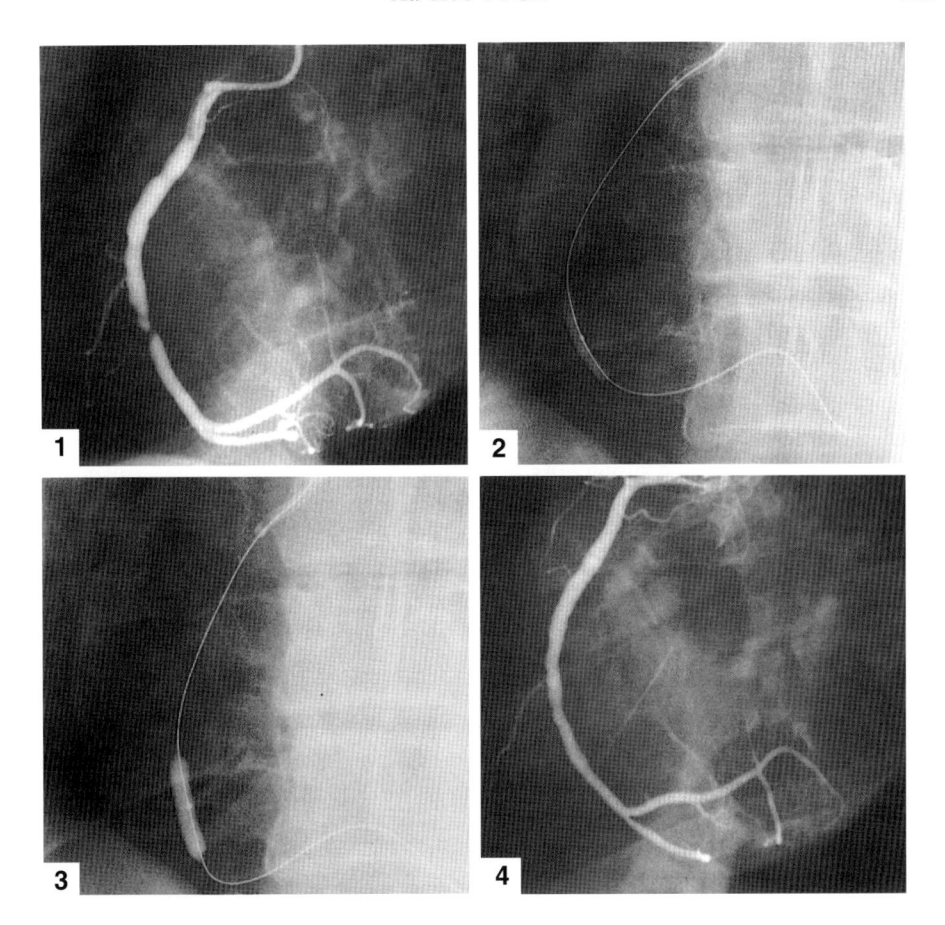

Angiogram 17.1. *Ad hoc PTCA of RCA lesion.* The patient gave a short two month history of angina, and the ECG was normal. There was 3 mm S-T depression at stage 2 of the Bruce Protocol. Diagnostic angiography with 6F catheters showed normal LV function and LCA, and a severe stenosis of a large calibre RCA (1). Angiography proceeded directly to PTCA using 7F right Amplatz I (AR1) guide catheter, 0.014" guidewire and pre-dilatation with a 2.5 mm balloon (2). A Palmaz-Schatz 15 mm (J & J CPS 153) stent was hand crimped onto a 4 mm Speedy balloon and deployed at 14 atmospheres pressure (3). The result is very satisfactory with no residual stenosis (4). 1 and (4) are LAO 60°. (2) and (3) were LAO 30°, which allowed screening of most of the RCA without the need for deep inspiration to lower the diaphragm below RCA.

patient and relatives is followed by scheduling the PTCA at a suitable time for the cardiological, catheter room and surgical staff.

Flushing the sheath with 5–10 ml of saline 4–6 hourly, helps maintain its patency. The value of adding a small dose of heparin, for example as a propietray heparin flush such as 'Hepsal', (C P Pharmaceuticals), which has 10 units of heparin per ml, is unproven. It is preferable to change the sheath (over a guide wire), for a new one at the time of PTCA, to reduce the risk of infection and of introducing old thrombus within the sheath into a guide catheter.

A further method much liked by the junior medical staff and nurses on the ward, is to insert a flexible obturator into the sheath, which then does not need flushing. When the obturator is removed for the PTCA, the sheath is patent.

Catheter Room Scheduling

If an ad hoc PTCA is scheduled, it is important to allow sufficient time to perform PTCA, i.e. a smaller number of cases be booked for the catheter session.

Patient Discussion

If ad hoc PTCA is to be considered, the patient and relatives should be informed that if an angiogram shows something that can be treated by PTCA, then the procedure will be performed all in the "same sitting". As the risks of PTCA will need to be explained, the initial consultation, discussions and obtaining consent, will take much longer than that needed for a routine angiogram.

Explain that if there is doubt whether PTCA can or should be done, it will be deferred to allow further discussion and review. However at times it is very clear that one, or two vessels, are the problem and have a lesion or lesions eminently suitable for PTCA. Diagnosis and treatment will both be given during the same procedure.

Anticipating ad hoc PTCA

For a patient with recent onset angina, without a previous history of myocardial infarction, there is a good chance that there will be single vessel disease with a stenosis rather than a total occlusion. If the patient's symptoms and investigations would warrant PTCA this can be scheduled as an ad hoc PTCA, i.e. angiogram, ? proceed (to PTCA).

If, on the otherhand, there is a long history over many years with recurrent myocardial infarctions, especially if the patient is elderly (over the age of 70), it is more likely that multivessel coronary artery disease will be shown and CABG be needed.

LAD Syndrome

There is a group of patients with features strongly suggesting single vessel LAD disease which may be suitable for PTCA. The features are:

a) Short history of angina ... less than 6 months, often presenting with unstable angina.
b) T-wave inversion over antero-septal leads (V1–V5), but no Q-waves (Figure 17.1).

The short history suggests single vessel disease. The absence of Q-waves and of transmural myocardial infarction, implies a stenosed (but patent) artery, rather than an occluded vessel. The distribution of ECG changes, i.e. of anterior subendocardial myocardial infarction implicates the LAD vessel.

Sometimes the ECG changes may involve leads I & AVL and there may be minor S-T elevation or biphasic T-waves.

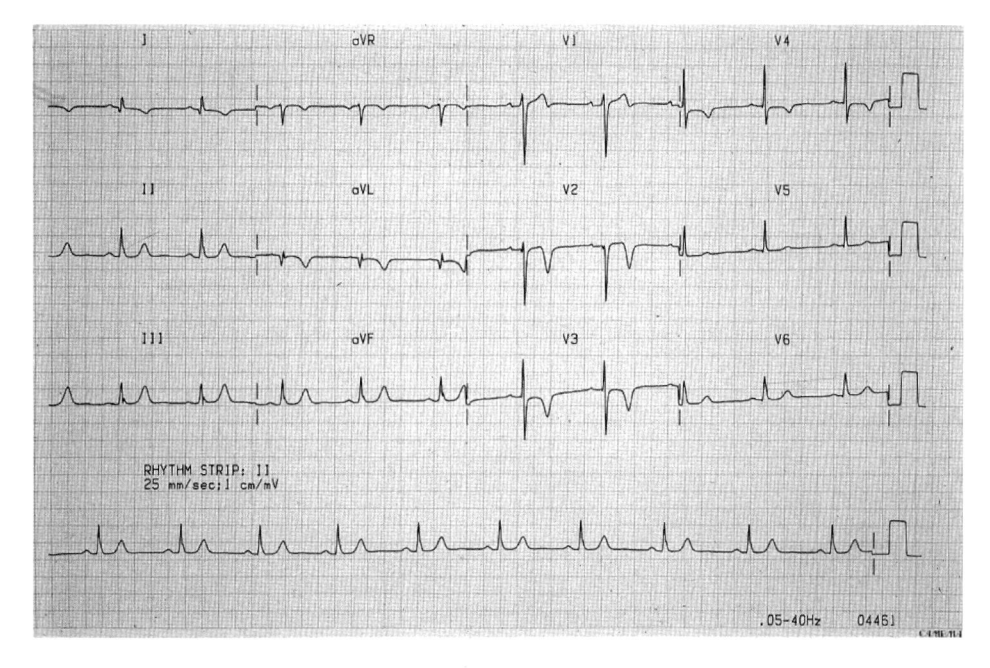

Figure 17.1. ECG of LAD Syndrome.

There may only be a history of recent onset angina, without any prolonged unstable episode. The T-wave changes may fluctuate, sometimes present but at other times the T-waves may be normal. This variation may occur both before and after, successful PTCA.

These patients nearly always have LAD disease as the culprit lesion, i.e. responsible for the recent onset angina. However there may also be disease elsewhere despite the short history. The extent of disease elsewhere will govern the management, from PTCA just of the culprit lesion, to revascularization of the LAD and other vessels by CABG or PTCA.

Conclusion

Most operators perform ad hoc PTCA for unstable angina and acute myocardial infarction. A few operators perform virtually all PTCAs as ad hoc procedures. The benefits of comfort and cost, need to be balanced by the problems of less adequate angiogram review and catheter room logistics.

18 Primary Angioplasty

History

Isolated cases of PTCA during the acute stages of MI (myocardial infarction) were soon reported after the introduction of PTCA. However it was Dr Geoffrey Hartzler of Kansas City, USA who first described the routine use of PTCA on all cases of MI as an alternative to thrombolysis. His results were impressive with an overall mortality of 7.8% and a low reinfarction rate. He described one important rule for this management, namely *angioplasty the infarct vessel ONLY.* Attempting PTCA of a severe lesion on a second vessel could be disastrous if this vessel occluded leading to yet further ischaemia of the left ventricle, in addition to the territory of the infarct.

As good as these results were, the findings were not based on a controlled trial. It was also considered more practical for PTCA to be performed some period after thrombolysis had been given. Hence 6–48 hours after thrombolysis an angiogram would be taken and if there was still a severe lesion then this would be dilated. Several trials however, such as the TAMI and SWIFT trials failed to show benefit of angioplasty at this stage after an MI. In fact the reverse was found — the PTCA patients had a higher mortality and a greater need for emergency CABG than those treated merely with an intravenous thrombolytic drug. One important reason for this lack of success, is that PTCA in the presence of a thrombolytic drug leads to an increased risk of haemorrhage in the wall of the dilated vessel. The risk of vessel closure is increased compared with routine PTCA. In other words, PTCA shortly after a thrombolytic drug has been given, may lead to a '*bloody dissection*' of the vessel at the site of dilatation. In the absence of stents, trying to deal with this can be very difficult.

Interventionists slept peacefully in their beds once more ... until 1994. Then the results of three moderately large and well conducted trials were published. These were the PAMI (Primary angioplasty in myocardial infarction) trial, the Dutch trial and the Mayo trial. In these trials the management returned to that described by Hartzler, i.e. angioplasty as an alternative to thrombolysis in the acute stages of a myocardial infarct. Primary angioplasty had a lower mortality, a lower reinfarction rate and a reduced incidence of stroke during the acute admission. Over the next year there was a lower incidence of death, reinfarction and need for revascularization procedures of PTCA and CABG.

The 30 day results of the three trials are summarized in Table 18.1.

Table 18.1

	1° PTCA	Thrombolytic Drug	p value
Number of patients	394	405	
Death	2.6%	6.4%	<0.0008
Recurrent MI	2%	7.9%	<0.001
Stroke	0.3%	2.5%	<0.007
Death or Recurrent MI	4.3%	13.1%	<0.00001

(after de Boer M-J, 1994).

There is controversy as to how effective thrombolysis and angioplasty are for the treatment of acute myocardial infarction. Angioplasty is only available at a small minority of hospitals admitting patients with acute MI. However, where these facilities and trained staff are available, primary PTCA is now an established treatment and some would argue the treatment of choice (see references at the end of the chapter).

PTCA and Myocardial Infarction

There are different times that PTCA can be performed following acute MI. The timings of the procedures have led to different names. These include:

Primary Angioplasty

PTCA is the first line treatment to reopen the artery, as an alternative to an i.v. thrombolytic drug.

Rescue or Salvage Angioplasty

When I.V. thrombolytic drugs have been unsuccessful at reopening the artery, angioplasty is then performed. The decision for angioplasty rests on clinical features such as continuing severe pain and no reduction of S-T segment elevation on the ECG. Ninety minutes may be the appropriate time to carefully reassess the MI patient and decide whether the thrombolytic drug has or has not worked. Unfortunately there is no simple, quick, reliable, non-invasive method to make the diagnosis of failed vessel reopening.

Angioplasty for continuing or recurrent ischaemic pain

This group merges with the rescue angioplasty group. However, it is mainly for patients whose pain largely settles and then recurs over the subsequent 6–72 hours. The patients do not settle and have further problems. They may receive a further thrombolytic agent, such as tPA, if streptokinase was given the first time. These patients are in a loose group of 'unstable angina post MI'.

Performing PTCA in the presence of a recently administered (<12 hours) thrombolytic drug will be more difficult and hazardous than primary angioplasty, or after the effects of a thrombolytic drug has cleared.

This chapter will continue to discuss the management of patients receiving primary angioplasty.

Advantages of Primary Angioplasty

The advantages of primary PTCA over an i.v. thrombolytic drug include:

1. Better reopening of the occluded vessel.
2. Less reclosure and recurrent MI.
3. Less risk of CVA.
4. Record a coronary arteriogram.

1. Better Reopening of the Occluded Vessel.

In the TIMI (Thrombolysis In Myocardial Infarction) trials blood flow after vessel reopening is graded as 0–4, where 0 is no flow, and 4 is completely normal flow. After PTCA, vessel reopening with normal flow (TIMI grades 3 or 4) to the distal artery is achieved in about 90% of cases. After I.V. thrombolytics no vessel reopening occurs at all in about 25% of cases. Some flow is re-established in most cases, but only in about 50% of cases is full normal flow (TIMI grades 3 or 4) re-established.

Some claim that reopening by PTCA is faster than thrombolytic drugs. Whilst this is probably true, it has to be balanced against a longer *'door to balloon time'* of PTCA compared to *'door to needle time'* of a thrombolytic drug.

2. Less Reclosure after PTCA

After primary PTCA the vessel over the next three months will remain patent in about 75% of cases compared with only 40–50% of patients given a thrombolytic drug. There is less recurrent infarction and angina and there is reduced damage to the left ventricle. The *'open artery'* theory suggests that later recovery and remodelling of the left ventricle, in the weeks and months following an MI, is improved if the artery is patent rather than occluded.

The improved reopening and sustained patency after primary PTCA compared to a thrombolytic drug, lead to less myocardial damage, lower acute mortality, and over the next year an improved prognosis with a reduced need for revascularization procedures.

3. Record a Coronary Arteriogram

There are significant advantages to determining the underlying coronary anatomy which include:

a) *Risk Stratification to at least three groups:*
   1. Those needing urgent CABG.
      The patients with extensive three vessel disease, or those with a severe (but patent) stenosis of the left main stem. These will not receive PTCA but go for early CABG.

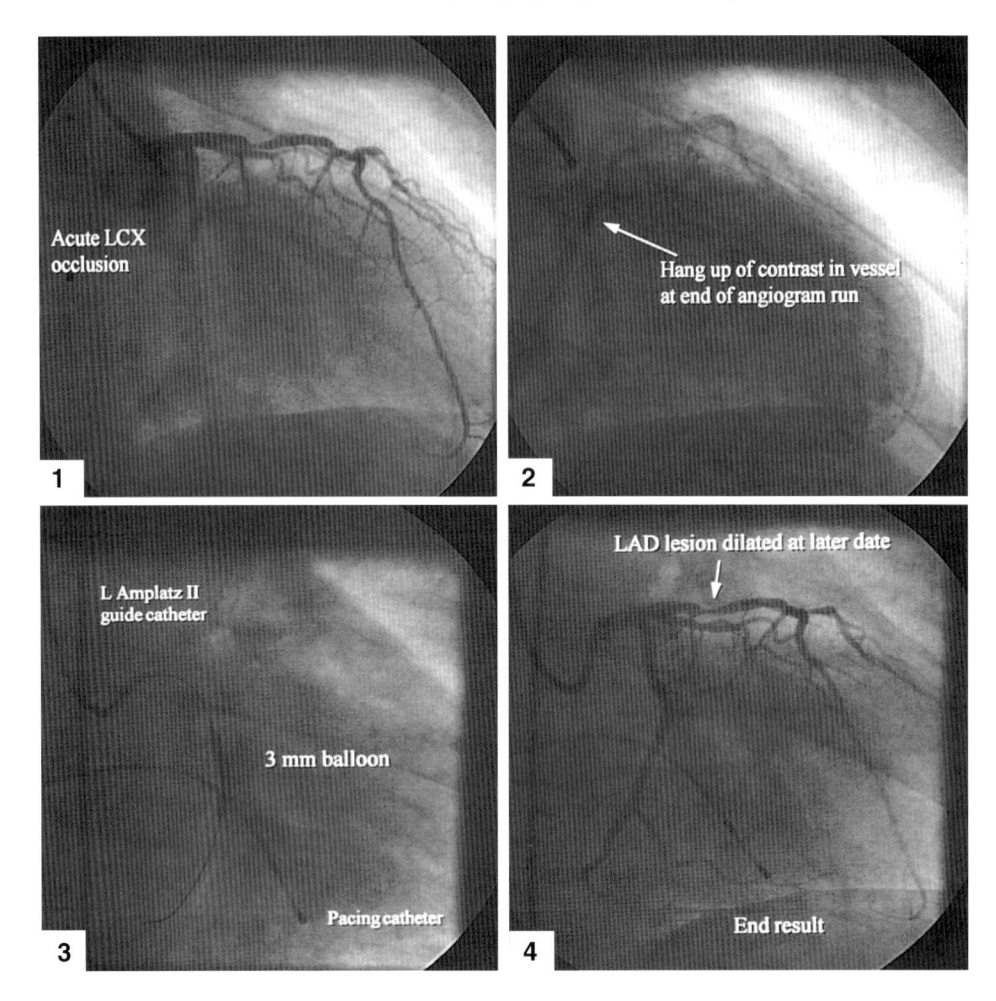

192   *Guide to Coronary Angioplasty and Stenting*

Angiogram 18.1. *Primary PTCA for acute LCX occlusion.* There is an acute occlusion of a dominant LCX artery (1), with hold up of contrast at the end of the angiogram (2). The occlusion was crossed with a routine soft tip guide wire (0.014 inch USCI Hi-Per Flex J wire) and dilated with a 3 mm balloon (3). The final result was satisfactory (4). Angioplasty of a significant LAD lesion was deferred to a later date.

> 2. Those with 2 or 3 vessel disease plus a culprit lesion.
>   PTCA is performed but later further revascularization will be needed.
> 3. Those with single vessel disease and an occluded vessel
>   PTCA can be curative for the disease shown at angiography.
> b) *Identification of a low risk category*
>   The patients from the single vessel disease category from above, will often be younger and have less severely damaged left ventricles. They should have a good prognosis. These patients can be mobilized quickly. They do not need to return to be managed in the CCU. They can discharged from hospital early i.e. about day 3 or 4 post MI.

c) *Reduce the need for subsequent tests*
Non invasive tests, to identify patients with more advanced CAD will not be needed. These investigations include exercise tests and thallium scans. Nor will a later coronary angiogram be required. Angiography is often performed after MI, at rates varying between different centres and countries. In the UK the rate over one year is about 30%, whereas in the USA it is nearer to 100%.

Disadvantages of Primary PTCA

There is *one major disadvantage* compared to thrombolytic drugs ... that of *logistics*. A thrombolytic drug can be given by any doctor (or paramedic), at any hospital, at any time of day or night. PTCA requires trained operators, in a hospital with angiography and angioplasty facilities. Primary PTCA interrupts the routine schedule of the catheter room during the day and places increased demands on the staff when needed outside routine hours.

To provide primary PTCA facilities nationwide has great logistic and financial implications. Three aspects relevant to this problem are:

1) *An experienced team of PTCA operators is needed.*
Whilst primary PTCA can be quick and simple, the patient is acutely ill and the procedure can be difficult and of high risk. Primary PTCA should not be performed by the 'occasional' operator. When starting a primary PTCA program, it is simpler to begin with cases admitted during routine hours as all the staff are already in the hospital.
2) *Surgery on site*
This is not mandatory but is very desirable to deal with acute emergencies arising in the catheter laboratory and to allow prompt surgery if CABG is needed.
3) *Transfer to a PTCA unit*
This can be arranged for higher risk and sicker patients and those in whom a thrombolytic drug is contraindicated (see below). Results in these patients seem to be as good as those patients admitted directly to the PTCA centre providing the travelling time is about 30 minutes or less.

Indications for Primary PTCA

These include:

1. Contra indications to thrombolytic drugs.
2. Cardiogenic shock.
3. Large anterior MI.
4. Others.

1. Contraindications to Thrombolytic Drugs

These include:

1. *Increased risk of bleeding from*:
   a) Haemorrhage at the time of the MI, e.g. gastrointestinal bleed.
   b) Head injury or fracture from a fall after loss of consciousness, occurring with an arrhythmia following the infarct.

c) Recent surgery, gastro-intestinal bleed, head injury, or stroke within the preceeding one to two weeks.

2. *Hypotension.*

If after pain relief with correction of a vaso vagal reaction and sinus bradycardia, the blood pressure is still low, i.e. with a systolic pressure of 80 mm of mercury or less, a thrombolytic is contraindicated. These drugs may lower the blood pressure further and in hypotensive patients are usually unable to reopen an occluded artery.

2. Cardiogenic Shock

These patients merge with those of the last section with hypotension as a contraindication to thrombolytic drugs. In cardiogenic shock thrombolytic drugs are ineffective. PTCA or CABG can approximately halve the very high mortality, i.e. from about 80% to 40%.

For revascularization to be of value it is essential that PTCA or CABG be given *early* i.e. within 12 and preferably within 6 hours from the onset of shock. Performing PTCA 24–36 hours after cardiogenic shock has set in, with the patient anuric, may give lead to a very good angiographic result but is very unlikely to prevent the patient's later demise.

3. Large Anterior MI

Patients with Q waves and S-T elevation on many or all of the V leads, are going to sustain a large anterior myocardial infarction unless the vessel is promptly and fully reopened. The same is probably true for an extensive inferior MI, particularly if the patient is hypotensive.

4. Other Indications

These include:

a) Older patients — over age of 70 years.
b) Previous CABG.
c) Previous MIs as opposed to the first MI.
d) Diabetics.

All these patients have a higher risk of dying from the MI and may be considered for Primary PTCA. However, they all carry a higher complication rate and mortality for the procedure. This is particularly true for very elderly patients over the age of 80, who may benefit greatly, but are likely to be technically more difficult and to be at greater risk. When starting a primary PTCA program, it is wiser to begin with the three basic indication groups, i.e. contra indications to thrombolytic drugs, cardiogenic shock and large anterior MIs.

Time Interval for Primary PTCA

As with thrombolytic drugs, the value of reopening a vessel will depend on how long it has been occluded and how much infarction of the myocardium has ensued. The shorter the duration of the occlusion the better.

Primary PTCA may be performed:
- <6 hours ... will give the greatest benefit
- 6–12 hours ... of benefit
- 12–24 hours ... still of benefit
- 24–48 hours ... consider the procedure only if the patient is still in pain.

Catheter Room Logistics

1. *Minimize the delays.*
   Aim to achieve a 'door to balloon time' of less than 1 hour.
2. *MI takes preference.*
   Despite interference with the schedule, the MI is an emergency and should displace the next patient on the list, or even the patient on the table if cannulation of the femoral (or brachial) artery has not yet occurred. Explain that 'it could be you tomorrow' and most patients will understand.
3. *On call team.*
   Arrangements need to be in place to achieve a prompt start to procedures outside routine hours. Faxing the ECG to the cardiologist on call, may aid the decision to initiate the call out process.

Don't Forget the Patient ... and the Relatives!

In all the rush to get the patient to the catheter room, there is a danger that the most important person is overlooked! Take care to adequately explain the diagnosis and to describe the proposed treatment with its benefits and potential complications, including emergency CABG .The operator should try to speak to the patient and not just rely on a consent form obtained by a junior doctor. In many hospitals primary PTCA is still relatively new and needs to be explained to the patient and if at all possible to the relatives too. If necessary speak to the relatives on the telephone, who will usually be very impressed and grateful that this effort has been made.

Drug Therapy prior to PTCA

a) *Aspirin*
   If the patient has not already been taking aspirin, two tablets of 300 mgm should be *chewed* and the fluid retained in the mouth as long as possible before swallowing. The aspirin should be taken as soon as the patient is seen and the diagnosis of myocardial ischaemia is suspected.
b) *Heparin*
   Heparin is not needed if transfer to the catheter room will be prompt. The chances that heparin will partially reopen an occluded artery are low. Cannulation of the femoral artery with the patient heparinized, will increase the risk of groin complications.
c) *Glyceryl Trinitrate*
   A nitrate may reduce coronary artery spasm and partially reopen a vessel. Usually, one or two puffs of GTN spray sublingually, or a buccal preparation is sufficient. A nitrate should not be given if the patient is hypotensive.

Catheter Room Procedure (Angiograms 18.1 and 18.2)

1. *Catheterize the infarct vessel first*
   If this confirms the diagnosis, assess which guide catheter and balloon size will be required. The assistant can be getting these ready whilst the non infarct vessel is catheterized.
2. *Perform LV angiogram*
   Document LV function at this stage, or at the end of the procedure. This can be very useful for comparison at a later date. If deferred to the end ... *don't forget to do it!* Some operators omit the LV angiogram in the interests of speed and possible safety.
3. *Choice of contrast agent*
   Most operators use *non ionic* contrasts as they cause less haemodynamic disturbance and are more pleasant to the patient. Dr Cindy Grines of Michigan USA, recommends *ionic* contrast media which have a weak anticoagulant effect and which may be safer in the context of acute MI.
4. *Aspirin*
   If there is doubt over its absorption from the gut, give 100–300 mgm i.v.
5. *Heparin*
   10,000 units as an i.v. bolus is given in the usual manner. Some operators use larger doses of heparin to achieve an ACT of 350–400 seconds, as opposed to the routine level of about 250–350 seconds for routine PTCA or stent patients. The increased anticoagulation may reduce risk of thrombus and vessel reclosure. However, there is no definite evidence for this view and the more aggressive anticoagulation will lead to more haemorrhagic and groin complications, see also page 162.
6. *Reopen the artery*
   Pass the GW and then the balloon across the occlusion (Angiograms 18.1 and 18.2). Usually this is easy and quickly done. Sometimes it may be difficult to negotiate the artery beyond the occlusion due to a stenosis at that level. Sometimes, the infarction lesion is distal to the occlusion, with retrograde thrombosis having occurred.

   Don't worry if the GW some distance beyond the occlusion ends up in a side branch, such as a diagonal rather than the main LAD. Usually it can safely stay there, but if necessary the wire position can be changed later once the vessel has been partially reopened and the anatomy of the distal vessel is clearer.
7. *Remember Hartzler's rule: Dilate the infarction vessel only.*
   Leave all other diseased arteries even those with straight forward (or 'juicy') lesions, until another procedure. When the acute MI has 'cooled down' and the damaged LV has had time to recover, angioplasty of other vessel(s) will be safer. This period should be at least 48–72 hours and perhaps 2–4 weeks if the patient is stable.

Problems that may arise:

a) *Reperfusion arrhythmias.*
   Bradycardia, nodal rhythm, idioventricular rhythm, ventricular ectopic beats and tachyarrhythmias and ventricular fibrillation are all to be expected. Except for VF, they are rarely a problem, are usually transient and do not usually require specific treatment. Complete heart block before or after vessel opening with RCA or LCX occlusion may need treatment with a temporary pacing wire.

Primary Angioplasty

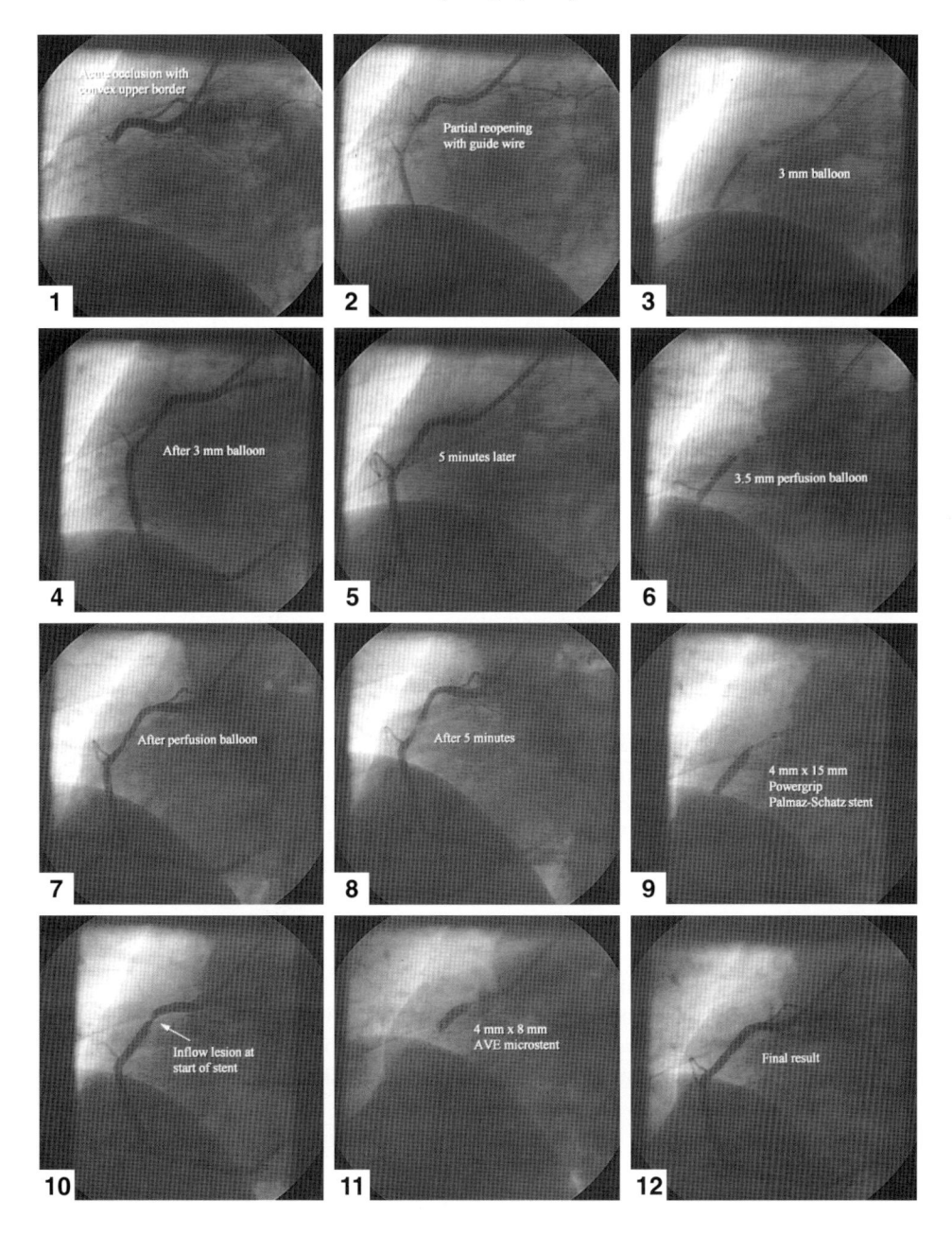

Angiogram 18.2. *Primary PTCA for acute RCA occlusion.* There is an acute occlusion of the RCA with no filling of the distal artery via collaterals (1). The occlusion was easily crossed with a soft tipped guide wire (0.014 inch High Torque Floppy II, ACS) (2). The lesion was dilated with a 3 mm balloon (3 and 4). After a 5 minute interval the lesion detiorated (5). A 3.5 mm perfusion balloon was inflated for 7 minutes (6). The appearance of the lesion improved (7), but this was not mantained (8). The lesion was stented (9), but there is an inflow lesion to the stent developed (10), so that a second stent was deployed (11). The final result was good (12).

This case illustrates that simple balloon angioplasty may not be sufficient for primary angioplasty, and stenting equipement and expertise may be required.

b) *Thrombus embolism*
   This occurs in about 10% of cases. The artery distally, or a branch beyond the bifurcation with the RCA, is seen to have developed a new 'lesion' or occlusion. Chase the embolus down the coronary artery! Pass the balloon to the distal site and dilate at low pressure. The embolus will usually pass on distally. Consider whether the same balloon or one of a smaller size should be used to dilate at progressively more distal sites. Once the embolus is relatively distal, such as in the distal third of the LAD or half away along the PDA or A-V branch of the RCA, it can be left and natural thrombolysis will usually take care of it adequately over the next few hours.

   One special form of embolism, is thrombus ending up in *another coronary artery*. For example, when reopening a proximal LAD occlusion, thrombus passes into the circumflex artery and obstructs it. This is particularly likely to occur when a balloon which has been used to dilate an LAD occlusion, is drawn back into the guide catheter. There may be clot on the balloon which is sheared off as the balloon re-enters the guide catheter. There is little that can be done to prevent this complication. Try to keep the number of withdrawals of the balloon into the guide catheter to as few as possible. Perhaps the risk may be less if the correct sized balloon is used from the start and it is not necessary to upsize the balloon. Be on the look out for this problem with very proximal LAD or LCX occlusions.

   Occasionally, there may be clot all along the coronary artery which doesn't clear with balloon inflations along the vessel. With these cases a small dose of TPA, such as 10 mgm into the coronary artery may be helpful. ReoPro (Abciximab) might also be tried.

c) *Persistent or recurrent lesion.*
   The lesion at the end of the procedure does not have to look perfect or 'stent-like'. However, it should have been well relieved and there should be good flow re-established. A continuing satisfactory result should be confirmed by a check angio after about 5–15 minutes. Sometimes the lesion can then be seen to have significantly deteriorated.

The management of an unsatisfactory residual lesion includes:

1) STENT — The Treatment of Choice
   If the vessel size and the course of the proximal artery will allow stent deployment, this will be the best solution. The presence of identifiable thrombus does NOT preclude the use of a stent. If good flow is re-established, thrombus will clear and there will not be an increased risk of stent thrombosis (Angiogram 18.2). ReoPro can be very helpful if thrombus reforms on the stent, (see page 162).

2) Prolonged Inflation
   An inflation for 5–10 minutes may successfully 'seal' an unstable flap. Usually a routine PTCA balloon rather than a perfusion balloon can be used. As the vessel was already occluded before the procedure started, the patient can usually tolerate a prolonged inflation.

3) Atherectomy
   This can be used to excise an unstable flap. For most cases where atherectomy can be performed, i.e. in large calibre relatively straight arteries, the lesion is also suitable for stenting.

d) *Continuing shock*

If the patient has cardiogenic shock before the procedure, start with the insertion of an intra aortic balloon pump (IABP).

If at the end of a successful reopening of an occluded artery, the blood pressure is still low, i.e. systolic pressure of 80 mm of mercury or less and angiographically or by the ECG changes, the patient has sustained a large MI especially an anterior one, insert an IABP. Have a low threshold to insert one, to tide the patient over the next 12–24 hours. Be careful to ensure that the patient continues on adequate amounts of heparin whilst the IABP is in the patient, to avoid limb ischaemia and the need for embolectomy.

Later Care on the Ward after Return from the Catheter Laboratory

1. *Sheath removal*
   In the majority of cases remove it at the routine time later that day or the next day. If the angioplasty result was only moderately good, 'reshooting' the coronary artery can be considered the next day and the sheath will be left in until that time.
2. *Heparin*
   For most cases no post procedure heparin is needed, i.e. none once the patient leaves the catheter lab. Some operators continue heparin for 24–48 hours to reduce the risk of vessel reclosure. The value of continuing heparin is uncertain and it will increase the risk of groin complications. It will also delay mobilization and early hospital discharge.
3. *Multivessel disease patients*
   A decision on their management will be needed; CABG or PTCA as appropriate. This may be required during the same admission, or the patient should be scheduled to return after about 2–4 weeks to get over the current MI.
4. *Low risk patients — Fast Track Discharge*
   If the patient is in this category (see page 192), he or she need not return to CCU and arrangements for early discharge on the 3rd or 4th day can be made.
5. *Drug therapy*
   Routine management post MI should include:
   a) Aspirin 75 or 150 mgm/day.
   b) ACE inhibitor for patients with large MI especially anterior.
   c) Beta blocker — to consider use, especially if the patient is hypertensive.
   d) Ticlopidine — if a stent has been used.
6. *Risk factors*
   These should be assessed and if the serum cholesterol is elevated a statin drug may be added.
7. *Information to the patient*
   Explain the amount of disease found, the severity of infarct sustained and the treatment that was given. Describe that the lesion may restenose or reocclude. *Give clear (and perhaps written) instructions as to what the patient should do and whom to contact, if there is an acute recurrence of pain.* It is usually best for the patient to telephone directly to the CCU.

Ensure that the drug regime is understood. It is valuable for the nursing staff or pharmacy to provide a written list of the drugs and the time that they should be taken.

Explanatory leaflets, audio and video tapes are very helpful as they allow the patient and the relatives to learn about myocardial infarction and its treatment at their own pace.

8. *Rehabilitation program*

   Though patients after primary PTCA are often able to be discharged early, rehabilitation is valuable for them too.

9. *Out patient visit*

   This should be in 4–8 weeks. The drug therapy should be reviewed. Ticlopidine should have been stopped 4 weeks after it was started (see page 154). Further revascularization procedures may need to be discussed.

Conclusion

Primary angioplasty is an exciting, relatively new development to the range of PTCA procedures. Primary PTCA is of proven value and is the treatment of choice for patients with acute MI arriving at a hospital with angioplasty facilities.

Sometimes primary PTCA can be quick and simple. More often it will be complicated and require a full range of angioplasty equipment to keep the reopened vessel widely patent. The patient is acutely ill and may develop cardiogenic shock. Primary PTCA requires a skilled interventionist and an experienced catheter room team.

References

Clinical debate. Should thrombolysis or primary angioplasty be the treatment of choice for acute myocardial infarction? Thrombolysis – the prefered treatment. Hillis LD and Lange RA. Primary angioplasty – the strategy of choice. Grines CL, *N Eng J Med* **335**, 1311–1318 (1996).

De Boer M-J, MD thesis. Primary angioplasty in acute myocardial infarction. Rotterdam University, 1994.

Gibbons RJ, Holmes DR, Reeder GS, *et al*. Immediate angioplasty compared with the administration of a thromboytic agent followed by conservative treatment for myocardial infarction. *N Engl J Med* **328**, 685–691 (1993).

Grines CL, Browne KR, Marco J, *et al*. A comparison of immediate angioplasty with thrombolytic therapy for acute myocardial infarction. *N Eng J med* **328**, 673–679 (1993).

Mueller HS, Cohen LS, Braunwald E, *et al*. for the TIMI Investigators. Predictors of early morbidity and mortality after thrombolytic therapy of acute myocardial infarction: analysis of patient subgroups in the Thrombolysis in Myocardial Infarction (TIMI) trial, phase II. *Circulation* **85**, 1254–1264 (1992).

O'Keefe JO, Bailey WL, Rutherford BD, Hartzler GO. Primary angioplasty for acute myocardial infarction in 1000 consecutive patients. *Am J Cardiol* **72**, 107G-115G (1993).

O'Neil WW. The evolution of Primary PTCA therapy for acute myocardial infarction. *J. Invas Cardiol* **7**, SuppF 2F-10F (1995).

Stone G, Grines CL, Topol EJ. Update on Percutaneous Transluminal Coronary Angioplasty for acute myocardial infarction. Current review of Interventional Cardiology, 2nd edition, pages 1–56. Editors: EJ Topol and PW Serruys. Current Medicine, Philadelphia, 1995.

Swift (Should We Intervene following Thrombolysis?). Trial Study Group. SWIFT Trial of delayed elective intervention v conservative treatment after thrombolysis with anistreplase in acute myocardial infarction. *Brit Med J* **302**, 555–60 (1991).

Topol EJ, Califf RM, George BS, *et al*. Thrombolysis And Acute Myocardial Infarction (TAMI) Trial. A randomized trial of immediate versus delayed elective angioplasty after intravenous tissue plasminogen activator in acute myocardial infarction. *N Engl J Med* **317**, 197–202 (1987).

Zijlstra F, DeBoer MJ, Hoorntje JC *et al*. A comparison of immediate coronary angioplasty with intravenous streptokinase in acute myocardial infarction. *N Engl J Med* **328**, 680–684 (1993).

19 PTCA of an Occluded Coronary Artery

An occlusion of a coronary artery or vein graft may be:

a) total or subtotal and of
b) recent onset or a chronic feature which has been present for months or even years.

A *subtotal occlusion* is a very tight stenosis where there is slow, often very slow, flow to the distal artery. With this type of occlusion it is virtually always possible to pass a guide wire across the lesion and then a balloon. It is doubtful whether a sub-total occlusion should be called an occlusion, rather than a severe stenosis. This type of lesion occurs with unstable angina, acute MI and late after an MI, often when there has been substantial myocardial damage.

With a *total occlusion*, there is no prograde flow across the lesion to the distal artery. Contrast is seen to come to a clear, complete and often abrupt halt at the lesion. There is a gap of varying length before the distal artery fills via collaterals from either another artery or from vessels arising before the occlusion ('bridge collaterals').

The more recent an occlusion has occurred, the easier it is to cross with a guide wire. After about 3 months the thrombus becomes quite firm and is then unable to be crossed with a soft flexible tip guide wire. A *chronic occlusion is defined as one more than 3 months old*. Sometimes it may not be known how long the occlusion has been present. At other times, especially with single vessel disease, the occlusion can be dated back to an acute MI or episode of unstable angina.

Recent Occlusion

The example par excellence of this lesion is an acute MI. There are two angiographic features to suggest that it is an acute occlusion:

1. Contrast held up in the proximal artery before the occlusion — i.e. it doesn't clear from the coronary artery as it does from the nearby vessels.

2. Absence of filling of the distal artery — via bridge collaterals progradely, or via collaterals from other coronary arteries.

Recent occlusions can usually be crossed without difficulty with a routine soft tip guide wire and angioplasty balloon. Sometimes with an acute MI. there may be retrograde thrombosis in the coronary artery, so that the causative lesion may be 2–3 cm more distal than the start of the occlusion. It may be difficult for the guide wire to negotiate this more distal lesion and care with patience should be taken to recognise and manage this problem. As with routine PTCA try to pass the guide wire as distally as possible. Sometimes inflating a balloon at the occlusion site may reopen the artery to then show a lesion more distally, which may also need treatment.

The soft thrombus of a recent occlusion may embolize when the vessel is reopened. The artery at a more distal site is seen to come to an abrupt end (see Angiogram 14.1). Pass a balloon of correct size for the vessel at that site and inflate to disperse or move the thrombus down the vessel. This process may need to be repeated until the thrombus ends up in a small distal section or branch which is less important. Here the thrombus will usually be spontaneously analysed over the next 24 hours to fully reopen the artery.

Chronic (Total) Occlusion

This is a complete occlusion to the coronary artery (or vein graft) which is believed to have been present for at least three months. It is difficult to cross the occlusion with a guide wire and a firm guide wire is needed. There is about 50% chance to cross and dilate the lesion. Rethrombosis leads to high restenosis or reocclusion rate of about 50%.

Features Favouring Lesion Crossing (Figure 19.1)

There are features seen on the diagnostic angiogram which favour the chances of a guide wire to cross a chronic occlusion. These are:

	Favourable	Unfavourable
1. Side branch arising at the occlusion site.	Absent.	Present.
2. Length of occlusion.	1–2 cm	More than 2 cm.
3. Bridge collaterals.	Absent.	Present.
4. Type of ending of the proximal vessel.	Tapering occlusion.	Square ended.
5. Proximal vessel tortuosity.	Little.	Prominent.
6. Amount of guide catheter back-up feasible.	More.	Less.

Features 1 and 2 are the more important. The ideal is a short occlusion with a taper into the occlusion without a side branch at the occlusion site. If such a side branch is present the guide wire tends to pass into it, rather than across the occlusion. The length of the occlusion is judged by the gap between where prograde flow stops and where retrograde flow ends in the distal vessel filled via collateral vessels.

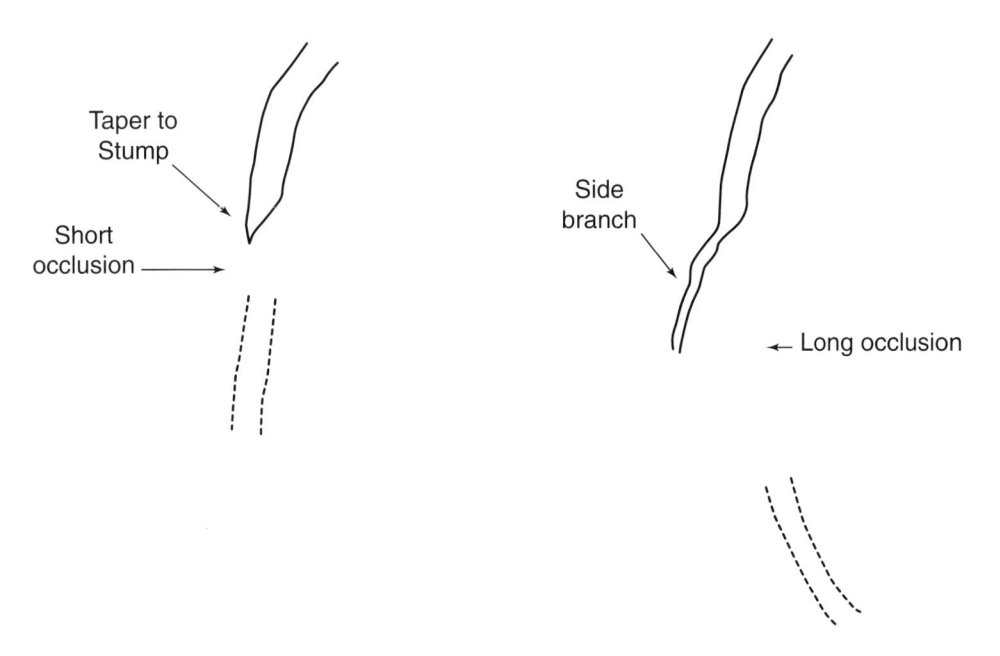

Figure 19.1. Chronic total occlusion: features influencing success to cross with a guide wire.

Is PTCA of Chronic Occlusions Worthwhile?

With an initial success rate of 50% (well below 80–90% of routine PTCA) and a restenosis/reocclusion rate also of about 50%, is PTCA cost effective? The answer is not a simple yes or no, but there are points to consider:

1. *How bad are the symptoms?*
   With a lower success rate, a more conservative approach should be given. Is medical treatment optimal?
2. *How much disease elsewhere is there?*
   If there is disease in other vessels, then CABG might be a better option.
3. *How easy is the lesion?*
   Is it a favourable or unfavourable form of occlusion.
4. *Newer regimes to improve results.*
   Stent placement, if vessel anatomy and calibre will allow, improves the long term result and lowers restenosis or reocclusion to about 20%. Without using a stent, oral anticoagulants started before the procedure and continued for 3 months may also reduce occlusion by lowering rethrombosis.

5. *LAST Procedure (Left Anterior Small Thoracotomy).*
   This mini CABG, performed via a thoracotomy using the LIMA, is very suitable for chronic occlusion of the LAD.
6. *Temporary reopening to cover PTCA elsewhere.*
   Some operators will attempt to reopen a chronically occluded artery, before attempting PTCA of another vessel, to give collateral support to the vessel during the PTCA. For example, a patient who had an inferior infarct five years previously, was then asymptomatic returns with a two month history of angina. The RCA is found to be chronically occluded and there is a new 'culprit' LAD lesion. Some operators will first attempt to reopen the RCA, before attempting the LAD lesion; aware that it may not remain open in the long term, but may provide collateral support during the LAD PTCA. However this approach takes longer and a complication may arise while attempting to reopen the RCA. It is simpler, quicker and probably safer, to dilate the LAD lesion and leave the RCA occlusion. If the RCA lesion has favourable features to reopen the occlusion, then the procedure would be a two vessel PTCA, the RCA followed by the LAD. (See also p. 86).

Risks of PTCA for Chronic Occlusion

It is sometimes assumed that if a vessel is totally occluded the risks of PTCA will be less than dilating a stenosed but still patent artery. The vessel is already occluded and therefore the need for emergency surgery would be low. However in practice the risk of problems and the rate of emergency surgery are similar to routine PTCA.

The risks of PTCA for chronic occlusion are:

1. *Vessel Perforation.*
   Even using a stiffer guide wire ('standard' or 'intermediate'), this complication is fortunately very rare. Providing the problem is recognised, it does not lead to haemorrhage or tamponade. Following the guide wire with a balloon which is then inflated, is quite another matter!
2. *Damage and Occlusion of the Proximal Vessel.*
   The proximal vessel can be dissected by the guide catheter, or rarely by the guide wire. The artery may then become occluded higher than the original lesion and may involve other branches. The worst scenario is a proximal LAD (or LCX) lesion leading to occlusion of the left main stem.

   One always feels regret and guilt after a vessel (and or a side branch) is damaged even before the target lesion is reached. There can be no doubt who was responsible!
3. *Embedding of a Guide Wire in the Occlusion.*
   It is possible for the guide wire to become embedded in the occlusion. The guide wire will then be unable to advance or to be withdrawn. On attempting to withdraw the guide wire it may uncoil, or even break off. If there is any suggestion that the guide wire has become stuck in the lesion ... *take care.* Extra support for the guide wire will be needed. This is provided by passing a balloon along the wire down to the occlusion. Try also to advance the guide catheter deeply, sometimes if feasible even down to near the lesion. Then withdraw all the equipment together, i.e. the guide

catheter, the balloon and the guide wire all as one unit. This nearly always frees a 'reluctant' guide wire!

Fracture of the guide wire tip in the lesion is very rare. It occurs more from repeated rotations of a guide wire in an occlusion, or in a branch at or near the occlusion. If the guide wire segment is small, no action (such as CABG) is needed — but the patient will retain a radiopaque souvenir of the procedure!
4. *Reocclusion of the Opened Artery.*
Reocclusion will usually be silent, with no acute episode and merely a return (or continuation) of the previous angina. Sometimes however acute ischaemia and further infarction may occur.
5. *Embolisation.*
With a chronically occluded vessel this is uncommon except in vein grafts.
6. *Vessel wall Dissection.*
This is relatively common with attempts to cross a chronic occlusion with a stiffer guide wire. The vessel beyond the occlusion has for varying lengths dissection and the true lumen of the artery is not reached. Usually there are no clinical consequences but the procedure has been unsuccessful.

Methods to Reopen a Chronic Occlusion

The problem with a chronic occlusion is to pass a wire across the lesion. If this is successful it is nearly always possible to follow with a balloon. For all techniques to cross an occlusion, good guide catheter support or backup is important. The methods used include:-

1. Firm or Stiff Guide Wire.
2. Magnum Wire.
3. Terumo Wire.
4. Rotacs Drill.
5. Laser Wire.

1. *Firm Guide Wire*
Instead of the very soft tip guide wires, an ACS intermediate or USCI standard guide wire is used. There are equivalent guide wires from other manufacturers. The tip can have a pre-shaped J shape, or one can be fashioned as required.

Though available in 0.014", 0.016" and 0.018" diameters, the 0.014" is usually employed, as most modern angioplasty balloons do not allow larger guide wires. The guide wire needs support to cross the lesion and this can be given by:-
a) PTCA balloon catheter taken nearly up to the end of the wire.
b) Non balloon catheter such as the 'Tracker 18' catheter (Target Therapeutics), or the 'Probing' catheter of Bard. These are fine catheters similar to a PTCA catheter but without a balloon. This is also taken up to near the tip of the guide wire. The original rationale for the use of this non balloon catheter was that it was cheaper than an angioplasty balloon catheter. As there is now little difference in price, it is simpler and quicker to use a small size PTCA balloon, e.g. 1.5 mm balloon.

2. *Magnum, Terumo and Laser Wires*
   These are all discussed in Chapter 3. The Magnum wire is specifically designed for use with chronic occlusions. Compared to a stiffer guide wire, the technique with the magnum wire is slightly more complicated and it is used only by a minority of operators.
3. *Rotacs (Rotational Angioplasty Catheter System) Drill* (P Osypka, GmbH)
   A battery powered unit drives a flexible stainless steel shaft with an olive shaped tip, 1.2–1.6 mm in diameter. The drive shaft rotates at a slow speed of up to 200 revolutions per minute. An 0.014 inch guide wire can pass through the hollow steel shaft to exit the olive. The olive drill is advanced across the occlusion with short bursts of rotation. The risks of vessel perforation are small, but vessel dissection and the tip becoming stuck within the occlusion, may occur. The technique is not widely used.

Techniques to Use for Typical Case of PTCA for Chronic Occlusion
(Angiogram 19.1)

1. *Good Guide Catheter Backup*
   Select a guide catheter for its good support, such as an Amplatz catheter. Ensure with the control angios that there is good guide catheter stability and support — "you are going to need it"! (See also Chapter 1 on guide catheters and page 89).
2. *Crossing of the Lesion with the Guide Wire*
   Using a firmer guide wire within a small size (or the smallest, 1.5 mm) balloon with as lower profile as possible, the system is advanced to the proximal vessel. The guide wire tip is taken to the lesion, followed by the balloon catheter to near the end of the guide wire tip. The tip is advanced and withdrawn, whilst being rotated also and may pass along into the lesion. Check in the working and backup radiographic views, that the course of the guide wire is along that of the vessel. Remember that a stiff guide wire emerging from a PTCA balloon is "like a dart" being thrown against the occlusion or the vessel wall. Perforation of the coronary artery is surprisingly rare, but more common is to proceed within and along the wall rather than the true lumen. After initial resistance, when the guide wire is judged to have reached the distal vessel, it should run freely, if it does not and it is still necessary to push quite hard to proceed, the guide wire is probably dissecting the vessel wall.
   Have a low threshold to stop. With the stiff guide wire technique, it will either cross relatively quickly (in 5–10 minutes) and 'work', or it will not. Prolonged attempts with several wires etc. will only lead to dissecting the coronary, or worse. Once the guide wire has crossed try to pass it as distally as possible. Prograde injections from the guide catheter will often fail to show the distal vessel. Check on other views to try and ensure the course for the distal vessel is correct e.g. the down, curve up and then down, of the track of the RCA in the LAO view (see Angiogram 15.1, page 170). Sometimes it turns out that the guide wire has passed down a diagonal branch rather than the main LAD. If the branch is some way from the occlusion the guide wire can be left there.

   Check with contrast injections to assess progress and the state of the distal artery. If an extensive dissection pattern is seen from the guide wire passing along the wall, rather than the true lumen, the vessel is unlikely to remain open and abandon the

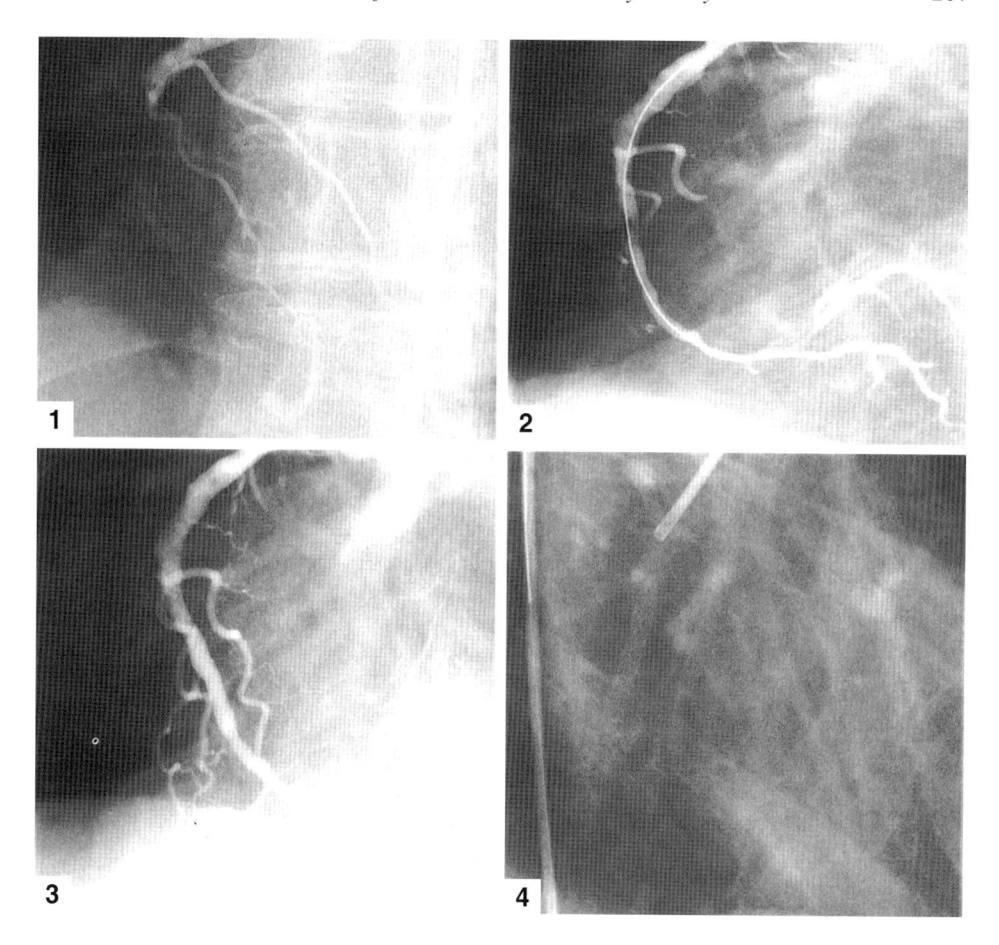

Angiogram 19.1. *PTCA for chronic occlusion of large calibre RCA.* The patient had sustained an inferior myocardial infarction six months earlier. A chronic occlusion of a large calibre RCA is seen beyond the marginal branch (1). There is no stub of normal vessel leading down into the occlusion. An 0.016 Standard guide wire (Bard) within a 1.5 mm balloon crossed the occlusion. After dilatation with a 3 mm balloon, a 15 mm Palmaz-Schatz stent (J & J CPS153) was delivered on a 3.5 mm Speedy balloon inflated to 16 atmospheres. There was a short (outflow) dissection at the distal end of the stent (2). A further short stent (half 15 mm Palmaz-Schatz stent) was delivered through the first stent overlapping its distal end. The second stent was inflated to 14 atmospheres and the final result is shown in (3). The overlapping stents (1 1/2 Palmaz-Schatz) were seen on fluoroscopy in the RAO projection (4).

procedure sooner rather than later. One possible way out in this situation is to consider the use of a long Wallstent to 'reconstruct' the artery.
3. *Crossing of the Balloon Catheter*
   Ensure optimal Guide catheter backup, if necessary deeply engage the guide catheter.
   Advance the balloon across the lesion. With modern low profile balloons, often the correct size for the vessel will cross. If it will not cross, go down to the smallest size, 1.5 mm and try again. Alternatively start with the 1.5 mm balloon and go up to the larger balloon.

If the procedure is successful, check the distal vessel as a mild lesion on the control angiogram may be more severe once prograde flow has been re-established. Check also there has been no distal embolisation.

If a non balloon catheter such as a Tracker 18 has been used to support the guide wire, attempt to advance this along the guide wire and across the lesion and often it will be possible. To replace this catheter with a balloon catheter, the guide wire can be extended, or the catheter can be "injected out" along the guide wire, using the Cumberland technique (see page 37).

4. *Consider Stent Deployment*

   If the vessel calibre and proximal anatomy will allow, consider the elective use of a stent, which will reduce vessel recoil and by maintaining a good coronary flow will reduce rethrombosis (Angiogram 19.1). The restenosis or reocclusion rate after stenting, is reduced compared to balloon angioplasty.

5. *Assess the Result of PTCA*

   If a stent is not suitable, assess the result after a 15 minute wait without the guide wire. Sometimes the vessel can already be seen to be closing down. If this occurs accept the inevitable, or consider redilatation and or reconsider the use of a stent.

   If the result remains satisfactory and a stent has not been used, consider IV heparin for 24 hours and or oral anticoagulation for 3 months to reduce risk of re-occlusion.

Follow-up after PTCA for Total Occlusion

Symptomatic progress may be sufficient. However re-occlusion may be silent and sometimes symptoms may be difficult to assess or be more severe than expected, especially with occlusion of a single coronary artery. Hence consider re-angiography at 4 months using small calibre 4 or 5F catheters, which can be a simple relatively quick and painless exercise to give a definitive opinion on the long term result.

Conclusion

If an occlusion is recent, PTCA is usually straight forward. For chronic total occlusion, the acute and long term success is much less favourable. Care is needed in the selection of cases to attempt angioplasty. If the guide wire does cross the occlusion, stent placement if feasible will improve the long term result.

20 PTCA Post CABG

Recurrent angina after previous coronary artery bypass surgery (CABG) is an increasing problem; about 10–20% of PTCAs are for this purpose.

Causes of Recurrent Angina Post CABG

1. *Old Vein Grafts*
   After one year following surgery, intimal hyperplasia, atheroma and thrombosis progressively develop, so that approximately 50% of vein grafts have closed within five years. A stenosis and or occlusion can occur at any site along the graft. The narrowings may be localised or diffuse. The atheroma is often very friable and prone to dislodgement and embolism.
2. *Early Post Operative (2–6 Months after Surgery).*
   A technical problem may occur with a vein graft or an internal mammary artery, with a stenosis at the anastomosis site of the graft with the native coronary artery. This type of lesion responds well to PTCA. Sometimes a problem occurs at a site of kinking along the shaft of the graft. Rarely the cause for early recurrent angina is inadequate revascularization, with failure of an important vessel to be grafted; this may or may not be amenable to PTCA.
3. *Progression of Native Coronary Artery Disease.*
   A vessel not previously grafted develops a severe stenosis. A grafted vessel develops distal disease beyond the anastomosis.

Frequently, 5–10 years post CABG, there is a new progressive disease of both grafts and native coronary vessels. Graft closure may be silent or present as unstable angina or acute MI. Often the patient will have more than one vessel or graft needing attention. Sometimes a clear cut 'culprit lesion' can be identified. A patient may have had mild angina for some months or even years, but is admitted with unstable angina. One vessel, a native coronary artery or a graft has a severe or critical stenosis and ECG changes may be in the territory supplied by the vessel.

This chapter will discuss the management of PTCA for the post CABG patient in general and specifically consider PTCA of saphenous vein grafts (SVGs). Chapter 21 will describe PTCA of the left internal mammary artery (LIMA) grafts.

Special Problems of Post CABG Patients

1. *Higher Risk Patients*
   The patients are older, have poorer LV function and more 3 vessel disease than the average PTCA patient.
2. *Emergency CABG is often Difficult or Impossible*
   After previous CABG, adhesions prevent a rapid exposure of the heart. There is a risk of damage to previous grafts, especially when there is an internal mammary artery graft. If a vessel occludes at PTCA it may be necessary to 'weather the storm' and accept a myocardial infarction. Emergency CABG for this group of patients is used in less than 1% of cases, compared to 2–3% of routine PTCA procedures.
3. *Risk of Vein Graft Embolism*
   The atheroma is very friable and prone to embolism during PTCA, especially with the use of stents.
4. *Technical Problems with PTCA Procedure*
   These include:
   a) Poor guide catheter back-up with some vein grafts.
   b) Long tortuous course of internal mammary arteries.
   c) Risk of damage to osteum of graft.
   d) Diffuse disease of grafts is common.
   e) Osteal stenosis is relatively common and is difficult technically to treat.
5. *Restenosis*
   In SVG's the rate is *higher* than in native coronary arteries, at about 50% compared to 30%. It also occurs over a *longer time frame* of 6–24 months, as opposed to 3–6 months after PTCA of native coronary arteries.
6. *Graft Disease is Progressive*
   Once lesions in old vein grafts (5–10 years post CABG) become a clinical problem, there is a high chance of further lesions and recurrent symptoms over the 2 years after successful PTCA. This risk has to be weighed against the increased surgical risk of 5–7% mortality for re-do CABG. It can be a difficult judgement sometimes whether to consider PTCA or re-do CABG.
7. *Single Remaining Artery*
   These patients with just one remaining vessel (graft or native coronary artery) have nearly always had previous CABG. They often have poor LV function and may have serious general medical conditions. The risks of PTCA (or CABG) will be high and these need to be explained to the patient and relatives.

Advantages of Post CABG Angioplasty

Every cloud has a silver lining and post CABG procedures are no exception. Advantages include:

1. *SVGs (saphenous vein grafts) are of large calibre.*
   SVGs are often 3.5–4.0 mm in calibre and allow stents to be used.
2. *Stent thrombosis is rare.*
   In most cases, elective stenting in SVG's carries the lowest risk for stent thrombosis, less than 0.5%. This may be due to the larger calibre of SVGs.
3. *No side branches.*
   SVGs have no side branches, are usually relatively straight and do not have overlapping branches from other vessels, as occurs in the left coronary artery. Unfortunately, the absence of side branches makes positioning of stents more difficult, as they are not available as land marks.
4. *Native coronary artery protected by a graft.*
   After CABG a left main stem lesion can be dilated if either the LAD or LCX has a well function graft. The same is true for dilatation of the LAD if there is a well functioning graft to the LCX, or vice versa.
5. *Less revascularization is acceptable.*
   In the older post CABG patient, it is often acceptable to reduce angina rather than to eliminate it completely.

Management of Post CABG Case

1. *Ad hoc PTCA*
   'Angiogram proceed directly to PTCA' can be considered, but as the anatomy and disease is likely to be complicated, these patients are less commonly candidates.
2. *Patient review*
   a) Carefully Assess Symptoms and Signs.
      Be on the lookout for signs of impaired LV function, renal impairment, carotid and peripheral vascular disease.
   b) Assess Severity of Symptoms.
      Assess life style and its interruption. Many of the patients are elderly and some take little exercise. Review the non invasive data, including the exercise test.
   c) Review Medical Treatment
      Ensure that the patient is on aspirin. Some patients are on warfarin to maintain graft patency, or because they have atrial fibrillation and reduced LV function. This drug will need to be reduced or stopped for a few days before the procedure.
   d) Discussion with Patient and Relatives.
      This should include the increased risks, possible use of stent and that emergency CABG may not be appropriate if vessel occludes.
3. *Review of all previous angiograms*
   Where possible review pre operative (CABG) angiogram and any subsequent angiograms where perhaps medical treatment was perused. Some patients have had several angiograms besides the latest diagnostic angiogram. An earlier angiogram may show that a vessel was of much larger calibre in the past than seen on the latest angio, i.e. it is more important and might take a larger balloon size or even a stent.
   Try to read the details of the operation notes. From all of these:
   a) *Decide on PTCA of SVG or native coronary vessel or both.*

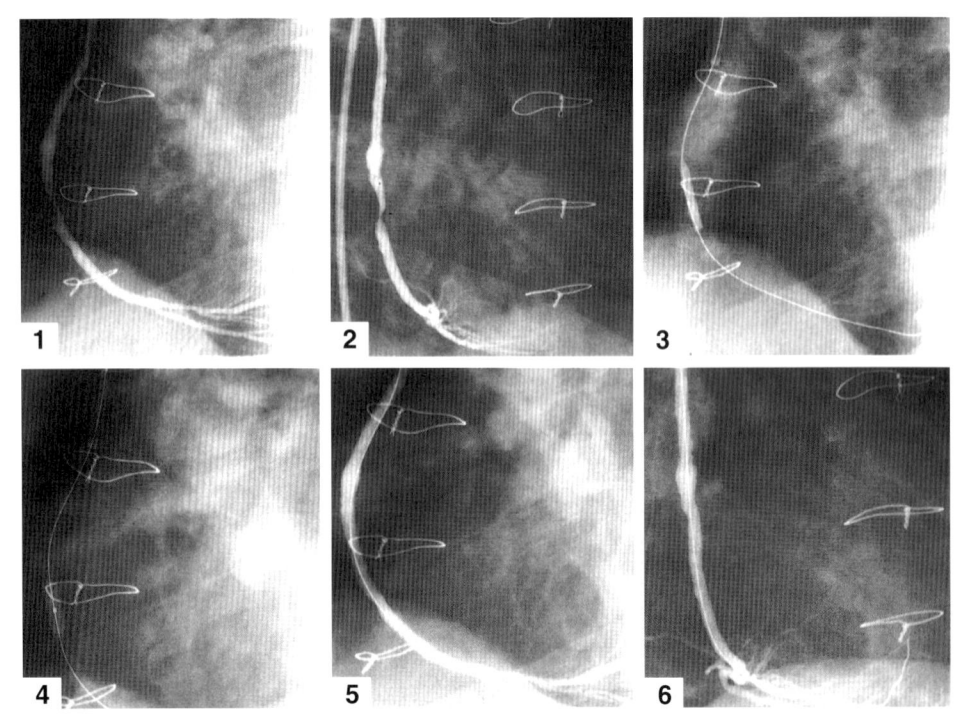

Angiogram 20.1. *PTCA and stenting of stenosis of RCA graft.* A short lesion in a seven year-old graft to RCA (1 and 2). Note relationship of the lesion to sternal wires, which are also very helpful to locate the osteum of the graft. The RCA graft, as is usual passes vertically downwards and is suitable to cannulate with a 7F Multipurpose (A-2) catheter (3). The lesion was easily crossed with an 0.014" guide wire and pre-dilated with a 3 mm balloon to 4 atmospheres. A 15 mm Palmaz-Schatz (PS153) stent was hand crimped onto the balloon and deployed at the lesion at 10 atmospheres. The stent was further dilated to 14 atmospheres with a 3.5 mm Chubby (Schneider) balloon (4) to give a very satisfactory final result (5 and 6). Note the presence of a mildly dilated segment probably respresenting a venous valve above the lesion. Above the dilated segment the vessel lumen is irregular both before and after stent delivery (2 and 6). The views are LAO 60° and RAO 30°.

b) *Stent deployment.*
1) Consider which type(s) and how many may be needed.
   Usually SVGs are of large calibre and can take a stent. The disease may be a short localised lesion, sufficient to be covered by one stent (see Angiogram 20.1). If the disease is long and diffuse, consider using a Wallstent (see Angiogram 20.2), or a longer version of other stents, or more than one stent.
2) Is there osteal disease? This will limit the placement a guide catheter in the graft. It will impede the passage of a stent down the graft to a lesion. However, stenting the osteum is a good form of treatment for osteal stenosis.
3) Is there proximal disease? Even mild disease may inhibit tracking of a stent and increase the risk of dislodgement of atheroma and distal embolism.
4) Is initial course of graft unfavourable? Sometimes an LAD or LCX graft can have a initial course which is tortuous and or has a right angle bend, making it difficult to track a rigid Palmaz-Schatz stent to the lesion.

c) *Locate the site of the origin of grafts*
Look carefully for the osteum of a graft, in relation to local landmarks, especially sternal wires, as seen in the LAO projection.

It can be frustrating (to say the least!) when unable to enter a graft with the guide catheter, that was clearly shown on the diagnostic angiogram. Sometimes this is due to a degree of osteal stenosis, allowing cannulation with a smaller diagnostic catheter but not with an angioplasty guide catheter.

d) *Select appropriate guide catheters*
For RCA graft a multipurpose or JR4 are often suitable.
For LAD and LCX grafts JR4 or Amplatz Right I (AR1) are often suitable.

e) *Assess Course of Graft and Possible Back-up.*
Has the initial course a severe bend?
How easy will it be to pass a stent?
Is there proximal disease prior to the lesion?

f) *Assess radiographic views for the procedure.*
These will need to be suitable for the vein graft(s) and or the native coronary arteries as necessary (see page 56).

4. *Have a plan for graft embolism* (see below, page 215)
Consider the arrangements for an IABP and the drugs which may be needed.
Consider the use of a small sheath (5F) for the contralateral femoral artery to give prompt access of an IABP ... one may be needed in a hurry!

5. *Discussion with surgeons*
Have a lower threshold to discuss the case. Have a joint view, if possible with the surgeon who did the original operation, that PTCA rather CABG is the appropriate treatment and whether emergency CABG will be an option during PTCA should the vessel occlude.

PTCA Graft Procedure

1. **Guide catheter.**
   a) *Consider the use of a long femoral sheath.*
   The patients are often older and may have tortuous iliac arteries and more manipulation of the guide catheter than usual may be needed for graft cannulation.
   b) *Attempt to achieve good back-up.*
   This can be difficult and a less than ideal amount of back-up and positioning of the guide catheter may have to be accepted. This may make passage of the stent more uncertain.
   c) *Care not to damage the osteum.*
   Be particularly gentle with the guide catheter as there is an increased risk to damage the osteum of SVGs.
   d) *RCA graft.*
   These often pass vertically down from the ascending aorta (Angiogram 20.1). They will allow a multipurpose or Judkins right 4 cm (JR4) to be passed down the graft to near the lesion. This gives very good backup and reduces the risk of dislodgement of atheroma particularly by a stent. However, the catheter may partially block the

graft and give ischaemia; this is rare as the grafts are usually of large calibre. The guide catheter itself may also dislodge atheroma. Deep passage of a guide catheter to near the lesion in a RCA graft often works very well, especially if smaller size guide catheters such as 7F or 6F are used.

2. **Guide Wire.**
   a) *Be on the lookout for graft embolism.*
      From start of the passage of guide wire, to the end of the case be ready to recognise and treat this complication ... and it probably then won't occur!
   b) *Guide wire passage.*
      This is usually easy as there are no side branches. Attempt to pass the guide wire as distally as possible, preferably into the native coronary artery. This will allow the stiffer proximal section of the guide wire to cover the lesion and aid tracking of the stent down the graft (see also page 133). If embolism occurs a guide wire into the native coronary vessel will prevent complete blockage by the embolus.

3. **Balloon.**
   a) *Assess tracking of balloon* i.e. how easy is it to pass the balloon down to the lesion. This can give some information as to how well the stent may later track.
   b) *Predilate the lesion.*
      With a 2.5 mm balloon to allow a stent to later cross the lesion.
   c) *Perfusion balloon.*
      Consider using one of these with a prolonged inflation (5–7 minutes), if the graft calibre is too small to deploy a stent, which is unusual. Against their use, is the fact that they are relatively bulky and perhaps at greater risk to cause graft embolism. Also ideally, the guide wire needs to be withdrawn proximal to the balloon during inflation, which is undesirable in graft cases with a risk of embolism. Often a prolonged inflation of 5–7 mins can be achieved with a routine balloon, especially if a long inflation is proceeded by 1 or 2 shorter ones (taking the benefit of preconditioning (see page 92).

4. **Stent.**
   a) *Risk of embolism.*
      This is greatest when passing a stent. The rigid metal cuts and displaces the graft debris, whereas a balloon catheter tends to slip through clefts.
   b) *Tracking of the stent.*
      This is often easy as grafts are usually relatively straight. Sometimes it can be very difficult, especially if the severity of 'minor' proximal disease has been underestimated. Resist the temptation to 'force' the stent down to the lesion. There is the risk both of dislodging the stent and of causing graft embolism.
   c) *Proximal and distal tears.*
      With SVGs there seems to be a greater incidence of a short dissection at either end of the stent. This will need treatment with deployment of a further short stent. If untreated, inflow or outflow obstruction to the stent will lead to stent closure. Sometimes redilatation with a balloon of the lesion may be successful. However redilatation may make matters worse and there is always doubt as to how successful merely ballooning the lesion has been. For dissection at an end of the stent, have a low threshold to electively deploy another stent.

5. **New Lesions — Spasm.**
   These are always worrying particularly with SVGs, as they may represent damage to the friable atheroma. However spasm is often the cause and it seems to be commoner just after a stent has been passed. It is more frequent with the stiffer 'extra backup' wires, but can also occur with routine guide wires. If the patient's condition is stable, without evidence of graft embolism, inject down the graft, 0.1–0.3 mgm of GTN or 1–3 mgm of isosorbide dinitrate.

6. **Graft Embolism — "No reflow Phenomenon".**
   This is the "feared" complication of graft PTCA, occurring in about 10% of cases. All the time one should be trying to prevent it by careful instrumentation within the graft. All the time be on the lookout for its development. A clear plan of action to treat this complication is needed.

   Cardiac surgeons performing redo CABG's, comment on how much debris or "gunge" is present within the lumen of old SVGs. The atheroma is very friable and "just waiting to embolize". It is amazing the embolism does not occur more often.

The severity of the syndrome will vary on the amount of embolism and as to how important is the distal coronary artery.

Typically there is:

1. *Intense chest pain.*
   This is often more severe and "sharper" than the usual anginal pain.
2. *Prominent S-T elevation on the ECG.*
3. *Varying haemodynamic consequences.*
   A fall in blood pressure is common. This can be profound leading to cardiac arrest.
4. *Arrhythmias.*
   These may occur induced by ischaemia. They are not particularly a problem. Bradycardias, secondary to the pain are more frequent than ventricular tachyarrhythmias.
5. *Angiograms showing a variety of pictures from:*
   a) Virtually nothing — graft and distal coronary arteries appear normal.
   b) Very poor flow into and clearance of contrast from the native coronary artery bed. This is due to intense coronary artery spasm and is known as the *"no reflow" phenomenon.*
   c) A clear filling defect in the distal coronary artery and or distal graft. This is unusual.

Natural History of Graft Embolism

After 30 mins to 2 hours the effects will often resolve completely and if the circulation can be supported, a full recovery is possible. Left untreated and sometimes despite treatment, myocardial infarction and severe hypotension can ensue.

Treatment

1. **Be prepared for it.**
   Be ready to recognise and treat it. Keep passage of balloons and stents to a minimum. Don't treat borderline lesions.

Have a list of drugs and doses available up on a wall of the catheter room, or given to the nurse before the start of the procedure.

2. **Verapamil**
   Verapamil given into the graft or intravenously is very helpful to relieve spasm. It may also act like a cardioplegia. The dose is 0.5–1.0 mgm, repeated as necessary to 3–4 mgm as necessary. Be on the lookout for heart block, especially if injected into a graft supplying the RCA.

3. **Nitrates**
   Nitrate boluses are given into the graft or intravenously using glycerlyl trinitrate (GTN) or isosorbide dinitrate (ISDN). For GTN, 0.1–0.3 mgm are given. Nitrocine with a sodium rather than potassium base is the preferred preparation of GTN. For ISDN 1–3 mgm is used.

   The bolus(es) are followed by a nitrate infusion such as GTN 1–10 mgm/hour, or ISDN 2–10 mgm/hour. (If an ampoule GTN contains 50 mgm in 10 ml. Draw up into a 50 ml syringe and add 40 ml of normal saline. The syringe then has 1 mgm of GTN/ml. Administer using an infusion pump).

4. **Adenosine**
   12 microgram boluses of adenosine can vasodilate the distal coronary bed. The effect is short-lived, 1–2 minutes or less and repeat doses can be given.

5. **Intravenous Fluids**
   Give dextrose saline to maintain the blood pressure, especially after vasodilatation caused by treatment with nitrates. Alternatively, use a plasma substitute such as Haemaccel (Hoechst, Marion, Roussel) or Dextran.

6. **Oxygen via face mask.**
   If the patient is not routinely receiving oxygen for the PTCA procedure, this should be started to maximise myocardial and tissue oxygenation.

7. **Dopamine infusion.**
   If the patient is hypotensive give dopamine at 5 micrograms/kg/min.
   (Prepare an infusion pump containing 200 mgm of dopamine in 5 ml + 45 ml of saline or 5% dextrose to give 4000 micrograms/ml.
   The formula for a 70 kgm patient commencing at 5 micrograms/kg/min is:
   $5 \times 70 \times 60$ = dose/body weight/hour
   $5 \times 70 \times 60$ divided by 4000 (strength of solution) = ml/hour = 5.2 ml/hour = approximately 5 ml/hour).

8. **Intra Aortic Balloon Pump.**
   Use this earlier rather than later. It may greatly improve the blood pressure and the clinical status of the patient.

9. **Consider Adrenaline**
   Give 50–100 micrograms intravenously or into the graft. (1 in 10,000 of adrenaline = 100 micrograms/ml. Give 0.5–1.0 ml = 50–100 micrograms.)
   This may help to improve myocardial contraction, but may also induce ventricular arrhythmias.

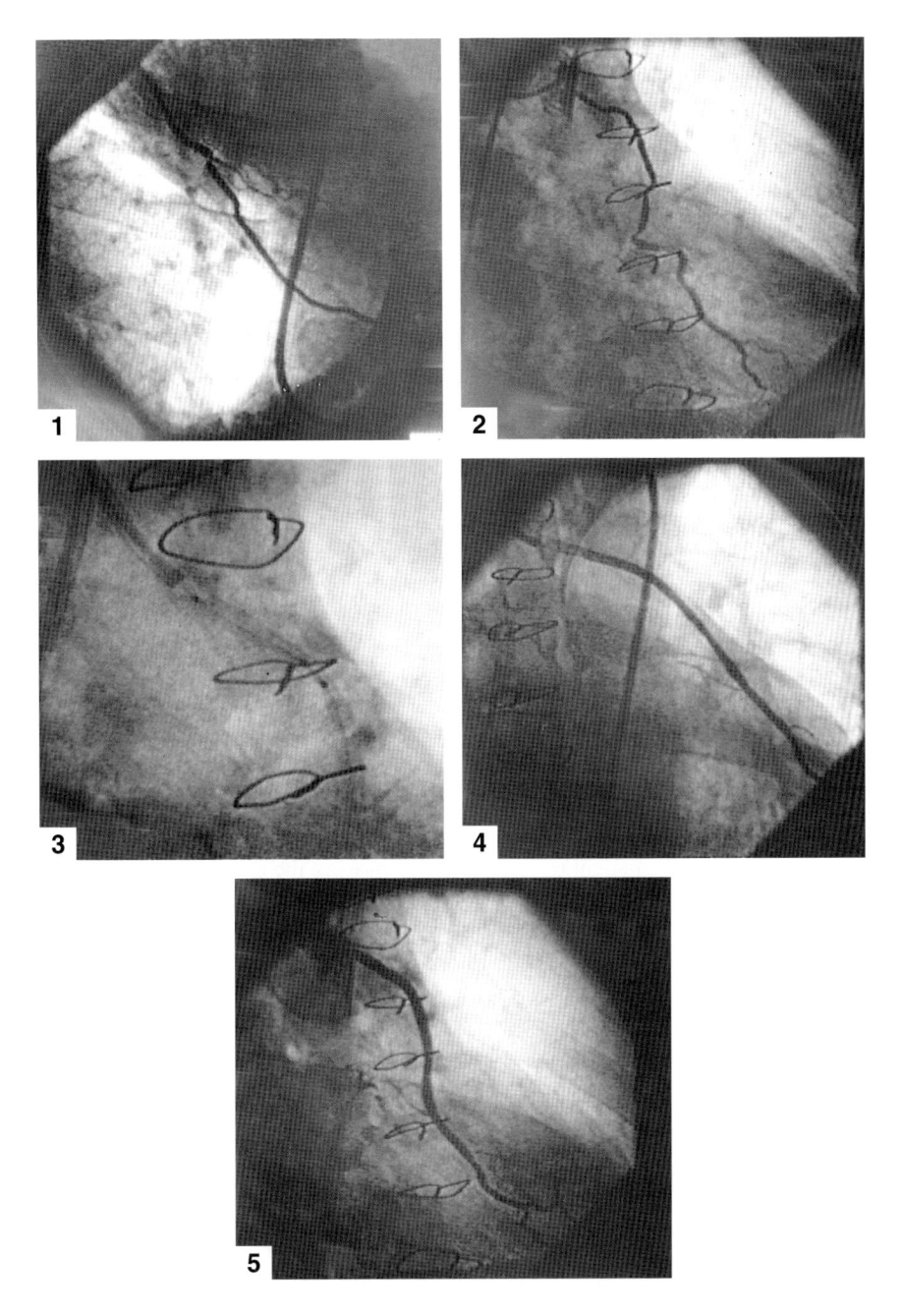

Angiogram 20.2. *PTCA for diffuse disease in a saphenous vein graft.* There is diffuse disease of the LCX graft, with a lesion at its start (which is not well seen), two lesions in the body and one at the anastomosis with the OM branch. The graft is shown in the PA and RAO caudal projections (1 and 2). With a S'port exchange guide wire the lesions were predilated with 2.5 and 3 mm balloons. A sheathed 3.5 mm × 15 mm ACS Multilink stent was placed at the origin of the vessel, followed by two overlapping Wallstents, 4.5 mm by 49 and 32 mm (3). The stents were postdilated with a 3.5 mm × 10 mm balloon to 10 atmospheres. The final result (4 and 5) is very good, and the whole LCX graft has been reconstructed. Angiogram kindly supplied by Dr Martyn Thomas, Kings College Hospital, London.

10. **Consider Vasoconstrictors**
    If the blood pressure remains low, especially after verapamil and nitrate boluses, whilst the IABP is being organised, a vasoconstricting drug can be helpful to maintain the blood pressure. Its effect will be short lasting, only 1–3 minutes.
    Give:
    Phenylephrine 0.1–0.3 mgm intravenously.
    (10 mg of phenylephrine in 1 ml. Take 0.1 ml into a 10 ml syringe of dextrose or saline. Give 1–3 ml).
    Noradrenaline 50–75 micrograms intravenously.
    (1 in 10,000 noradrenaline = 100 micrograms per ml. Give 0.5–0.75 ml).

11. **Anaesthetic assistance.**
    The patient may arrest, or to be near to it, having deteriorated seriously. An anaesthetist can be very helpful, supervising the airway and the administration of drugs.

12. **Pacing catheter.**
    Be prepared for heart block, but a pacing catheter only needs to be inserted if there is a specific need.
    Sometimes the vessel being dilated, e.g. an RCA graft will have an increased risk of heart block if occlusion occurs. In this situation a prophylactic pacing wire inserted via the femoral vein at the start of the procedure may be considered.

Weather the Storm

It usually takes about 40 minutes for the features of graft embolism to recede. The chest pain eases, the S-T elevation settles and the blood pressure rises. There is little or no advantage in referring the patient to surgery, as by-passing the embolized coronary artery is not usually helpful or easily achieved with speed. The main benefit from surgery may be a period on cardiopulmonary bypass and support.

The patient may sustain a myocardial infarct but more usually, perhaps in about 60% of cases, a transmural infarction with new Q-waves is avoided.

PTCA of the Native Coronary Artery

If this can be performed, it is usually simpler than PTCA of a graft. If the lesion can be approached along the native coronary artery, the procedure is that of a routine PTCA. Sometimes a grafted vessel which is occluded proximal to the graft, has a lesion a short distance down from the anastomosis site. The lesion may only be approached via the graft. Usually this will be straight forward to dilate via the graft. Use of a stent will increase the risk, as it may dislodge atheroma in the graft as it tracks down to the lesion. RCA grafts in particular seem to be associated with lesions a short distance beyond the anastomosis and usually do very well with PTCA.

Post PTCA Procedure

There is nothing special from the routine procedure described on pages 74 and 153. Reinforcement of measures to reduce risk factors should be given. Review serum lipids and treat if the cholesterol is above 5.0 mmol/litre. If the patient has received a stent, ensure that he or she knows what to do if stent thrombosis occurs and about the treatment with Ticlopidine if this has been given (see page 154).

Old Vein Grafts? Warfarin

There is anecdotal evidence suggesting that long term warfarin may reduce the risk of subsequent SVG occlusion where there is moderate or diffuse disease. Low dose warfarin is not sufficient and if used the dose of warfarin needs to achieve an INR of 2.5–3.5:1.

Conclusion

PTCA post CABG is an important and increasing indication for the procedure. The patients are of higher risk and emergency CABG is often not appropriate. PTCA of a native coronary artery is a routine procedure. PTCA of a SVG has the specific serious complication of graft embolism. Patients who receive PTCA and a stent for a diseased vein graft usually do well in the short term, but have a moderately high risk for further problems due to progressive disease in the grafts elsewhere.

For recurrent angina post CABG usually both the patient and the surgeon prefer PTCA rather than redo CABG ... and the cardiologist is only too happy to oblige!

21 LIMA PTCA

When the LAD is bypassed with the left internal mammary artery (LIMA) as the graft, its long term patency is much improved compared to after a saphenous vein graft (SVG). The increased patency is due to atheroma rarely developing within the internal mammary artery. CABG now routinely involves the LIMA for grafting of the LAD. Often the right internal mammary artery (RIMA) is used for the RCA or LCX. Sometimes other arterial conduits are used such as a segment of radial artery, or the gastroepiploic artery to distal RCA.

This chapter will discuss LIMA angioplasty, but the same principles will apply to PTCA of a RIMA graft.

The commonest situation requiring PTCA is early post-operative recurrent angina, 1–6 months post CABG, with a stenosis at the insertion site of the LIMA into the native LAD.

LIMA angioplasty is more complicated than routine PTCA, partly because it is performed less frequently. The special problems include:

1. Cannulation of LIMA.
2. Poor guide catheter backup.
3. Damage to the osteum.
4. Long tortuous course.

Cannulation of LIMA

This can be difficult, but may be achieved in three stages (see Figure 21.1 and Angiogram 21.1):

1. *In Shallow LAO 10°–20°*
   Pass a straight 0.032" or 0.035" guide wire through the LIMA guide catheter so that its floppy tip is protruding about 1 cm from the end of the catheter. With the catheter

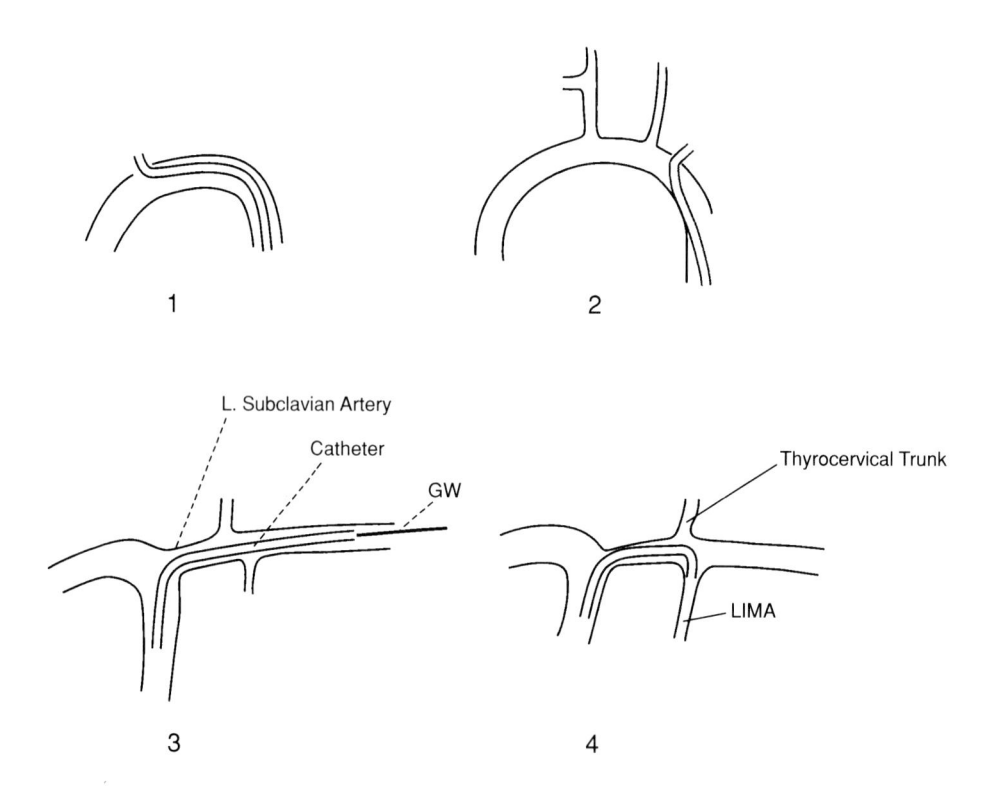

Figure 21.1. *Cannulation of LIMA.* 1) LAO 10–20°. Pull back LIMA catheter with GW protruding one cm, and tip of catheter facing upwards. Catheter may enter Innominate or L. carotid artery. 2) Pull catheter back until it "pops" into L. subclavian artery. 3) RAO 10–20°. Advance guide wire (GW) along vessel and well down into subclavian artery. 4) Remove GW. Slowly withdraw LIMA catheter, injecting small amounts of contrast. When LIMA vessel is seen or "ghosts", rotate catheter anticlockwise until tip falls into orifice of LIMA.

in the ascending aorta and its tip pointing to the aortic valve, withdraw and rotate the catheter anticlockwise so that the tip faces upwards. As the catheter is withdrawn along the arch of the aorta, avoid or pull out the catheter tip from the innominate or left carotid arteries. The catheter tip will slip into the third artery along, i.e. the left subclavian artery.

2. *Turn to Shallow RAO 10°–20°*

   Pass the guide wire well down into the left subclavian artery i.e. 4–5" (5–10 cm) along. If the guide wire will not pass into the distal subclavian artery beyond the branches (vertebral artery, thyro-cervical trunk, and costo-cervical trunk), change it to an 0.035" Wholey Wire which has very good torque control (Wholey HiTorque Modified J Guide Wire System. 0.035 inch. 145 cm. Malinckrodt). Advance the LIMA catheter along the guide wire, well down into the subclavian artery.

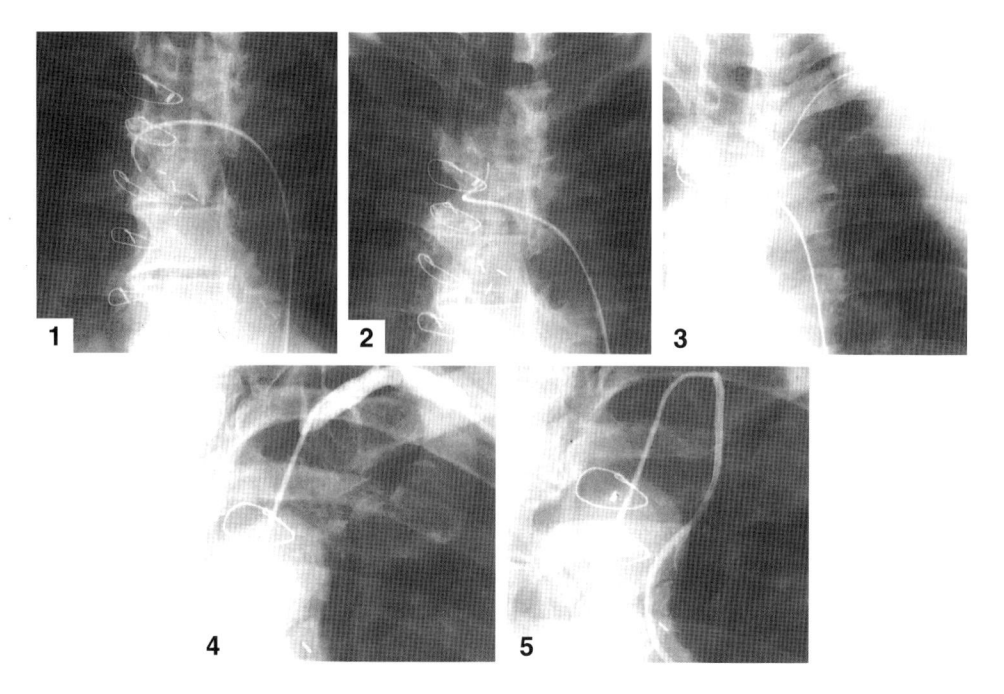

Angiogram 21.1. *Catheterization of the left internal mammary artery (LIMA).* In a shallow LAO 10° projection the LIMA (or JR4) catheter is passed to the top of the ascending aorta (1). An 0.035" guide wire protrudes for about 1 cm from the tip of the catheter. The tip of the catheter is rotated to point upwards to the great arteries (2). The catheter is then withdrawn along the arch of the aorta until the left subclavian artery is entered. The guide wire is advanced along the artery beyond the thyro-cervical trunk into the distal artery (3). If negotiating the guide wire to the distal subclavian artery is difficult, it is changed to a Wholey wire which is easier to pass distally. The guide catheter is advanced along the guide wire into the distal subclavian artery. The guide wire is removed and in shallow RAO°, the catheter is slowly withdrawn as injections are made until the LIMA begins to 'ghost' (4). The catheter tip is rotated and withdrawn gently to intubate the LIMA (5).

3. *Withdraw Slowly LIMA Catheter*
   Give small test dose injections until the LIMA is seen to fill or 'ghost'. Rotate the catheter with small movements usually anti clockwise, but sometimes clockwise, to engage the LIMA.

   Preferably use a 7F or 6F catheter rather than 8F especially in women. This will allow easier cannulation, as the LIMA is relatively small. The LIMA may become blocked by the catheter, and this is less likely with the smaller catheter sizes. GTN sublingually, or into the LIMA, may reduce spasm induced by the catheter.
   If cannulation of the *subclavian* artery is difficult, it may be easier to start with a 6F or 7F JR4 diagnostic catheter. Having entered the left subclavian artery the JR4 is exchanged over a long (260 cm) wire for the LIMA catheter. This is "fiddly" and best avoided if possible.

Poor Guide Catheter Backup

The shape of the LIMA catheter often gives very poor backup. Because of its curved shape it is not advisable to slide or deeply engage the catheter into the LIMA. There is often not much that can be done about poor guide catheter support.

Damage to the Osteum

The LIMA is a relatively small and fragile vessel, whilst the LIMA catheter itself is hooked shaped. Hence damage to the osteum may easily be produced and extra care and attention are needed to avoid this complication. As with dissection of the proximal RCA by a guide catheter, there can be no doubt that it was the operator who has been responsible for the dissection of the LIMA osteum … it cannot be blamed on to bad luck after inflating a balloon across a lesion!

Long Tortuous Course

The anatomy of the LIMA is quite variable. It is often very tortuous and sometimes extremely so, undergoing several "corkscrew" like turns. The tortuosity makes guide wire manipulation difficult, especially trying to rotate the tip away from a septal perforator once the guide wire has reached the LAD. If manipulation is a problem this may be eased by using a nitinol (Microvena), Terumo or a Choice PT plus (SciMed) wire (see pages 37, 38 and 35), which have very good trackability along a tortuous vessel. Another technique is to give extra support to the guide wire by passing it through a Tracker 18 catheter (see page 205).

The tortuosity and length may make tracking of the balloon difficult. With the modern low profile balloons this is now not usually a problem. If there is difficulty, including attempts to cross the lesion, one of the following may help:

1. Use the smallest (1.5 mm) lowest profile balloon available. Once the dilatation has been successful with this balloon, move up to the appropriate sized balloon.
2. Use a stiffer guide wire, such as an extra backup guide wire, or a standard/intermediate guide wire. These will all tend to straighten out the curves and aid tracking. Spasm in segments of the LIMA may be induced. As the LIMA is usually of small calibre, 2–3 mm, a coronary stent is not usually considered. The very tortuous course would also limit some stents such as the Palmaz-Schatz from being used.

    Sometimes because of the length and tortuosity of the LIMA, the balloon catheter is nearly at its hub by the time the tip has reached the LIMA/LAD anastomosis site. A special *long length shaft balloon* may be needed, and this should be anticipated (and ordered) when reviewing the diagnostic angiogram.
3. Use a fixed wire balloon such as the Probe (Bard), the Ace (Scimed), or the Lightning (Cordis).

Restenosis after LIMA PTCA

Anastomotic lesions at the junction site of LIMA and LAD do well and seem to have a low rate of restenosis. Hence though LIMA angioplasty is "fiddly", it is usually well worth while if the procedure is successful.

Other Arterial Conduits

All that has been written applies equally to the RIMA, apart from a slightly different method of cannulation, where the innominate artery is entered rather than the left subclavian artery.

For the gastro-epiploic artery, it is recommended that a joint procedure with a vascular radiologist be considered ... use someone else's experience (and previously climbed learning curve)!

Conclusion

LIMA angioplasty is more difficult as the procedures are infrequent, and the vessel is more difficult to cannulate, very tortuous and prone to spasm. The commonest lesion at the anastomosis site with the native LAD, usually responds well to angioplasty.

22 Osteal Lesions, Lesions on Bends and Undilatable Lesions

Osteal Lesions

An *osteal lesion* is one at the mouth or the very start of a coronary vessel. They occur at two sites:

a) *At the origin of a vessel arising from the aorta*
   These include osteal lesions of the RCA, LCA, saphenous venous grafts (SVGs) and the internal mammary artery.

b) *At the origin of a branch arsing from a larger coronary artery*
   These include the origin of the LAD or LCX from the main left coronary artery, or the posterior descending artery from the RCA, or a diagonal branch off the LAD. These osteal narrowings are really forms of bifurcation lesions, which are discussed in Chapter 23.

This chapter will discuss osteal lesions of vessels as they arise from the aorta. The commonest ones treated by PTCA are those on the RCA or a SVG.

Problems with Osteal Lesions

These include:

1. Difficulty to cannulate the vessel.
2. Instability of the whole PTCA system.
3. Difficulty to pass the guide wire.
4. Difficulty to dilate the lesion.
5. Difficulties to deploy a stent.
6. High restenosis rate.
7. Infrequency of the procedure.

1. **Difficulty to Cannulate the Vessel**

   The vessel is difficult to find and cannulate, as the osteum is stenosed. Once intubated, the recorded pressure is almost certain to damp off as the artery becomes occluded by the catheter. This can be partially relieved by use of a catheter with side holes, but often ischaemia still develops.

2. **Instability of the Whole PTCA System**

   To dilate the osteum it is necessary to withdraw the guide catheter out into the aorta. This is always a risky manoeuvre, as the guide catheter may then retract up the aorta, pulling with it the guide wire and the balloon catheter out of the artery, like a strand of spaghetti. Great care (and some luck) are needed as the guide catheter is withdrawn a short distance out of the vessel into the aorta.

3. **Difficulty to Pass the Guide Wire**

   As the guide catheter is barely across the lesion, it may be difficult to pass the guide wire across the osteum down into the main vessel. If the guide wire starts to buckle, withdraw it and readvance with a rotatory movement until the wire crosses and passes freely to the distal artery. Try to advance it as distally as possible.

4. **Difficulty to Dilate the Lesion**

   Attempting to pass the correct sized balloon may be difficult and will risk the guide wire prolapsing out of the vessel. Predilate with the smallest sized balloon available, usually of 1.5 mm diameter. When the correct sized balloon for the vessel is passed across the lesion and inflated, it may be seen to be fully expanded. However, when the balloon is deflated the lesion may still be there with very little improvement. Osteal lesions often have considerable *elastic recoil*, perhaps reflecting that the pathology lies in the aortic wall rather than in the vessel arising from it. This is particularly so for RCA and LCA lesions and less so for those of SVGs. Recoil of the lesion may be treated by using a stent, atherectomy, or rotoblator.

5. **Difficulties to Deploy a Stent**

   To position a stent accurately across an osteal lesion and without dropping it, is quite a challenge! The tasks include:

   a) *To Ensure Accurate Placement of the Stent*
   With the guide catheter outside the coronary artery, contrast injections show very poorly if at all, the osteum and where to place the stent. This breaks a 'rule of stenting', that the lesion should be well identifiable and visible before considering their use. It is better to err with the stent protruding out of the orifice into the aorta, rather than positioning it too far down the vessel and missing the true osteum. It is very helpful to use a stent mounted on a balloon with end markers to show *each end* of the stent, such as the AVE Micro or NIR stents.

   b) *To Avoid Damaging the Stent with the Guide Catheter*
   There is a great risk of damaging the stent with the tip guide catheter after it has been deployed. The guide catheter may 'snow plough' into the stent. Particular care is needed with the final angiograms after delivering the stent.

c) *Need to Use a Strong Stent*
   Strong radial strength is required for a stent to prevent the elastic recoil. The more rigid Palmaz-Schatz PS153 is ideal, but less easy to deploy.

6. High Restenosis Rate

The restenosis rate for an osteal lesion after simple balloon angioplasty is about 50%. Even using a stent restenosis is commoner, at about 20–30%, than when stenting a lesion further down the vessel.

7. Infrequency of the Procedure

Osteal lesions account for only about 2% of PTCA procedures and hence experience is limited ... one never quite ascends the learning curve!

The difficulties with osteal lesions lead more often to failure of the procedure, rather than emergency CABG. Before the procedure these cases are best reviewed with a surgeon and the reduced success rate explained to the patient and relatives.

Right Coronary Artery Osteal Lesions

These whilst a challenge, can be very rewarding to perform (Angiogram 22.1).

1. *Guide Catheter*
   The choice of the guide catheter is important. The aim is to select one that can more easily be retracted out of the coronary artery along the guide wire, to reduce the risk of pulling the guide wire out too. If the start of the RCA is straight or downward pointing, use a multipurpose (A-1 or A-2) shaped catheter which has a smooth final curve, reserving the JR4 or Amplatz right catheters if the RCA cannot be entered with the multipurpose catheter. If the RCA is upward pointing, PTCA will be even more difficult. An Arani catheter may be tried (see page 10).
2. *Guide wire and Balloon*
   The guide catheter should have side holes to reduce the problem of catheter induced ischaemia (see above, page 228). If, despite side-holes, ischaemia develops easily, have the guide wire and balloon already loaded in the guide catheter and on entering the RCA pass the guide wire as quickly (but also as carefully) as possible to the distal vessel and then withdraw the guide catheter. Predilate with a small balloon and then move up to the balloon size appropriate for the artery. Pass the balloon along the guide wire to a short distance beyond the osteum. Retract the guide catheter slowly and gently out of the RCA orifice. As this done also withdraw the balloon to position it correctly across the osteum. If the balloon is positioned at the osteum before withdrawal of the guide catheter, it too may be withdrawn and miss the osteum. The proximal end of the balloon is often near the tip of the guide catheter, but avoid the balloon lying within the tip and dilating the guide catheter too.

   After balloon dilatation there is often only minor improvement of the lesion as prominent elastic recoil is common.
3. *Stent*
   A similar technique is used to position the stent. With the tip of the guide catheter in the artery, the stent mounted balloon is passed into the proximal RCA beyond the

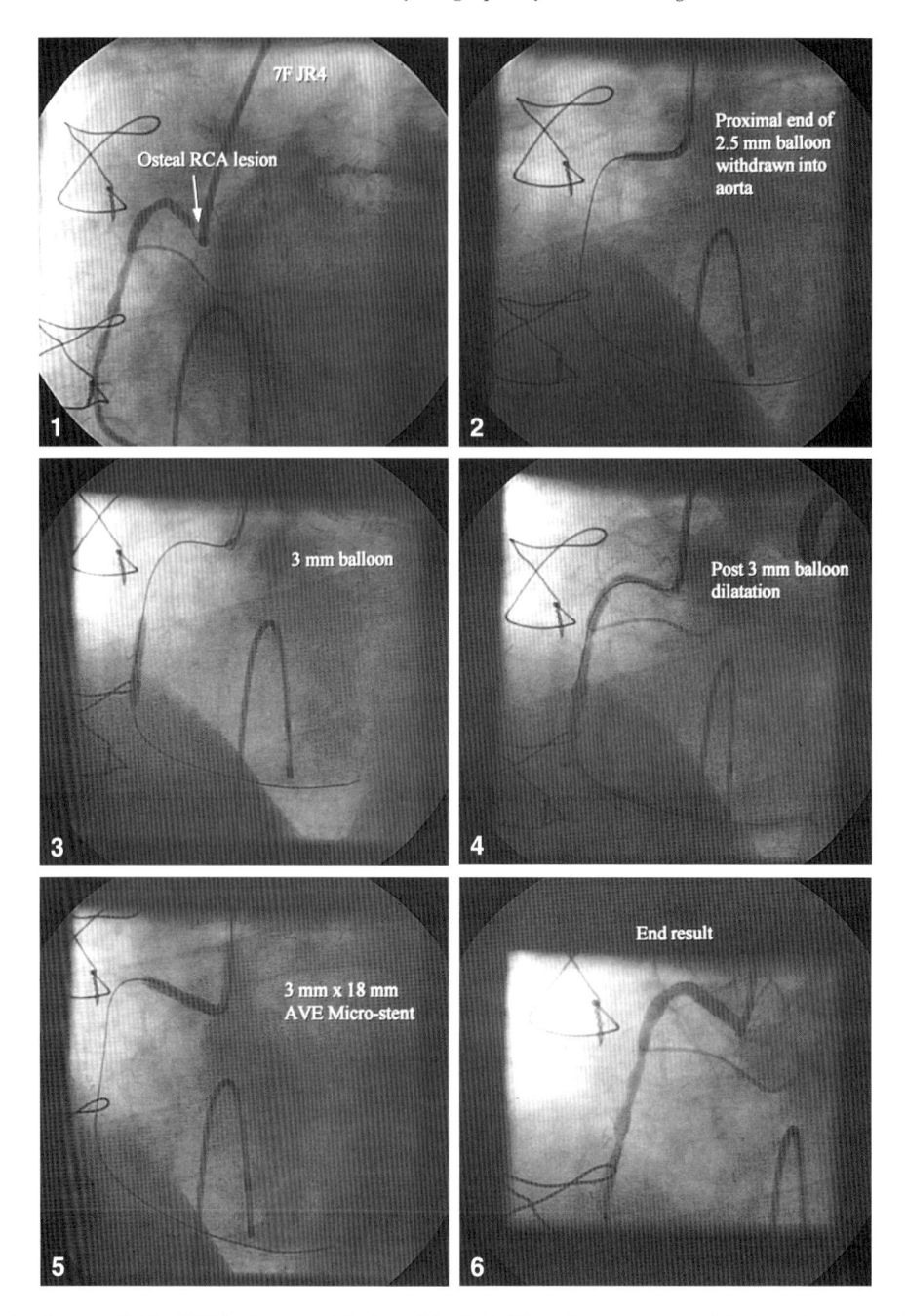

Angiogram 22.1. *PTCA of an osteal lesion of the RCA.* There is a severe osteal lesion with a second lesion in the mid portion of the RCA beyond a short ectatic segment (1). CABG had been performed to all three arteries but the RCA graft given for an osteal stenosis had occluded. PTCA was performed twenty three months after CABG. The osteal lesion was dilated with 1.5, 2.5, and 3 mm balloons inflated across the osteum into the aorta (2). The mid RCA lesion was dilated with the 2.5 and 3 mm balloons (3). The progress reached at that stage is shown in (4). A 3 mm × 18 mm stent was deployed at the osteum (5), to give the final result shown in (6).

osteum. Ever so gently the guide catheter plus the balloon are withdrawn along the guide wire, until it is estimated that the stent is covering the osteum with a portion of the stent protruding into the aorta. The risk is for the stent to be deployed too distally and miss the osteum. Inflate the balloon to the *maximum* pressure that might be needed, as redilating with another balloon risks damaging the proximal end of the stent as the balloon enters the stent. The stent requires good radial strength to overcome the elastic recoil and a Palmaz-Schatz PS153 or AVE Micro stent or NIR, Multilink, or Palmaz-Schatz Crown stents are suitable.

4. *Post Stent deployment*

After deploying the stent, withdraw the balloon carefully, so as disturb the stent as little as possible. Thereafter it is VERY IMPORTANT to keep the guide catheter AWAY FROM THE STENT, as it is very easy to damage the stent with the tip of the guide catheter. Do not try to re-enter the stent with the guide catheter for the post PTCA angiogram record. Instead assess an injection with the catheter tip a short distance back from the stent; this usually is unsatisfactory. Preferably withdraw the guide catheter and guide wire from the RCA and pass a small diagnostic 4, 5 or 6F multipurpose or NIH catheter to near the stent and record the angiogram. A further possibility is to do an aortogram in the LAO projection to show the RCA osteum. Returning 4–6 weeks later, it is much safer to intubate the stent with a diagnostic catheter, such as a JR4 shape, as by then the stent has become covered and strengthened by an endothelial lining.

Osteal Lesions of Saphenous Vein Grafts (SVGs)

These are relatively common and may be truly osteal, but more often involve the osteum and the initial 0.5–1 cm of the graft. The techniques are essentially the same as those described for an RCA osteal lesion. Selection of the guide catheter is important. For an RCA graft, which is usually downward pointing, a multipurpose A-2 or a JR4 catheter may be used. For LCX and LAD grafts, JR4 or AR1 shaped catheters are usually suitable.

With the longer amount of guide wire in the vein graft passing to the native coronary artery, there is less risk of the guide wire and balloon prolapsing out when the guide catheter is retracted from the osteum. Elastic recoil is usually less prominent and predilation of the lesion is often unnecessary.

Usually SVG, osteal lesions are less difficult than those of the RCA, as they are often moderate rather than very tight and may be slightly distal to the true osteum, allowing easier intubation of the vessel. There are usually fewer problems with the guide wire, balloon dilatation and with positioning of a stent.

Sometimes a mild osteal lesion may require dilatation before a stent can be passed to treat a culprit lesion in the body of a graft. Consider stenting the osteum too, once the lesion in the body has been treated satisfactorily.

Osteal Left Main Stem (protected LMS)

For a patient with previous CABG and left main stem stenosis, if a graft to either the LAD or LCX is occluded but the graft to the other LCA branch is still healthy, the left main stem is said to be "protected". The vessel with the occluded graft may be treated by dilatation of the left main stem. The number of cases in this category is very small. The technique is similar to that used for an RCA osteal stenosis (see above page 229). For the guide catheter, a JL4 or Voda shape may be used. The left Amplatz shape is not suitable, as it is difficult to withdraw it a short distance out of the LCA to allow dilatation and stenting the osteum. The Amplatz guide tends retract up the aorta pulling with it the guide wire and balloon. The Amplatz shape is also more traumatic to the left main stem than other catheter shapes (see page 9).

Lesions on Bends

A lesion on a bend has an increased risk of dissection as the vessel is straightened out by the balloon during dilatation. Unfortunately, by their nature coronary vessels are tortuous and frequently have a bend. If the bend is a mild one of less than 45°, the risks of dissection are small (see page 84). In about 25% of PTCA cases the lesion to be dilated is on a bend of varying magnitude. *Elective stenting* if the vessel is of sufficient calibre is often the best method to treat the lesion and avoid the risk of dissection.

Three lesions on bends warrant further discussion, one for each coronary artery and for at least two of them stenting is often the answer.

1. First corner on the RCA

With the proximal RCA, the vessel often first passes horizontally or downwards. After 2–4 cm the vessel takes a bend, or sometimes two, as it turns nearly vertically downwards. The bend may be better appreciated in the RAO projection (see Angiogram 15.2, page 173). The initial course may be truly sinusoidal with 2–3 bends. With a single bend, the angle between the first more section and the next more vertical part, varies but is often 60°–90°, or more. A lesion at this site (Angiogram 22.2) may be approached by:

a) *Pre dilatation* with a small (2 or 2.5 mm) balloon followed by,
b) *Placing a stent*
   An elective stent will usually prevent a dissection and straightens out the bend. A Wiktor stent and some second generation stents such as the ACS Multilink or the NIR stent are more flexible and conform to the shape of the bend in the vessel. There is risk of a tear or minor dissection at either end of the stent, especially the distal end. A further short stent overlapping the end of the first stent may be needed.
c) *Simple Balloon Dilatation*
   Following the initial small balloon with another balloon which is slightly undersized and avoiding high inflation pressures (i.e. above 8 atmospheres), often produces a satisfactory result. If a dissection does occur it may be a long one and a Wallstent may then be considered. Simple balloon dilatation should first be tried if the RCA is of small calibre, making it less suitable to stent.

   A short balloon (9 mm long, e.g. a Chubby balloon) or a fixed wire balloon may reduce the risk of dissection. Sometimes a short balloon will jump to either side of the lesion as the balloon is inflated.

   If there is a tight lesion at the apex of a sharp shepherd's crook bend on the RCA, the risks of dissection will be very high and even passing a stent to the lesion may not be possible. Discretion may suggest that CABG will be more suitable than PTCA.

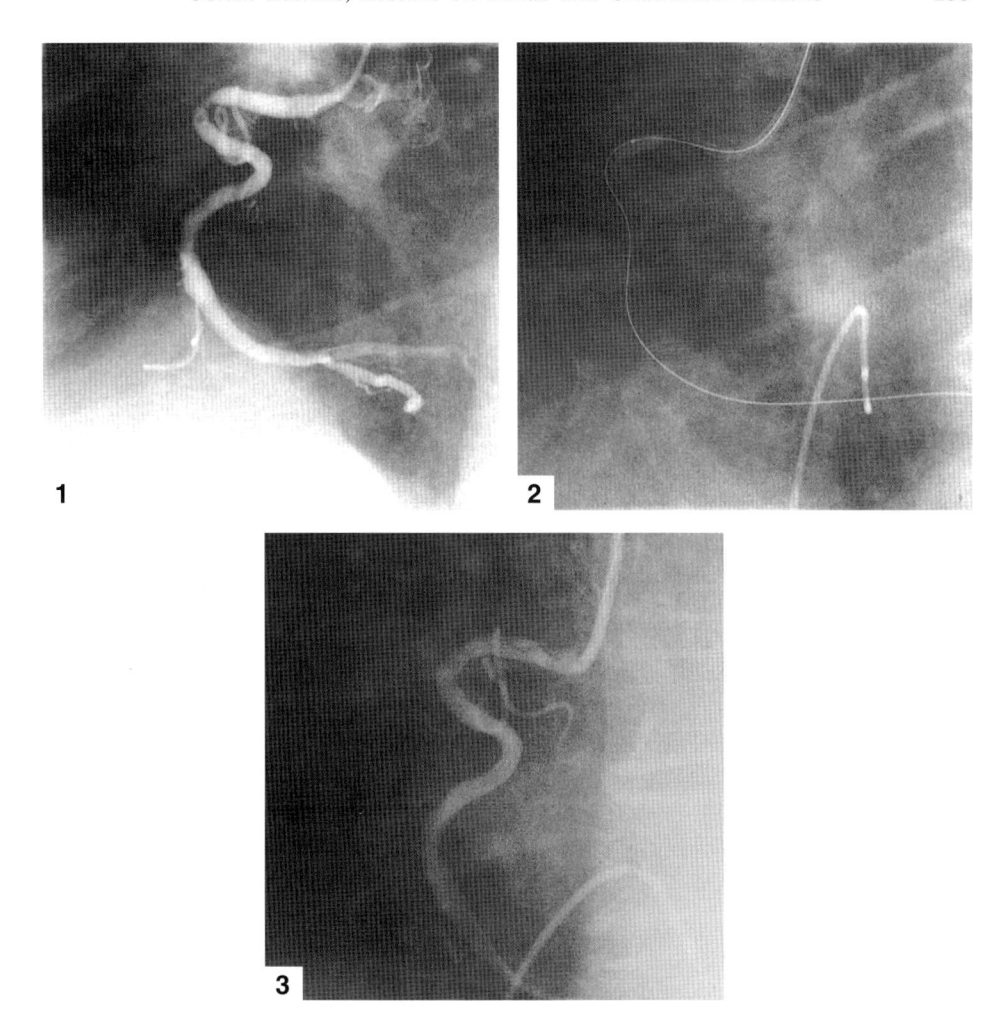

Osteal Lesions, Lesions on Bends and Undilatable Lesions 233

Angiogram 22.2. *PTCA of a lesion on a sharp bend of the RCA.* Very tortuous, snake-like RCA, with a lesion on a sharp 180° bend (1). The lesion was predilated with a 2 mm short balloon (Chubby). The result was better than expected, so a decision to attempt PTCA before or instead of stenting was made. The lesion was redilated with a a 3.5 mm Chubby balloon (2). The final result is satisfactory (3).

2. Dog-Legged Bend on the Left Circumflex Artery

The circumflex artery is prone to develop a lesion on a step-like bend in its proximal half (see Angiogram 8.2, page 94). The lesion besides being at increased risk for dissection, can posses prominent elastic recoil and can also be very resistant to dilatation despite using high pressures. A stent with strong radial force e.g. a Palmaz-Schatz is needed to treat the lesion, which is usually straightened out by the stent. Good guide catheter support is essential to pass a stent across the lesion despite predilatation. An Amplatz catheter is recommended.

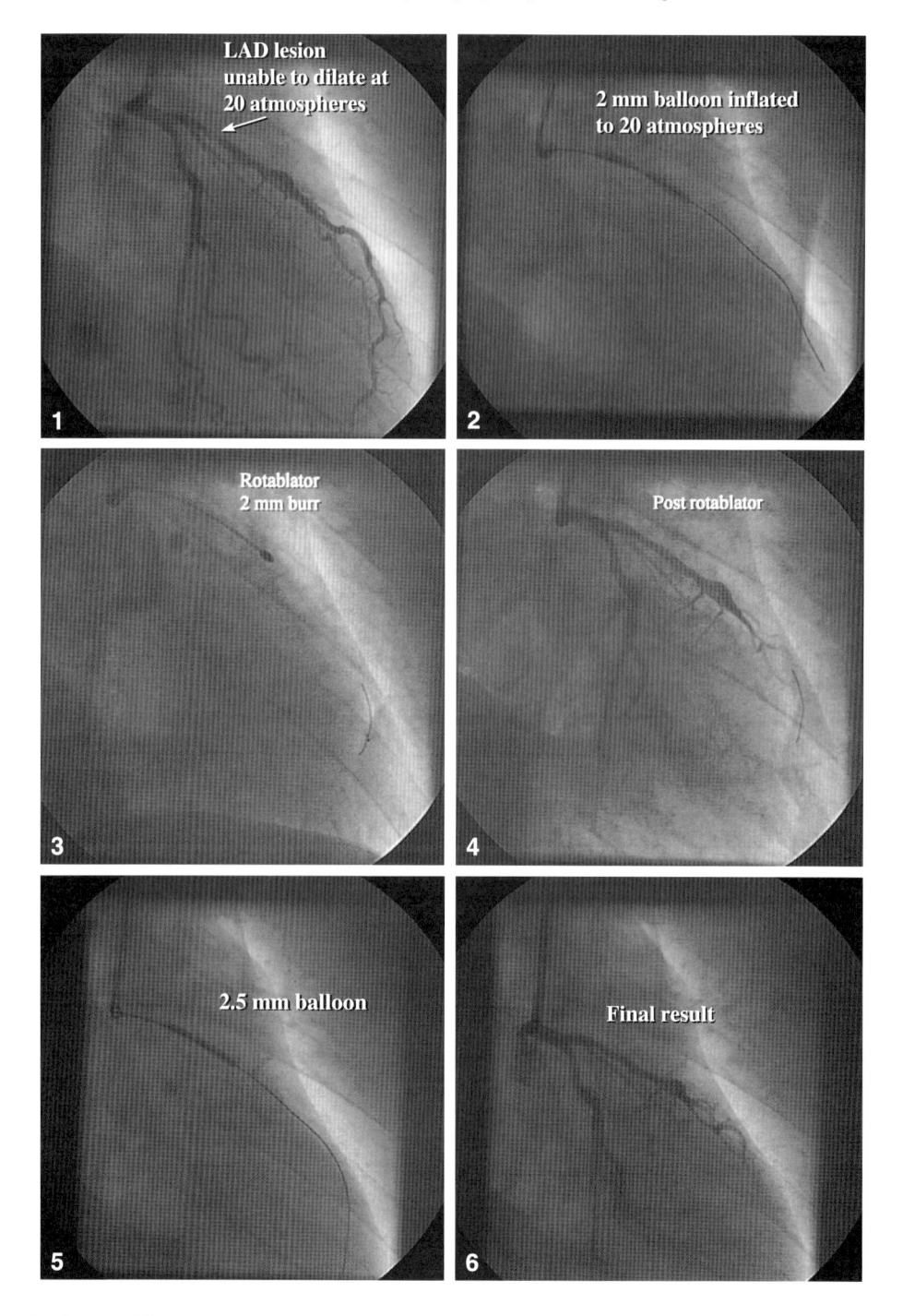

234				Guide to Coronary Angioplasty and Stenting

Angiogram 22.3. *Undilatable lesion on the LAD.* It was not possible to dilate the LAD lesion (1), despite using a 2 mm balloon inflated to 20 atmospheres (2), when the balloon ruptured. A 2 mm Rotablator burr was passed (3 and 4), after which a 2.5 mm balloon could easily be fully inflated to 6 atmospheres (5). The final result was good (6).

The dog-legged bend on the circumflex artery may respond to a prolonged inflation of 10–20 minutes with a perfusion balloon. Even a lesion with considerable elastic recoil may be fully relieved with little or no dissection. A perfusion balloon is an alternative strategy to elective use of a stent, or if a stent cannot cross the lesion.

3. **Round the Corner LAD Bend** (Angiogram 7.1 and 7.2, pages 80 and 82)

Towards the end of the middle third of the LAD, the vessel turns to run straight down the front of the heart in the interventricular groove. Stenoses on the LAD are common before this portion of the vessel is reached. If there is a lesion on this bend, a stent may be unsuitable as the calibre of the artery by this stage is often small at 2.5 mm or less. Balloon dilatation with a regular PTCA balloon should first be attempted, with stenting or a perfusion balloon kept in reserve.

Undilatable Lesion

This is a lesion which cannot be dilated with a balloon despite using high pressures (Angiogram 22.3). The dumb-bell appearance to the balloon persists and the lesion cannot be 'cracked'. There is a danger that inflating the balloon to higher and higher pressures, will enlarge the balloon on either side of the lesion to such an extent as to cause dissection. These lesions are rare and may be treated with the following methods:

1. *Downsize the balloon*
   The balloon size is reduced to a 2 mm balloon. This can usually be safely inflated to high pressures up to 20 atmospheres without the worry of balloon expansion at the ends leading to dissection. Be prepared for balloon rupture and coronary artery spasm being induced (see also pages 141 and 164).
2. *Use Prolonged Inflation*
   This technique is only rarely successful, but can be tried using a routine balloon or a perfusion balloon inflated for 2–5 minutes.
3. *Use of Rotablator*
   An undilatable lesion is 'the' indication for the use of the Rotablator (North West Technologies). Other techniques usually do not work, whereas the Rotablator can be practically guaranteed to be successful. An undilatable lesion has nearly always a ring of calcification over most of the circumference of the lesion and the Rotablator fractures the calcium and opens a channel. The lesion will then respond to balloon dilatation (see Angiogram 22.3).

Conclusion

An osteal lesion is always a challenge and a lesion on a moderate or severe bend 'spells trouble' from an increased risk of dissection. A strategy to manage these lesions needs to be considered before (starting) the procedure. Elective stenting for both these types of lesions has considerably improved the results from PTCA. Undilatable lesions are rare, but respond well to rotational atherectomy with the Rotablator.

23 Bifurcation Lesions

Bifurcation lesions are some of the most challenging and interesting lesions to tackle by angioplasty, but they can also be very frustrating.

Though surgically and prognostically this lesion is described as single vessel disease, to the interventionist it is certainly not a straightforward procedure involving one vessel. In fact most operators would prefer lesions on two separate arteries rather than one bifurcation lesion. Surgically, often the lesion will be treated with two grafts (one perhaps a jump graft), rather than a single graft.

PTCA of bifurcation lesions can be a lengthy procedure with an unpredictable outcome and a less than complete success for each of the branches. Even stents are not the complete answer for these lesions.

Sites of Bifurcation Lesions

The three common sites requiring PTCA are:

1. *LAD and Diagonal*
   This is by far the commonest lesion, accounting for about 90% of cases. They are usually in the proximal or early middle third of the LAD.
2. *Obtuse Marginal and Main Circumflex*
   Often the OM is the larger branch, with the main circumflex artery continuing down the atrio-ventriculat groove as a smaller vessel to give off one or more smaller OM vessels.
3. *RCA bifurcation*
   A lesion involving the bifurcation of RCA into posterior descending artery and atrio-ventricular branch is uncommon, as lesions requiring PTCA usually occur more proximally in the vessel. Sometimes the lesion may be at an early bifurcation of the RCA in the mid portion of the vessel.

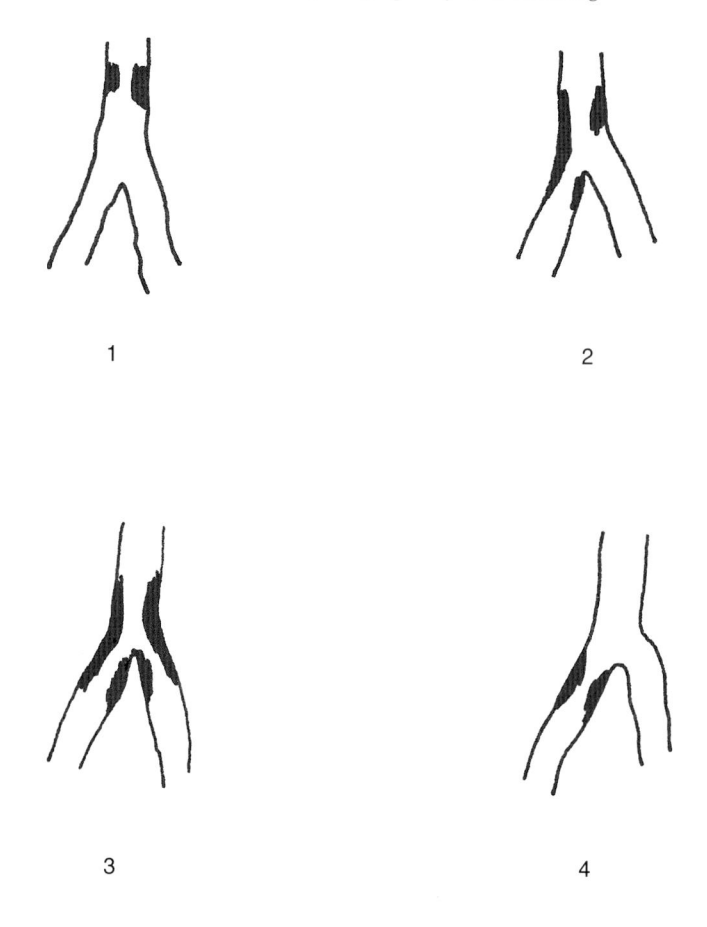

238   *Guide to Coronary Angioplasty and Stenting*

1. Lesion Proximal to Bifurcation
2. Lesion at Bifurcation but not involving side branch
3. 'True' Bifurcation Lesion
4. Lesion Just Distal to the Bifurcation

Figure 23.1. Types of Bifurcation lesions.

Types of Bifurcation Lesions

A variety of lesions are sometimes grouped together under the term 'bifurcation lesion'. Some are much less risky or troublesome than others (see Figure 23.1).

1) *Lesion proximal to the bifurcation*
   The lesion is close, but is definitely separate from the bifurcation. Problems are infrequent (see Angiogram 7.1, page 80).
2) *Lesion at the bifurcation but not involving the side branch*
   The side branch seems to be 'clean'. Risks are less high.

3) *'True' Bifurcation lesion* (Angiogram 23.1, page 246)
   The narrowing starts before the bifurcation and extends down into the start of each of the branches. This form carries the greatest risk.
4) *Lesion just distal to the bifurcation*
   The main artery or its branch has a lesion just beyond the bifurcation. This again is less risky, with the main concern being that a dissection from a branch vessel might extend retrogradely and involve the more important main artery.

Problems with Bifurcation Lesions

What makes these lesions more difficult and hazardous for PTCA? Some of the features are:

1. Squeezing atheroma from one branch to the other.
2. Need for two guide wires.
3. Greater risks for dissection.
4. Increased risk for emergency CABG.
5. Stent jail.
6. Increased restenosis.

1. Squeezing atheroma from one branch to the other

Usually one branch is dilatated at a time e.g. a wire and a balloon in the LAD which is then is dilatated. Next the balloon is taken off the LAD wire and passed along the wire in the diagonal artery to dilate its lesion. After this a good result may have been obtained with the diagonal lesion, but atheroma at the bifurcation may have been squeezed into the LAD, narrowing or even blocking it. On redilatating the LAD the reverse may occur, with nipping at the origin of the diagonal. With repeated dilatations of the branches, a ping pong shift of athereroma between them can occur. Usually repeated dilatation of the branches will not relieve this problem of 'snow-ploughing' the atheroma from one branch to the other.

Despite the angiogram showing compromised flow to the side branch or even the main channel, often ischaemic pain or ECG changes are mild or absent at least during the procedure.

To surmount this problem of shifting atheroma, consider:

1) **Sacrifice the smaller vessel**
   The side branch may be relatively small and supply only a small area of myocardium. Its blockage at most will lead to only a small myocardial infarction. Emergency CABG is not warranted and the vessel anyway might be too small to graft. Its loss will have to be accepted. Sometimes the branch may later reopen ... but by then a small MI may have occurred.

2) **Kissing balloon technique**
   This technique is described in textbooks and articles but is rarely used in practice. A balloon on *each* wire is positioned across the lesion into *each* branch. This requires a larger sized guide catheter (8F) to allow the two balloons to pass along the lumen of the guide catheter easily. However with the modern very low profile

balloon catheters with very thin shafts, such as the Goldie (Schneider), Viva (SciMed) and Worldpass (Cordis), two balloon catheters can travel down within a 7F guide catheter.

Another method to pass two balloons down the same guide catheter, is to have one of them as a fixed wire balloon, as these have a very low profile shaft (see page 19). The fixed wire balloon is tracked along side the guide wire of the less important branch. The guide wire is then removed. A routine balloon is then passed along the guide wire within the main artery. This can be a fiddly, difficult procedure especially if fixed wire balloons are rarely used.

Both balloons are inflated across the lesion simultaneously. As two balloons are across the lesion and in the proximal vessel, there is a moderate risk of dissection at or proximal to the bifurcation.

3) **Stenting**
A variety of procedures can be used. However stenting bifurcation lesions is difficult and still leaves problems to be answered, not the least being risk of restenosis. The approaches can be:

a) *Stent the main artery*
Secure the main artery and sacrifice the smaller side branch. It is preferable to withdraw the guide wire from side branch before stenting across it.

b) *Stent the main artery and dilate the branch*
If a Wallstent or Palmaz-Schatz PS153 or the Modified Spiral Palmaz-Schatz stent is placed in the main artery it is very difficult to pass a guide wire and then a balloon through the stent into the side branch, which is then described as '*jailed*'. Entrance into the branch will be prevented during the procedure and any subsequent one in the future. If however a stent with a more open design of struts such as a coiled stent e.g. a Gianturco-Roubin (Angiogram 23.1, page 246), Wiktor or Cordis CrossFlex stent is used, or with an AVE Micro stent, it is relatively easy to pass a guide wire and then follow with a balloon through the struts into the side branch. One version of the Jo-stent (see page 112), has reduced struts at the centre to make it easier for a guide wire to cross the stent into a side branch.

It is better to *leave* the guide wire in the side branch as the stent in the main artery is deployed, (Angiogram 23.1). Surprisingly, it will slip out with ease as traction is applied when it needs to be withdrawn. Deploy the stent to routine pressures, i.e. to 8–10 atmospheres. Defer any high pressure inflations until the initial side-branch guide wire has been withdrawn.

With the guide wire already in place passing to the side branch, this aids the tracking of the second wire along the branch once it has crossed the stent of the main artery. The first guide wire may then be withdrawn. A small balloon, followed by the correct sized balloon for the calibre of the branch, are then inflated in turn across the origin of the branch.

This technique is often successful when the origin of the side branch is nipped by shift of atheroma between the branches, rather than dissection at the start of the side branch. Usually the stent prevents the atheroma shifting back into the main artery.

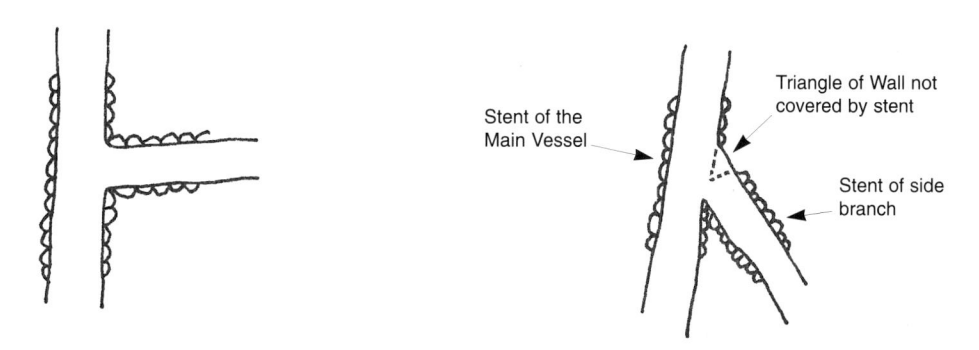

Figure 23.2. Double stenting for bifurcation lesion.

Crossing the stent with a balloon is usually easy, but *withdrawal* of the *balloon* after it has been inflated may be *difficult* and the balloon quite reluctant to leave! This can be rather worrying (!!), but ensuring full negative pressure on the balloon and persevering with manipulation and traction on the balloon, it will (or should!) come back.

c) *Stent the main artery and the side branch*
   If despite balloon dilatation, the origin of the side branch remains pinched or dissected, a stent can be passed to the branch. Positioning the second stent is important but difficult. For an LAD/diagonal lesion, the LAO cranial projection, (see page 52) is usually the clearest. Ensure that the second stent is sufficiently proximal to cover the osteum of the side branch. If after the second stent is in position, the main artery becomes narrowed, a kissing balloon technique (see above), with one balloon across each stent may be needed. This will be a challenge!

   Two stents are still not the whole answer, as side branches rarely arise at right angles to the main artery. Instead they usually come off obliquely, which leaves a triangle of wall of the side branch which is not stented (see Figure 23.2). Atheroma at this site can still narrow the origin of the side branch and can ping pong back into the main artery if the side branch is dilatated with a balloon.

d) *Use of two stents overlapping in the main channel*
   Particularly with two coiled stents, it is feasible to stent the main vessel (e.g. LAD), pass a stent through the first stent into the branch (e.g. diagonal) and ensure that the proximal end of the second stent overlaps the bifurcation and is in the main channel proximal to the bifurcation. Blood flow to the distal segment of the main artery will need to cross the struts of the second stent, which may lead to an increased risk of stent thrombosis. The distal main artery is to a varying extent 'jailed' by the sidebranch stent.

e) *Emergency CABG*
   If both the branches are of significant size then surgery will bail out the problem and remove the risk of restenosis in the short term. A decision *before* the procedure should be made, whether sacrifice of a branch or emergency CABG are appropriate possible managements. Avoid endless attempts at redilation to

try and 'fix' the problem, while the myocardium becomes progressively more ischaemic.

If the patient goes to surgery, remove the wire from the patent or open branch keeping the guide wire down the partially occluded artery, which will help to maintain some flow down it until it is bypassed. Sometimes little or no ischaemia is apparent and surgery can be arranged electively for the next free operative slot. Whist waiting the patient may go to the surgical ITU.

2. Two Guide Wires

Placing two wires, one in each branch makes the procedure more complicated and prolonged. With two wires:

a) *The Lesion is more Difficult to Assess*

If two guide wires with long (8–10 cm) terminal radiopaque sections are used, where they cross will show the bifurcation site very precisely, but may tend to obscure the lesion itself. This is not usually a problem and also most operators use wires with only a short (2–3 cm) radiopaque section.

b) *Difficulty of Passing Two Wires*

Passing two wires is more difficult and time consuming. It does not matter which branch is entered first, but ideally the initial attempt should be to the larger or more important vessel e.g. the main LAD. The second wire tends to 'follow' or track along side the first guide wire and the second branch is more difficult to enter. A short sharp bend of about 70–90° over 2–4 mm to the tip of the guide wire aids pointing it to and entering the desired branch (see page 31). However, the more pronounced tip will make subsequent passage down the artery beyond the lesion more difficult, as the tip tends to catch on small branches. If the balloon is brought up to near the tip (i.e. 1–2 cm back), it will support the guide wire and aid manipulation of the tip.

c) *Guide Wires Entwining*

The second wire may twist round the first before entering its branch. This is not apparent until a balloon is passed along one of the wires, when it will not track further than the bifurcation. With guide wires which have a longer radiopaque section they will be seen to buckle and to move, as attempts to pass the balloon are made.

It is surprising that entwining doesn't happen more frequently. Try to keep manipulation of the second guide wire to a minimum ... this is largely wishful thinking, as either the guide wire passes to the second branch easily, or it does not when more manipulation will be needed.

Be on the *look-out* for this problem when passing a balloon across the lesion for the *first* time. If the balloon will not cross, entwining may be the problem and persisting with the attempt may cause dissection by the guide wires acting as cheese cutters at the bifurcation.

d) *Greater Risk for Thrombus Formation*

With two guide wires and a balloon, there is more 'hardware' down the artery than is usual during PTCA. This probably leads to a higher risk of thrombus formation. Ensure that sufficient heparin is given to raise the ACT to above 250 seconds and preferably above 300 seconds.

e) *Risk of Moving the Wrong Guide Wire*
With two guide wires there is a risk of manipulating or withdrawing the *wrong* guide wire. When the guide wire doesn't move it may be withdrawn further and only then is it realised that the *other* guide wire (to the one wished), has been manipulated and may even have come back past the lesion. Have a small towel over the guide wire not currently in use, to help to prevent this accident. Using one radiopaque and one non radiopaque guide wire, also helps to distinguish between the wires.

In view of all these difficulties with two guide wires, some operators will nearly always use only one guide wire. If the smaller branch occludes, it is either left (sacrificed), or an attempt is then made to enter it (which may or may not be possible), or emergency CABG is considered.

3. Greater Risk for Dissection

Dissection and occlusion may occur from:

1) *Oversizing the Balloon for the Distal Artery*
It may be difficult to know the true size of the artery beyond the bifurcation which is usually smaller than the vessel before the bifurcation. Start dilatations with a balloon size appropriate for artery distal to the lesion and go up in size as necessary if the distal vessel opens up. IVUS can be helpful to show the correct size of all relevant sections of the main vessel and branches, but will also prolong an already complicated procedure.

2) *Manipulation of the Guide Wires*
As there are two guide wires being manipulated across a complicated lesion, there is a greater risk of raising an intimal flap with a wire and starting a dissection. Be particularly careful and gentle with guide wire manipulation for a bifurcation lesion.

4. Increased Risk for Emergency CABG

For the reasons already described, i.e. alternating branch closure, lesion dissection and thrombus on the guide wire, there is about twice the routine rate for emergency surgery. Prior discussion of the case with a surgeon is preferable but not essential.

5. Stent Jail

As explained above (see page 240), if stenting of the main artery (e.g. the LAD) is performed, access to a side branch (e.g. a diagonal) will be restricted and the branch 'jailed'. This concern has largely been removed by using stents with a more open meshwork than the original Palmaz-Schatz stents. Gianturco-Roubin, Wiktor and Crossflex stents allow relatively easy access through the struts to a side branch. One version of the Jo-stent is designed for bifurcation lesions (see above on page 240). With patience it also possible to cross some 'second generation' tubular mesh stents, such as the NIR, Multilink and the Palmaz-Schatz Crown stent. The 7 mm cell design of the NIR stent has a more open mesh with larger spaces between the struts, making it easier to cross with a guide wire (see page 111).

If the two branches are large and important, e.g. an LAD and significant sized diagonal branch, consider preplanned elective CABG if the PTCA result is not entirely satisfactory. The patient can go straight to theatre and PTCA is a procedure that may or may not be successful, before surgery is performed.

6. Increased Restenosis

Despite all the hard work one may be rewarded by restenosis which is slightly commoner with this type of lesion. If restenosis does occur, carefully consider the options and CABG or continued medical treatment may be preferable to redilation.

Management of a Typical Case of LAD/Diagonal Bifurcation Lesion

This is the commonest bifurcation lesion treated and the principles and methods used will be similar for circumflex and RCA lesions.

1. Review of the Diagnostic Angiogram

Decide whether it is 'a one or two wire job', (see Angiograms 7.1 and 23.1, on pages 80 and 246). Look carefully as to the exact site of the lesion and whether it above the bifurcation or whether it is involving one or both branches. Decide on the importance of the diagonal branch and whether it should be protected with its own guide wire and whether CABG will be offered if it occludes. Assess the size of the branches to select balloon sizes and consider which guide catheter may be used to give good back-up. A Voda guide catheter may be very helpful.

2. Discussion with Patient Relatives

Remember to explain the increased complexity, risks of emergency CABG and restenosis.

3. Equipment

    a) *Double Y-Connector* (see page 18)
       This is needed to allow the use of two guide wires.
    b) *Wire Introducer*
       A hollow needle-like probe through which an uncovered (by balloon) guide wire is passed safely into the Y-connector and the guide catheter.
    c) *Torquer*
       Even if this is not routinely used to manipulate a guide wire, it may be helpful in this type of case.
    d) *Guide Catheter*
       Use a larger size to accommodate the increased amount of hardware, i.e. instead of 6 or 7F, consider using 8F sized guide catheter. Ensure a stable position for the guide catheter to allow optimal visualization with injections and secure back-up.
    e) *Guide Wire*
       Use the guide wire(s) which you use routinely (and are most happy with) and fashion a short 70–90° bend to the tip. Consider one wire at least, having a short radiopaque terminal section.

f) *Balloon*

Try to use balloons with a low profile shaft which will leave more room in the guide catheter for the guide wires and allow easier contrast injections.

4. Technique

After the control angiograms, pass one guide wire into the proximal LAD using a projection showing the left main stem and its bifurcation, such as an RAO caudal view. To cross the lesion, the LAO cranial, or RAO cranial views are usually the most helpful. Be very careful and gentle with the guide wire manipulation and aim to first enter the LAD. If the guide wire passes first into the diagonal, leave it there unless the flow to the distal LAD appears very poor. If the balloon is brought down to near the end of the guide wire it will provide support to assist the wire to cross the lesion.

Once beyond the lesion, the sharp bend on the tip may inhibit the guide wire passing down the vessel, as it will tend to catch on branches. As the guide wire is passed distally, a U-shaped loop may form at its terminal section. With the loop advance the guide wire as distally as possible. Then withdraw and rotate a short amount of the wire and the loop will often come out. If it does not it is usually safe to leave the looped guide wire in the distal artery. It is worth trying to pass the guide wire as distally as possible to improve guide wire support (see page 29) and to allow the wire to come back an amount during manipulations, yet remain well distal to the lesion.

Next pass the second guide wire into the diagonal artery. Often this wire will track or follow the first wire into the proximal LAD and then across the lesion into the distal LAD. With a prominent bend to the tip of the guide wire, rotate the tip to face and then enter the diagonal artery. Try to manipulate the second guide wire as little as possible, to avoid entwining it around the first wire.

With both guide wires in place, consider predilating with a small balloon, or use the smaller balloon if the diagonal artery is smaller than the LAD branch. Pass the balloon down the LAD wire being on the look out for buckling of the guide wires if the balloon has difficulty crossing the lesion; this would suggest entwining of the guide wires (see above on page 242). Dilate first the LAD, then slip the balloon off the LAD wire and replace it on the diagonal wire to dilate this branch. Redilate as required with balloon sizes appropriate to the calibre of the vessels.

If there is lesion recoil or the result of the LAD distal or proximal to the lesion is unsatisfactory, stent the LAD branch. A Gianturco-Roubin or another stent may be considered (see above page 240). Note with Gianturco-Roubin II stent (see page 113), the gold marker on either end of the stent is a short way back from the marker at each end of the delivery balloon (see Angiogram 23.1). To avoid missing the end of the lesion, it is necessary to have the distal balloon marker well clear of the end of the stenosis.

There is about a 30% chance that atheroma will be dislodged between the branches, in which case consider the options discussed earlier (see page 239). Be aware that the procedure may become quite prolonged. Don't forget to check ACT readings and give top-up doses of heparin as necessary.

When the results of the procedure are considered satisfactory, remove the diagonal wire and then LAD wire. Dawdle in the catheter room for about 5–10 minutes to ensure that the good angiographic result is maintained.

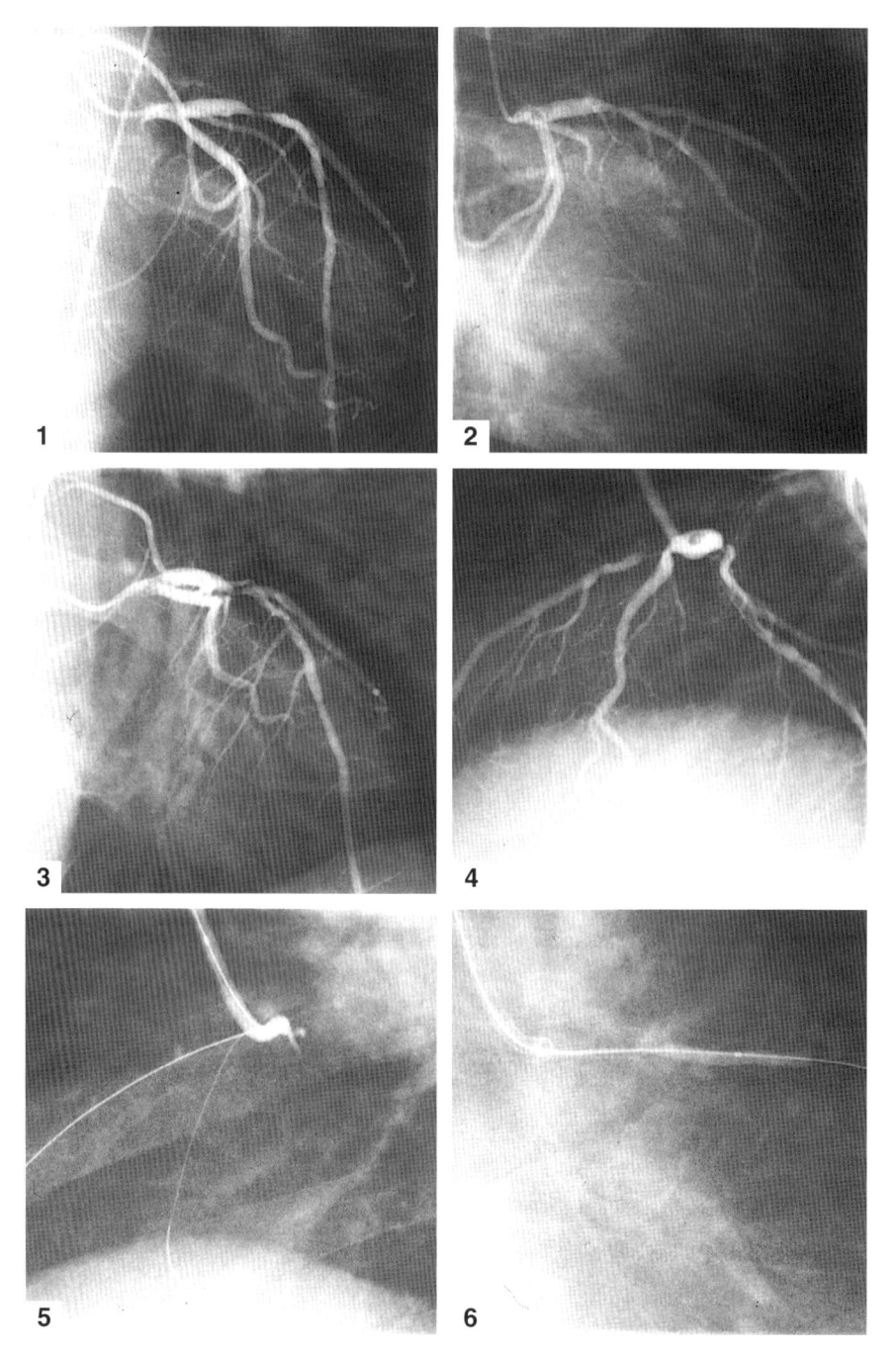

246   *Guide to Coronary Angioplasty and Stenting*

Angiogram 23.1. *PTCA of LAD Bifurcation lesion.* (next page) The LAD lesion is shown on the PA projection to start before the bifurcation (1), and involves the start of both the LAD and diagonal branches (2–4). In the RAO Caudal view the LAD is higher and the diagonal is the lower vessel (2). In the RAO Cranial view the LCX and diagonal vessels are raised higher, so that the diagonal branch is above the LAD (3). The Left Lateral with 10° Cranial, shows the severe narrowing at the start of the LAD branch (4). Figure five shows both the branches wired, the LAD wire with a long radiopaque section (0.014" hi-per flex, Bard), and the diagonal with an ACS 0.014" High Torque Floppy II, with a short radiopaque terminal section. The LAD (6) and the diagonal and the

Bifurcation Lesions 247

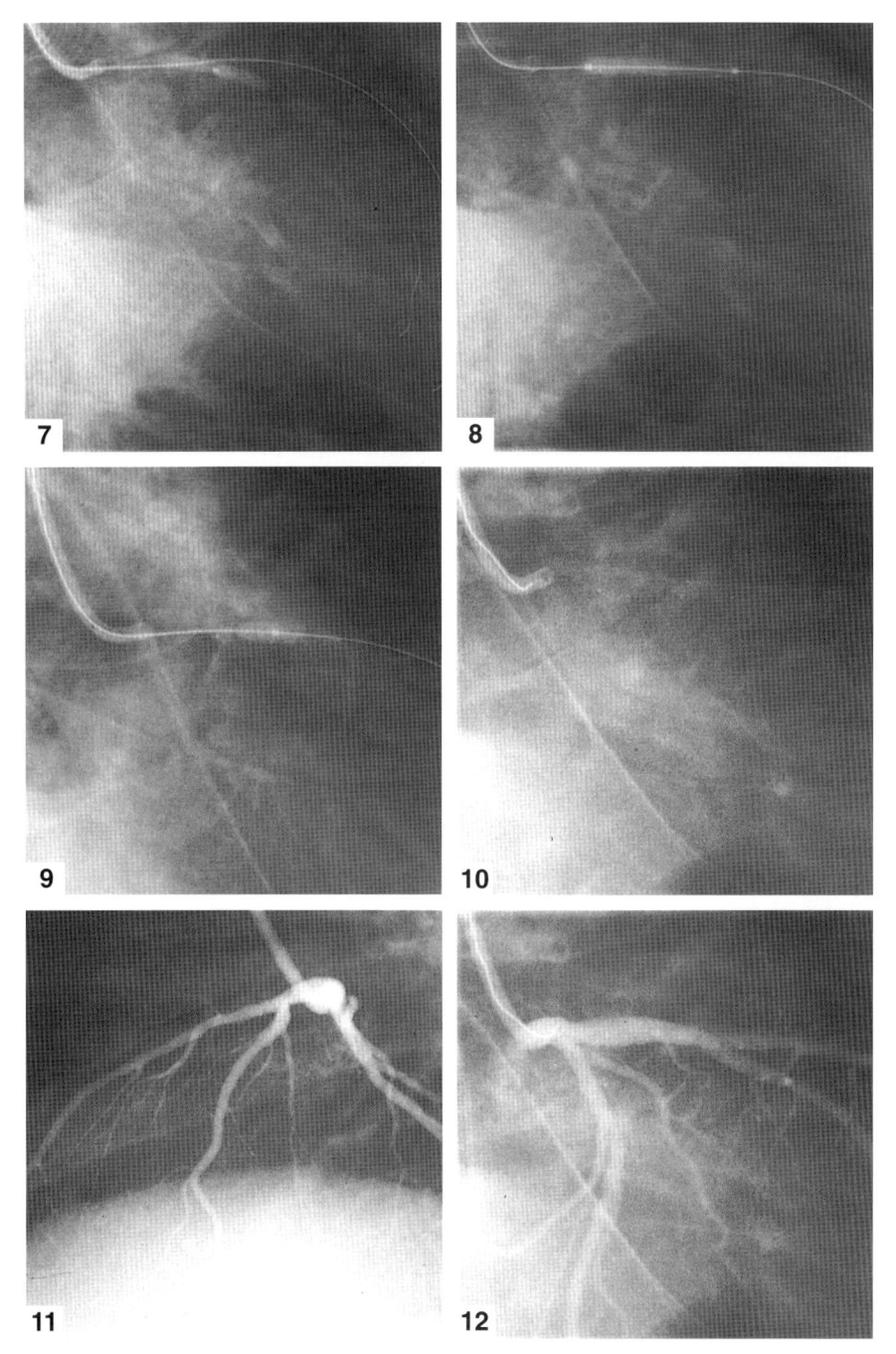

7	8
9	10
11	12

diagonal (7), are dilated with 2.5 mm then 3mm Europass balloons. A Gianturco-Roubin 3.0 mm × 20 mm. stent is deployed at the lesion on the LAD wire (8). The diagonal wire is then withdrawn and the stent re-dilated with a 3.5 mm Chubby balloon inflated to 8 atmospheres (9). The two radiopaque gold dots identify each end of the stent (10). They can just also be seen internal to the balloon end markers when the stent is deployed (8), where the distal dot can be indentified. The final result is shown in 11 and 12. There was good relief of the milder narrowing at the start of the diagonal branch. There was no displacement or 'snow ploughing' of atheroma from the LAD to the diagonal branch when the LAD was dilated and then given a stent.

There are no special features for the post-op care and intravenous heparin is not needed. If a stent or stents have been deployed, the routine post stent management is followed. Usually this will merely involve aspirin and ticlopidine. Sometimes intravenous heparin may be continued over night, especially if a check angiogram the following day is to be performed.

On discharge the risk of restenosis should again be discussed with the patient. Arrange an exercise test prior to a routine follow up appointment in 4–8 weeks.

Circumflex Artery Bifurcation Lesion

Often the OM is the more important branch, with the main circumflex the smaller artery. If atheroma is being dislodged from one branch to the other, at surgery it is easier to graft the OM rather than the main circumflex artery which continues down the atrio-ventricular groove. Hence there may be an argument, that before the patient goes to surgery, to retain flow along the main circumflex artery, allowing the atheroma to nip the origin of the OM branch. On the other hand if the OM branch is the larger vessel, keeping this artery fully open will minimize myocardial ischaemia whilst awaiting emergency CABG.

RCA Bifurcation Lesion

Often one of the branches after the bifurcation of the RCA is smaller and less important, so that a two wire technique is rarely needed. The lesion is relatively distal and back-up is often poor. Good guide catheter support and a low profile balloon are needed. If the artery is a large calibre dominant vessel, consider inserting a temporary pacing wire.

Conclusion

Bifurcation lesions are reasonably frequent, especially of the LAD and diagonal artery. PTCA of these lesions can be challenging, lengthy and unpredictable. After all one's efforts you may be 'rewarded' with restenosis, when the surgical option may then be considered. Stents have not had the major impact on the management of bifurcation lesions as they have had elsewhere. There is under development a trouser or Y-stent, which may yet be the 'answer' to bifurcation lesions.

24 Restenosis

Restenosis has been described as the Achilles' Heal of angioplasty. What use is the procedure if one third of the arteries renarrow within three months? The immediate answer is that two thirds of vessels *do not renarrow* and that to repeat PTCA is a *relatively simple process* (compared to CABG).

Immense research efforts have been devoted to study the mechanisms and prevention of restenosis. Trials of over twenty different drugs have all been unsuccessful in patients.

There are at least three components to restenosis:

1. Elastic recoil.
2. Amount of residual plaque.
3. Intimal hyperplasia or scarring.

Elastic Recoil

When a lesion is dilated, an angioplasty balloon may be fully expanded and measured to be approximately 3 mm in calibre. When the balloon is deflated and removed, the vessel size often reduces to approximately 2.2 mm. There has been recoil of the artery (see Figure 11.1, page 125).

Recoil occurs not only at the time of the angioplasty procedure, but continues for several weeks following it. Different processes are operating at the varying time intervals:

1. *Immediately Following Deflation of the Balloon*
   The balloon ceases to stretch the wall and compress the lesion. The muscle and elastic tissues of the media and the adventitia recoil or relax. The plaque tissue of the lesion gradually expands and unfolds into the lumen.
2. *Subsequent 24-48 Hours*
   Repeat angiography shows a further 20% lumen loss occurring over this interval, after which it remains the same until …

3. *One to Three Months*
   When a further reduction occurs, probably due to shrinkage of the vessel wall from scar contraction within the intima, media and adventitia, so called *remodelling*. Recent IVUS studies suggest that this an important mechanism.

Residual Plaque

IVUS studies have also shown that the amount of residual plaque tissue after PTCA is an important predictor of restenosis. After stenting, the plaque tissue is squeezed behind the stent and out of the lumen. With atherectomy, if sufficient plaque tissue is removed to produce a large lumen size, low restenosis rates similar to those after stents may be achieved.

Intimal Hyperplasia or Scarring

This used to be thought of as the main cause of restenosis and hence many drugs reducing intimal hyperplasia in animal models were assessed in patients, but without success. Intimal hyperplasia varies greatly between cases, from profuse thickening to a very thin layer. The hyperplasia is probably a healing process, which starts with platelet rich thrombus deposited at the lesion immediately after angioplasty. The cells of the intima proliferate and are joined by new cells from the media which have changed or morphosed from smooth muscle cells. The cells in the intima actively divide. At a certain stage the whole process slows down and stops.

The amount of intimal hyperplasia may be related to the degree of vessel wall damage produced by the balloon dilatation. Tears extending through the media to the adventitia induce greater intimal hyperplasia (and vessel wall shrinkage). With atherectomy if the tissue specimens contain adventitia, restenosis is more common.

Bigger is Better

This 'theory' was proposed by Professor Don Baim of Boston, USA to explain the success of stents at lowering restenosis (see page 124). A stent greatly reduces or prevents vessel wall recoil, so that a larger lumen is initially obtained than after balloon angioplasty. The larger lumen persists despite increased intimal hyperplasia after stenting. Hence if an initial *bigger* or *larger* lumen is achieved, the long term result will be *better* with less restenosis (see Figure 11.1, page 125).

If sufficient plaque tissue can be removed at atherectomy to give a lumen size similar to that of a stent, then the restenosis rate may be as low too. Professor Paul Yock of Stamford University, California, USA describes this as *'less is best'*.

Frequency and Time Course of Restenosis

The restenosis rate of about 30% over three months is a convenient figure to give to patients. In some studies the angiographic restenosis rate is nearer 40%. Restenosis presenting as recurrent angina, peaks at 1-2 months, falls by 3 months and is rare after 6 months. In vein grafts the restenosis rate is about 50% and occurs over a longer time course of up to 24 months.

It is *fortunate* that restenosis with native coronary arteries does occur *early* after PTCA. During this period the patient is in "limbo" or "on parole", uncertain what the lottery of restenosis will bring. Will the patient be lucky, or will further angioplasty or perhaps CABG be needed? At least within 3 months and certainly by 6 months, the period of uncertainty has passed.

Recurrent angina is expected to occur at 1-2 month after PTCA. Angina recurring very early after PTCA e.g. during the first week, is unlikely to be due to restenosis. It may be due to a poor PTCA result, or that the pain is non-cardiac and due to anxiety. Rarely, early recurrence of angina is caused by progression of disease in another coronary artery. This can also be the cause of angina at the usual time of presentation of restenosis. If the dilated vessel has not restenosed, inject the other coronary artery and check that another vessel has not developed a tight lesion.

Late presentation at 6-12 months can still be due to restenosis, as initially angina may be mild and gradually worsen later.

Clinical Restenosis less than Angiographic Restenosis

Though the angiographic restenosis rate is about 30%, the clinical recurrence of angina is less, at about 20%. It uncertain why a patient with a severe restenosis lesion should be asymptomatic. The stenosis may be less severe than the original lesion. PTCA is often performed for patients with unstable angina, who even without PTCA can "settle down" and become asymptomatic despite having a severe stenosis. The development of collateral vessels is involved in some patients.

Recurrent Angina, not Myocardial Infarction

It is fortunate that restenosis rarely leads to acute myocardial infarction. It usually presents as gradually returning angina, sometimes unstable angina. The reasons why MI is rare with restenosis may include:

1. *Intimal hyperplasia and scarring.*
   This thickened layer may be less likely to fracture, ulcerate, or develop a fissure, than a lesion before angioplasty.
2. *New cells of the intima*
   These cells are rich in tissue plasminogen activator and perhaps other compounds inhibiting thrombosis.

Whatever the reasons, the infrequency of myocardial infarction contrasts sharply with that of stents, where thrombosis may present with acute MI which may be fatal.

Predictors of Restenosis

The factors associated with an increased risk of restenosis include:

1. *Long diffuse lesions.*
2. *Lesions in vein grafts.*
3. *Osteal stenosis.*
4. *Diabetes.*
5. *Unstable angina.*
6. *Proximal LAD lesion.*
7. *Soft lesion* i.e. one which is easy to dilate at low pressures.
8. *Small calibre vessel, 2.5 mm or less.*
9. *Bifurcation lesions.*
10. *Amount of residual plaque shown on IVUS,* (see above, page 250).

Management of Patient with Restenosis

This will be described under the following headings:

1. Angiography ? Proceed to PTCA.
2. Risks of Repeat PTCA.
3. Redilatation with a Balloon
4. Stent ... the treatment of choice.
5. Atherectomy.
6. How Many Time to Redilate?

1. Angiography? Proceed to PTCA.

The repeat angioplasty starts with an angiogram using a diagnostic catheter. If restenosis is believed to be likely a 6F or 7F sheath is used. If restenosis is considered unlikely a small 4F or 5F sheath can be used. If the vessel has restenosed the small sheath can easily be changed to a larger one for the angioplasty guide catheter.

2. Risks of Repeat PTCA.

Redilatation with a balloon is often simpler, quicker and safer than the first procedure for a number of reasons.

a) *If the first PTCA was particularly difficult*
Then a repeat procedure will not be considered. Instead at end of the first PTCA record on the angiogram report: "if lesion restenoses, not for repeat PTCA ? for CABG or continued medical Rx".

b) *You have been there before*
   The radiographic views, guide catheter and any problems such as entering LAD from the left main stem with the guide wire, will all be known from the previous procedure.
c) *Choice of balloon*
   The size used will be known. If the lesion was believed to have been underdilated then a slightly larger balloon may be chosen.
d) *Restenosis lesions can be simpler*
   Whilst this is sometimes true, at other times the reverse occurs, with the restenosis lesion being longer and more complex than the pre PTCA lesion. Rarely, the PTCA lesion has progressed to a total occlusion.

The frequency of emergency CABG with PTCA for a restenosis lesion is about half that of a "de novo" lesion, i.e. at about 1%. However, vessel occlusion and emergency CABG do still occur and the patient and relatives still need to be forewarned.

3. Stent the Treatment of Choice

After a second balloon dilatation, the restenosis rate is again about 30% over 3 months and these figures remain true for all subsequent redilatations for restenosis. Hence it is very desirable to offer a technique which has a lower restenosis rate than with the first PTCA. Stents reduce the restenosis rate by a similar amount to "de novo" lesions, i.e. to about 20% with a clinical recurrence of angina of about 10%. When reviewing the angiogram of the previous procedure the main question is whether the lesion and the vessel are suitable for a stent (Angiogram 24.1). The principal issues are vessel size (3 mm or more), course and or disease of proximal vessel and length of the lesion.

If the vessel is too small, or too tortuous, or has very diffuse disease, stenting will probably not be feasible. If tortuosity is the problem, consider a Cordis CrossFlex, NIR or ACS Multilink. Stents for smaller vessels (2.5 mm) are now becoming available and their restenosis rates will become established.

4. Redilatation with a Balloon

If it is to be a POBA (plain old balloon angioplasty) again, consider:

a) *Bigger is better*
   Try to get as large as lumen as possible, as good result as possible. Consider upsizing to the next balloon size to that previously used.
b) *Use of IVUS*
   IVUS may be helpful in assessing the mechanism of restenosis. There may be a ring lesion of calcium which was not "cracked" last time at PTCA. The vessel size may be larger than appears from the lumen shown on the angiogram. The vessel may be able to take a stent after all (see page 59).

If repeating balloon angioplasty, take a little longer time ... not just one inflation of the balloon and away! If not a "stent like" result, at least aim for a *very good* PTCA result.

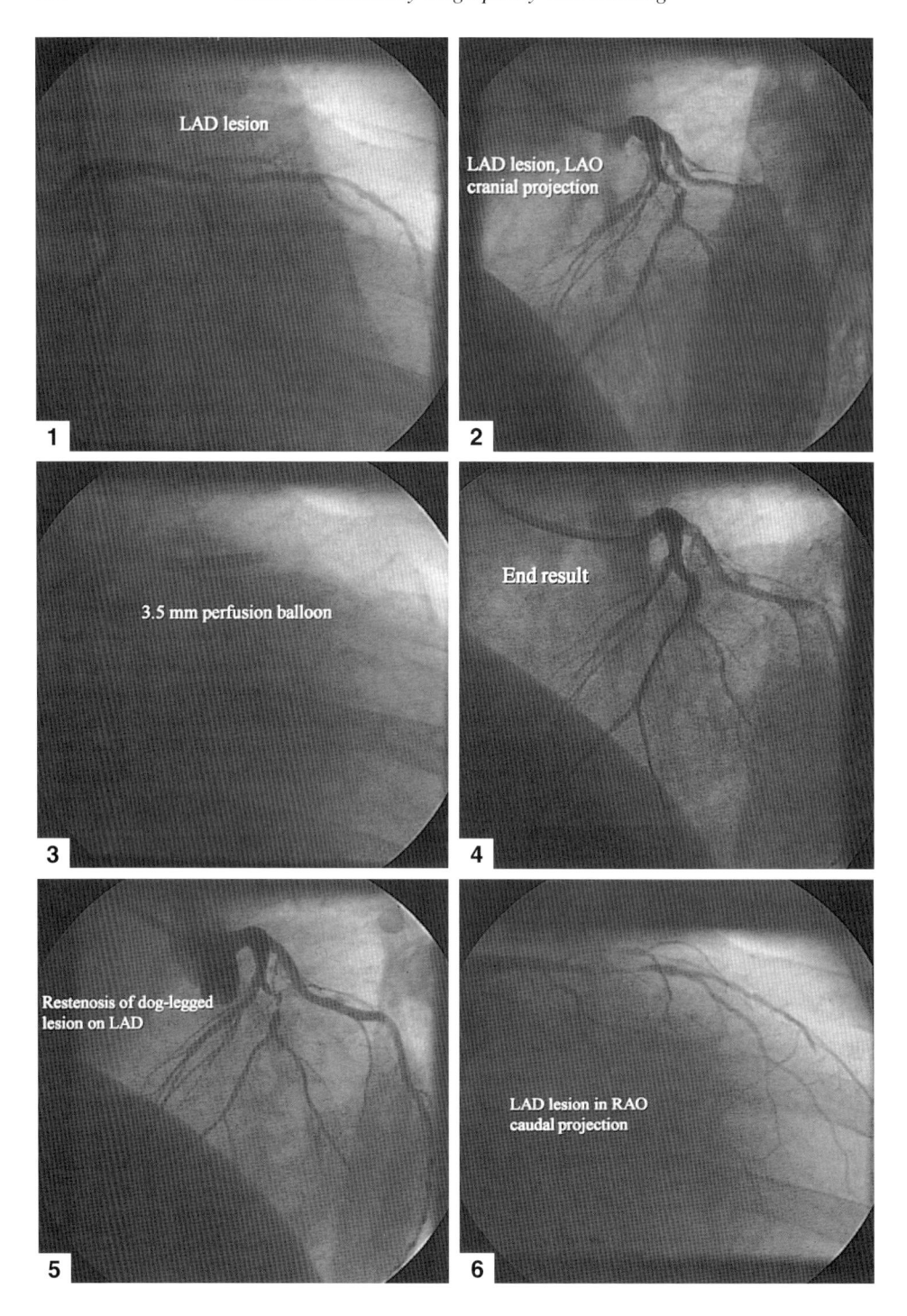

1. LAD lesion
2. LAD lesion, LAO cranial projection
3. 3.5 mm perfusion balloon
4. End result
5. Restenosis of dog-legged lesion on LAD
6. LAD lesion in RAO caudal projection

Restenosis 255

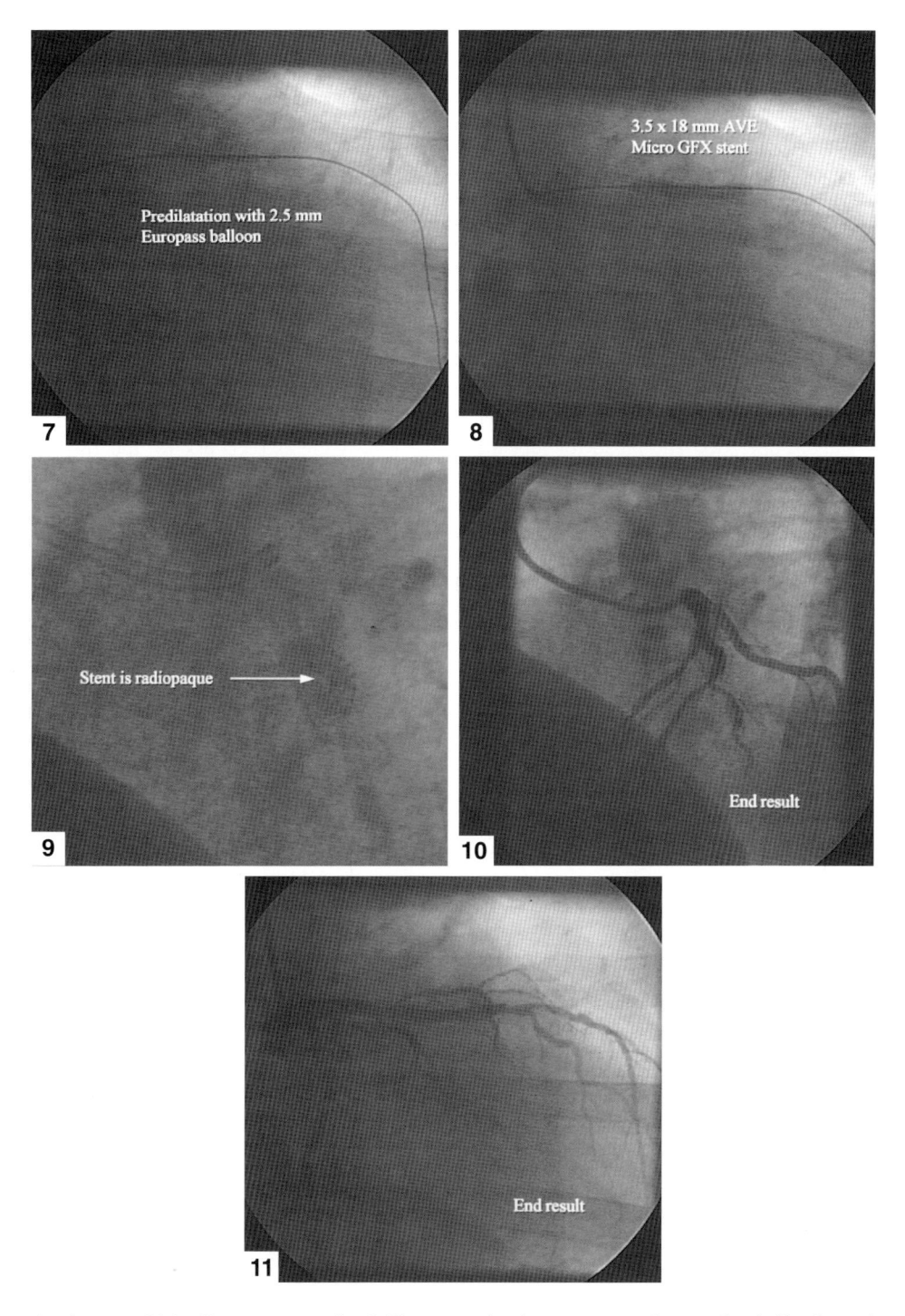

Angiogram 24.1. *Coronary stent for LAD restenosis.* A severe stenosis on a bend (dog-legged lesion) is seen in the proximal LAD of a patient presenting with unstable angina (1 and 2). It was dilated with a 3.5 mm perfusion balloon inflated for 7 minutes (3), with a good result (4). Two months later the lesion had restenosed (5 and 6). After predilatation with a 2.5 mm balloon (7), and delivery of a 3.5 mm AVE Microstent (8 and 9), the final result was satisfactory (10 and 11).

5. Atherectomy

This is a possibility in large calibre straight vessels. However, earlier studies on "de novo" and restenotic lesions showed no reduction of restenosis by atherectomy over balloon angioplasty. Hence the use of atherectomy has declined, but may be revived if on going studies aiming to remove more atheroma and achieve a larger lumen, show a reduction of restenosis. Atherectomy has been a valuable research tool allowing removal of tissues from restenotic lesions.

6. How Many Times to Redilate?

In other words, how many times before CABG? The answer lies in the frame of mind of the operator and the preference of the patient. Some operators take it as a personal challenge to "defeat restenosis" and go on and on redilating until the lesion, the patient, or the medical insurance company get fed up! Some patients are desperately keen to avoid operation and plead for repeat PTCA. Other patients soon ask for the "proper operation" to sort them out permanently.

Most operators offer a patient a second PTCA and will sometimes agree to perform a third. If PTCA does not seem to be working, there is a very successful alternative, i.e. CABG. Some patients may continue with medical treatment.

Restenosis Within Stents

Though the rate of restenosis is much less in stents, it still does occur (Angiogram 24.2) with a clinical return of angina of about 10%. As the rate is so low, have a greater reluctance to re-angiogram the patient after stent insertion, especially if the procedure was an elective one in a large calibre vessel. Carefully assess the history and even if the patient comes in with "unstable angina" consider an exercise test. If the history is atypical and the exercise test is negative, a stented lesion is very unlikely to have restenosed.

Redilatation for restenosis within a stent is usually straight forward. Dissection is rare as the stent protects the wall, but may still occur at either end of the stent. If using the same sized balloon as delivered the stent, higher pressures may be tried. Alternatively consider upsizing to the next balloon size.

IVUS can be helpful to assess the cause of restenosis. It may show that the original stent was not fully expanded, or was smaller that the true size of the vessel, or that restenosis is due intimal hyperplasia. Debulking procedures such as rotational atherectomy with the Rotablator, may be helpful for intimal hyperplasia.

Since the thrombotic risks with stents are now very low, restenosis has become one of the most important of the problems associated with stents. For further details on the management of stent restenosis (see page 144).

"Stent-like" Result from PTCA

The success of stents has made operators more careful in reviewing the result following a balloon angioplasty. Results that in the past would have been acceptable, are no longer passed. "Unsatisfactory PTCA result" is a frequent indication for stenting.

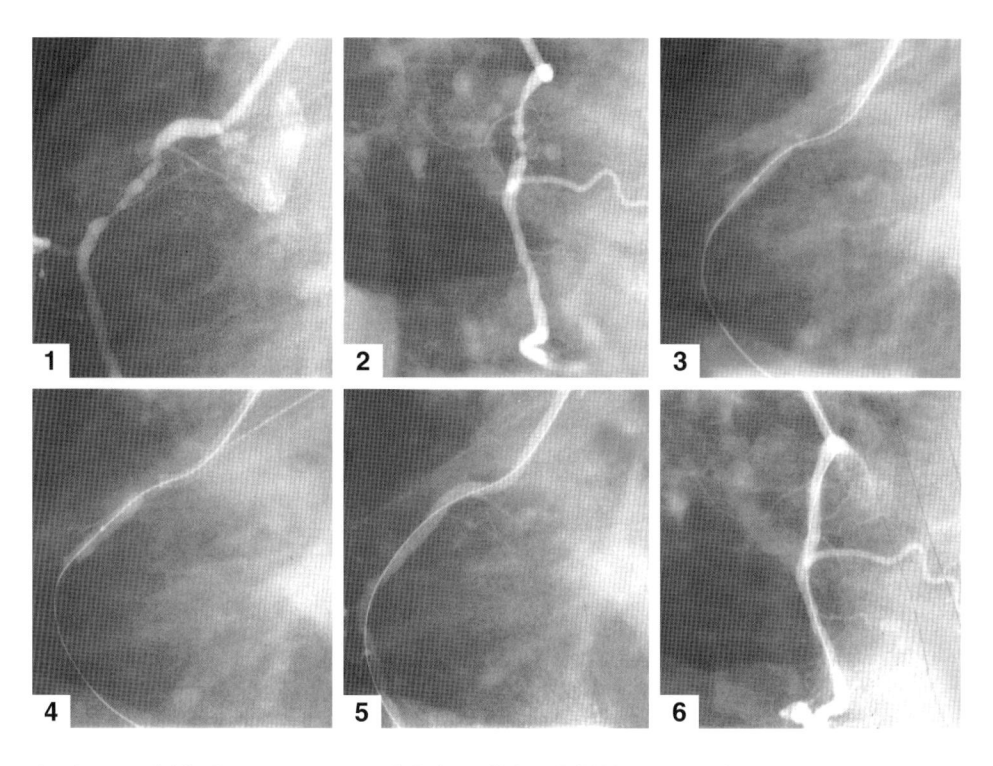

Angiogram 24.2. *Instent restenosis.* A Palmaz Schatz PS153 stent was inserted as a bail-our for acute occlusion at PTCA, see Angiogram 16.1. Five months later in-stent restenosis is shown in LAO 30° and RAO 30° projections (1 and 2). It was dilated with 3.0, and 3.5 mm balloons (3 and 4) to achieve a satisfactory result (5 and 6). No further restenosis occurred.

IVUS is also allowing the results from PTCA to be more carefully scrutinised (see page 250). From these twin approaches to improve angioplasty results, restenosis rates may tend to fall.

Restenosis the Achilles' Heel of PTCA

This is the description given to the weak point or downside of angioplasty. Well, if restenosis is the Achilles' Heel, then stenting is the *splint* for the Achilles' heel. However this *splint* does not come cheap!

Conclusion

For the first decade after the introduction of angioplasty, intimal hyperplasia was considered to be the main mechanism for restenosis; many antiproliferative drugs were assessed, but were not successful in patients. Recoil of the lesion and the amount of residual plaque are now believed to be the important processes. The larger the lumen ('bigger is better') hyposthesis supports the importance of these two mechanisms. The success of stents is primarily due to their ability to produce immediately after deployment, a much larger lumen than can be obtained after balloon angioplasty. Intimal hyperplasia has however not gone away and is the most important cause of instent restenosis.

Reference

Foley, D.P., Serruys, P.W. The changing face of restenosis. Chapter 14, pp. 249–268. Practical Interventional Cardiology. Edited by E.D. Grech and D.R. Ramsdale. Martin Dunitz Ltd, London, 1997.

25 PTCA Quotes

1. *Be Prepared.*
   'To be prepared is to be forearmed' ... and 'well begun is half done'. Time spent planning the PTCA and considering the strategy for possible complications, will reap dividends during the procedure in the catheter room.

2. *Catheter Room Dawdle.*
   This phrase was used by Grüntzig and describes that at the end of a difficult PTCA, or one where the result is less good than usual, stay a while with the patient in the catheter room. Have a chat with the patient and discuss the procedure and its progress. At the end of a 5–15 minute period 'reshoot' the dilated vessel(s) to confirm all is well. It is much better to detect in the catheter room that the lesion (and or the patient), are beginning to deteriorate, rather than have the patient 'go off' shortly after returning to the ward.

3. *Don't have everything stacked against you.*
   Don't attempt the impossible. For example hesitate before accepting for PTCA a complex lesion where guide catheter back-up will be poor, where there is proximal and distal disease, in a vessel which is the last remaining artery, for a patient who has very poor left ventricular function.
   For a high risk patient, such as one with a single remaining artery, consider PTCA if the lesion and the vessel look "straight forward" for PTCA. If not, think carefully before taking on the case for PTCA.

4. *It is not good practice to first meet the patient on the catheter room table.*
   Time spent properly assessing the patient may prevent hours of time in medical litigation. An exception to this rule is the emergency patient, with acute myocardial infarction for primary PTCA, or one developing an acute occlusion during diagnostic angiography. Patients with unstable angina being considered for ad hoc PTCA need a careful clinical assessment, including a discussion of the benefits and risks with the relatives.

5. *It's not a crime to send a patient for surgery.*
   It is better to refer a patient for an elective CABG, than to send the patient in the middle of a PTCA which has failed. Sometimes a patient can be potentially be treated either by a difficult or complex PTCA, or by a straight forward elective CABG. You have nothing to lose (except perhaps some pride), if after reviewing the angiogram before the procedure, you wish to change your mind and refer the patient instead for CABG. The patient will not be upset if you explain the reasons, even if it means discharge from hospital and joining a surgical waiting list. Try then to encourage the surgeon to give the patient priority for operation.

   During PTCA if the vessel occludes it is better to send the case *earlier* for emergency CABG, than trying repeatedly one technique after another to bail the patient (or yourself) out of the problem. Often all that will be achieved, is a more infarcted myocardium, a sicker patient and a higher angioplasty bill.

6. *Do the infarct (or culprit) vessel only.*
   The recommendation ('rule') of Hartzler for Primary PTCA is to *treat the infarction vessel only*. Do not attempt PTCA of another vessel, for if it goes wrong and occludes, the additional ischaemia on top of the infarction may be too great for the heart and patient to sustain. Restrain enthusiasm at primary PTCA procedures. Defer elective PTCA of other vessels for a few days or weeks as necessary.

7. *PTCA can be awfully simple or simply awful.*
   Aim to achieve the former!

8. *KISS (keep it simple and safe).*
   This is not always possible, but for example if there is a clear culprit lesion, deal with this first and consider whether PTCA of other vessels is really needed. Balloon angioplasty, perhaps with a prolonged inflation, may be much simpler for some lesions and vessels than trying to deploy a stent.

9. *Perfection is the enemy of good.*
   Sometimes more and more attempts to achieve an excellent result may lead to a complication, especially dissection. If after balloon dilatation there is a mild residual lesion, this may be acceptable. By returning with a larger sized balloon redilation may lead to dissection. Sometimes by trying too hard, you may end up '*snatching disaster from the jaws of success*'.

   Whilst the above is true, attempting to obtain a *good* angioplasty result should be the aim. Often in the past indifferent angioplasty results were accepted and restenosis was not a surprising later result.

   For stents, aim for an excellent result, with no residual stenosis and no inflow or outflow obstruction ... in fact aim for a 'stent-like' result!

10. *Err on the side of safety.*
    One can always go up a size of balloon ... but not down after a dissection. If the vessel size is uncertain between 2.5 and 3 mm, start with a 2.5 mm balloon.

11. *Restenosis is the "Achilles' Heel" of PTCA.*
    Then stenting is the "splint" for the Achilles' heel!

12. *Bigger is better and less is best.*
    The bigger the lumen after PTCA, the lower the rate of restenosis. After stenting elastic recoil of the wall is largely prevented so that the lumen is larger than that after balloon angioplasty. The lower the amount of residual plaque, the better will be the final lumen size and probably the lower will be the restenosis rate. See Chapters 11 and 24.

13. *Stents are the "second wind of PTCA".*
    Stents have changed and significantly improved the practice of PTCA.

14. *PTCA stands for ... "put that catheter away".*
    Don't be tempted to dilate unnecessary or mild lesions ... *if in doubt, don't.* Consider whether a significant stenosis on a *small* artery really is causing the patient's symptoms and whether it really does warrant intervention.
    Resist the *"occulo-dilatory reflex"* ... i.e. a stenosis seen by an interventionist leads to the desire to dilate it. On the other hand, a lesion very suitable for PTCA will have a lower risk for complications and it *is correct* to have a lower threshold to recommend PTCA.

15. *Stick with your friends that you know well.*
    Use known and trusted equipment, rather than always be trying out something new. Of course assess new equipment to compare with your 'work horse' version. However for a difficult case don't end up trying out a new guide catheter, a new guide wire, a new balloon and a stent that you have never used before!

26 Angioplasty Formulary

The formulary includes a list of less commonly used drugs, or preparations of drugs, that may be needed for angioplasty patients.

Abbreviations:
i.v.   intravenous
i/c.   intracoronary (or into SVG, saphevenous vein graft)
i.m.   intramuscular
s.cut   subcutaneously

Abciximab — see ReoPro

Adenosine
   i/c or into SVG, or i.v. 12 microgram boluses. The effects are short-lived, 1–2 minutes or less. Repeat boluses can be given.

Adrenaline
   Saphevenous vein graft embolism 50–100 µgm i.v. or into the graft.
   (1:10,000 of adrenaline = 100 micrograms per ml).
   Anaphylactic reaction, 0.5–1.0 mgm i.m., or s.cut (0.5–1.0 ml of 1:1000 solution).
   Note the different strengths of adrenaline used for these two indications.

Amiodarone
   5 mgm/kgm in 250 ml 5% dextrose i.v. over 20 mins–2 hours, followed by 1200 mgm in 500 ml of 5% dextrose over 12 hours.
   Note that drug should be administered in glucose as it is *incompatible with saline*.

Aprotinin (Trasylol)
   Test dose of 50,000 units (5 ml) i.v. slowly over 5 minutes.
   Then 2 million units (200 ml) i.v. over 20–30 minutes. Further doses of aprotinin 200,00–500,000 units i.v. per hour may be needed. Note that there is uncertainty over

the correct dose of aprotinin to reverse the effects of thrombolytic drugs (e.g. streptokinase or tPA), and the amount given is as needed.

Aspirin
100–300 mgm i.v.

Dextran
200–500 ml i.v. infusion over 15–30 minutes and then as necessary. The drug may lead to pulmonary oedema and hypersensitivity reaction.

Diamorphine
2.5 mgm i.v.

Diazemuls
5–10 mgm i.v.

Dopamine
5 µgm/kg/min.
Use an infusion pump containing 200 mgm of dopamine in 5 ml plus 45 ml of saline or 5% dextrose, to give a solution of 4000 micrograms per ml.
Formula for a 70 kgm patient at 5 micrograms/kg/min is:
5 × 70 × 60 = dose/body weight/hour
5 × 70 × 60 divided by 4000 (strength of solution) = ml per hour
= 5.2 ml/hour = approximately 5 ml/hour.

Flumazenil
100–200 µgm i.v.
To reverse the effects, e.g. respiratory depression of benzodiazpines. The drug may cause convulsions.

Glyceryl Trinitrate (GTN)
Intracoronary 0.1–0.3 mgm i/c bolus(es). Use sodium based preparation (Nitrocine) which is safer than the preparations with a potassium base.
I.V. infusion 1–10 mgm per hour. 50 mgm GTN ampoule is made up to 50 ml with 5% dextrose or normal saline, (1 mgm/ml). Give by an infusion pump.

Haemaccel
Plasma Substitute, 100–500 ml i.v. over 15–30 minutes, and then as necessary.

Hydrocortisone
100 mgm i.v.

Isosorbide Dinitrate (ISDN)
Intracoronary 1–3 mgm i/c. bolus(es)
I.V. infusion 1–10 mgm per hour.
A 50 mgm ampoule is made up to 50 ml with 5% dextrose or normal saline, (1 mgm/ml), and given by an infusion pump.

Metoclopramide (Maxolon)
10 mgm i.v.

Midazolam
2.5–5 mgm i.v.

Noradrenaline (Norepinephrine)
50–70 μgm i.v.
(1:10,000 of noradrenaline = 100 micrograms per ml). Give 0.5–0.7 ml.

Norepinephrine (*see noradrenaline*)

Phenyl Ephrine
0.1–0.3 mgm i.v. 10 mgm in 1 ml.
Take 0.1 ml into 10 ml syringe of 5% dextrose or saline. Give 1–3 ml.

Prochlorperazine (Stemetil)
5 mgm i.v.

Protamine
1 mgm neutralizes 100 units of heparin.
Dose of protamine should be that to neutralize half previous dose of heparin. Give drug i.v. slowly, 5 mgm or less per minute. Maximum dose of 50 mgm.

ReoPro (Abcixmab)
bolus dose i.v. 0.25 mgm/kgm over 5 minutes followed by,
infusion i.v. 10 μgm/min over 12 hours.
ReoPro preparation contains 10 mgm in 5 ml.
Bolus dose needed = 1 ml ReoPro per 8 kgm body weight of patient.
Note no heparin to be given after the ReoPro.
If ReoPro is used electively, give a reduced heparin dose at the start of the angioplasty procedure (50–70 units/kgm to achieve ACT of 200–250 seconds).
If the patient starts to bleed actively, stop the ReoPro, and give 5 units of platelets. Reverse the heparin if it is still active (ACT greater than 150 seconds), with protamine.

Stemetil (Prochlorperazine)
5 mgm i.v.

Streptokinase
i/c. 100,000 units over 5 minutes.

Ticlopidine
250 mgm dose is 250 mgm b.d. orally, to reduce the risk of stent thrombosis.
It is preferably to start this 2–3 days before the stent procedure. If a stent is only *possibly* needed, start the drug the night before procedure. Continue ticlopidine 2–4 weeks after stent deployment. It is preferable to check a full blood count and platelet level after 2 weeks on treatment, as the drug may cause bone marrow depression.

TPA or tPA (Tissue Plasminogen Activator)
   i/c. 20–40 mgm over 2–5 minutes, followed by 20–50 mgm over 3–6 hours i.v., or into the coronary artery via a small infusion catheter.

Tranexamic Acid
   1–5 gm by slow i.v. injection over 5 minutes, followed by 1 gm i.v. per hour as needed. This drug is to reverse the effects of thrombolytic drugs.

Trasylol (*see aprotinin*)

Verapamil
   i/c or into SVG, 0.5–1.0 mgm bolus, to 3–4 mgm. (*Be on the look out for heart block*).

Further Reading

Original Papers/Abstracts on PTCA

Grüntzig A, Myler R, Hanna E, Turina M. *Circulation* **84**, Abstracts III55–56 (1997).
Grüntzig A. Transluminal dilatation of Coronary Artery Stenosis. *Lancet* (**1**), 263 (1978).

AHA/ACC Classification of Coronary Artery Lesions

Ryan TJ, Faxon DP, Gunnar RM, *et al*. Guidelines for percutaneous transluminal coronary angioplasty. *J Am Coll Cardiol* **12**, 529–545 (1998).

Prevention of Groin Complications

Hasdai D, Holmes DR, King SB, Chronos N. Prevention of Groin Vascular Complications Associated with Percutaneous Procedures. *J Invas Cardiol* **9**, 119–125 (1997).

Primary Angioplasty and Thrombolysis

Clinical debate. Should thrombolysis or primary angioplasty be the treatment of choice for acute myocardial infarction? Thrombolysis – the prefered treatment. Hillis LD and Lange RA. Primary angioplasty – the strategy of choice. Grines CL, *N Eng J Med* **335**, 1311–1318 (1996).
De Boer M-J, MD thesis. Primary angioplasty in acute myocardial infarction. Rotterdam University, 1994.
Gibbons RJ, Holmes DR, Reeder GS, *et al*. Immediate angioplasty compared with the administration of a thromboytic agent followed by conservative treatment for myocardial infarction. *N Engl J Med* **328**, 685–691 (1993).
Grines CL, Browne KR, Marco J, *et al*. A comparison of immediate angioplasty with thrombolytic therapy for acute myocardial infarction. *N Eng J med* **328**, 673–679 (1993).
Mueller HS, Cohen LS, Braunwald E, *et al*. for the TIMI Investigators. Predictors of early morbidity and mortality after thrombolytic therapy of acute myocardial infarction: analysis of patient subgroups in the Thrombolysis in Myocardial Infarction (TIMI) trial, phase II. *Circulation* **85**, 1254–1264 (1992).
O'Keefe JO, Bailey WL, Rutherford BD, Hartzler GO. Primary angioplasty for acute myocardial infarction in 1000 consecutive patients. *Am J Cardiol* **72**, 107G–115G (1993).
O'Neil WW. The evolution of Primary PTCA therapy for acute myocardial infarction. *J. Invas Cardiol* **7**, SuppF 2F–10F (1995).
Stone G, Grines CL, Topol EJ. Update on Percutaneous Transluminal Coronary Angioplasty for acute myocardial infarction. Current review of Interventional Cardiology, 2nd edition, pages 1–56. Editors: EJ Topol and PW Serruys. Current Medicine, Philadelphia, 1995.

Swift (Should We Intervene following Thrombolysis?). Trial Study Group. SWIFT Trial of delayed elective intervention v conservative treatment after thrombolysis with anistreplase in acute myocardial infarction. *Brit Med J* **302**, 555–60 (1991).

Topol EJ, Califf RM, George BS, *et al*. Thrombolysis And Acute Myocardial Infarction (TAMI) Trial. A randomized trial of immediate versus delayed elective angioplasty after intravenous tissue plasminogen activator in acute myocardial infarction. *N Engl J Med* **317**, 197–202 (1987).

Zijlstra F, DeBoer MJ, Hoorntje JC *et al*. A comparison of immediate coronary angioplasty with intravenous streptokinase in acute myocardial infarction. *N Engl J Med* **328**, 680–684 (1993).

Radial Artery Angioplasty

Kiemeneij F, Laarman GJ. Percutaneous transradial artery approach for coronary stent implantation. *Cath Cardiovasc Diagn.* **30**, 173–178 (1993).

Kiemeneij F. Transradial artery coronary stenting. In 'Endoluminal Stenting', pp. 306–310. Edited by Ulrich Sigwart. WB Saunders Co Ltd, 1996.

Lowe MD, Ludman PF. Cardiac Catheterization via the radial artery. *Brit J Cardiol* **4**, 71–74 (1997).

Initial Paper on Coronary Artery Stenting

Sigwart U, Puel J, Mirkovitch V, *et al*. Intravascular stents to prevent occlusion and restenosis after angioplasty. *N Engl J Med* **316**, 701–706 (1987).

Studies of Restenosis after Coronary Artery Stenting

Benestent Trial

Serruys PW, de Jaegere P, Kiemeneij F, *et al*. A comparison of balloon expandable stent with balloon angioplasty in patients with coronary artery disease. *N Engl J Med* **331**, 489–495 (1994).

Stress Trial

Fischman D, Leon MB, Baim D, Schatz RA, *et al*. A randomized comparison of coronary stent placement and balloon angioplasty in the treatment of coronary artery disease. *N Engl J Med* **331**, 496–501 (1994).

Coronary Artery Stenting Without Oral Anticoagulants

Colombo A, Hall P, Nakamura S, *et al*. Intracoronary stenting without anticoagulation accomplished with intravascular ultrasound guidance. *Circulation* **91**, 1676–1688 (1995).

Case Report of an Infected Stent

Gunther H-U, Strupp G, Volmar J, *et al*. Coronary stent implantation: Infection and myocardial abscess with lethal outcome. *Zeitschrift für Kardiologie* **82**, 521–525 (1993).

Intravascular Ultrasound (IVUS)

Intravascular Ultrasound Imaging. Jonathan Tobis and Paul Yock. Churchill-Livingstone Inc., New York, 1992.
An introduction to Intravascular Ultrasound. Neal Uren. Remedica, Oxford, 1996.

Glycoprotein IIb/IIIb Antagonist (ReoPro)

The EPIC Investigators: Use of a monoclonal antibody directed against the platelet glycoprotein IIb/IIIa receptor in high risk coronary angioplasty, *N Engl J Med* **330**, 956–61 (1994).

The EPILOG Investigators: Platelet glycoprotein IIb/IIIa receptor blockade and low dose heparin during percutaneous coronary revascularization, *N Engl J Med* **336**, 1689–1696 (1997).

Review on Restenosis

Foley, D.P., Serruys, P.W. The changing face of restenosis. Chapter 14, pp. 249–268. Practical Intervention Cardiology. Edited by E.D. Grech and D.R. Ramsdale. Martin Dunitz. London 1997.

Reviews on Coronary Angioplasty

Atlas of International Cardiology. Jeffrey J Popma, Martin B Leon and Eric J Topol. W.B. Saunders Co. Philadelphia. USA. 1994.

Current Review of Interventional Cardiology, Second Edition. Editors EJ Topol and PW Serruys. Churchill-Livingstone, 1995.

The New Manual of Interventional Cardiology. Mark Freed, Cindy Grines and Robert D Safian. Physicians Press, Michigan. USA. 1996.

Practical Interventional Cardiology. Ever D Grech and David R Ramsdale. Martin Dunitz Ltd, London. UK. 1997

Reviews on Coronary Stenting

Endoluminal Stenting. Edited by Ulrich Sigwart. WB Saunders Co Ltd, London. 1996.
Handbook of Coronary Stents. Editor in chief: Patrick W Serruys. Martin Dunitz, London. 1997.

Manufacturers of Equipment

Manufacturers are mentioned throughout the book. Some produce a wide range of angioplasty equipment, whereas others manufacture a specific item(s) mentioned in the text. The base or head office is listed, but there will often be a local address for other countries.

ACS
See Guidant

AngioDynamics, Glen Falls, NY, USA.
Angiostent.

Arrow International Inc., Reading, PA, USA.
Radial Artery Catheterization Set.

Arterial Vascular Engineering, Inc., Santa Rosa, CA, USA.
AVE Micro stent.

C R Bard Inc., Billerica, MA, USA.

Baxter Edwards, Irvine, CA, USA.
Angioscopy catheter.

Boehringer-Mannheim Corp.,Indianopolis, IN, USA.
CoaguChek Plus, Coagulation Monitor for APTT/PTTK testing.

Boston Scientific Northwest, Redmond, WA, USA.

Cardiometrics, Mountain View, CA, USA.
This manufacturer of the FloWire, is now part of Cordis.

Cardiovascular Dynamics, Irvine, CA, USA.
CAT balloon.

Centocor, Malvern, PA, USA.
ReoPro (abciximab).

Cook, Inc., Bloomington, IN, USA.
Gianturco-Roubin stent.

C P Pharmaceuticals, Wrexham, UK.
Hepsal heparin flushes.

Cordis, a Johnson & Johnson Comany, Warren, NJ, USA.

CVIS Boston Scientific, Orchard Park Way, San Jose, CA, USA.
IVUS equipment.

Datascope Corp., Collagen Products Division, Montvale, NJ, USA.
Vasoseal femoral arterial closure kit.

Eli Lilly & Company, Indianapolis, Indiana, USA.
ReoPro (abciximab).

Endosonics Corp., Rancho Cordova, CA USA.
IVUS equipment.

Guidant/Advanced Cardiovascular Systems, Santa Clara, CA USA.

Hewlett Packard, Palo Alto, CA, USA.
IVUS equipment.

Hoechst, Marion, Roussel Ltd., Broadwater Park, Denham, Middlesex, UK.
Haemaccel, iv fluid, for vein graft embolism.

InterVentional Technologies, Inc., San Diego, CA, USA.
Cutting Balloon.

Johnson and Johnson, Warren, NJ, USA.

Jo-Med International AB, Drottninggatan 92, Helsingborg, Sweden.
Jo-stent.

Malinckrodt Medical. St Louis. MO, USA.
Wholey HiTorque Guide Wire.

Medtronic Inc., Minneapolis, MN, USA.

Microvena Inc., White Bear Lake, MN, USA.
Nitinol guide wire.

North West Technologies Boston Scientific, Redmond, Washington, USA.
Rotablator, rotational atherectomy equipment.

Perclose Inc., Menlo Park, CA, USA.
Perclose, femoral arterial closure kit.

P Osypka GmbH, Germany
Rotacs (Rotational Angioplasty Catheter System) Drill.

Progressive Angioplasty Systems Inc., Menlo Park, CA, USA.
ACT-One Stent.

Radi Medical Systems, Uppsala, Sweden.
Fem Stop, femoral arterial closure kit.

Schneider AG, Bulach, Switzerland.

Schwarz Pharma, Monheim, Germany.
Nitrocine, sodium based preparation of glyceryl trinitrate.

SciMed Live Systems, Maple Grove, Mininesota, USA.

Sherwood Medical International, Stent Louis, MO, USA.
Angio-seal, femoral arterial closure kit.

Target Therapeutics, Fremont, CA, USA.
Tracker 18 catheter.

Technidyne Corporation, Edison, New Jersey, USA.
Haemochron machine ACT machine.

Terumo Corporation, Tokyo, Japan.
Terumo guide wire.

USCI
See Bard.

Index

A

Abciximab, (*see ReoPro*)
ACE inhibitor, 199
Achille's heal, of PTCA, 103, 124, 257
Acoustic shadow, 62
ACT (Activated Clotting Time), 73
ACT-One stent, 112, 140
Ad-Hoc PTCA, 183–7, 211
   After M.I. (*see primary angioplasty*)
Adenosine, 216, 263
Adrenaline, 164, 216, 263
Allen test, 100
Amiodarone, 263
Amplatz Goose-neck snare, 135
Amplatz guide catheter, 8, 81, 133, 172, 206, 229, 233
Anaesthetist, 70, 164, 181
Anchor exchange device, 34
Angina,
   Post M.I., 190
   Stable, 67
   Unstable, 184
Angiogram review, 70, 79, 88, 148
Angiographic views, 41–58, 246
Angioplasty, 1, 67
   Primary, 189–200
   Rescue or Salvage, 190
Angioscopy, 64
Angioseal, 97
Angiostent, 114
Anticoagulants, 2, 103, 129, 131, 179
Antiplatelet drugs, 130
Aprotinin, 179, 263
Arani guide catheter, 10, 229
Arrhythmias, reperfusion, 196
Arterio-venous fistula, 176
Aspirin, 72, 73, 130, 195, 199, 248, 264
Atherectomy, 2, 145, 175, 199, 256
Atmosphere, balloon inflation pressure, 14
Audit, 180

B

Back-up for guide catheter, 81, 133, 206, 213
Back-up view for angiography, 43, 153, 206
Bail-out for failed PTCA, 22, 169, 174, 181
Baim, Prof. Don, 125, 250
Balloon,
   catheters, 13–26
   inflation, 93, 173
   long length shaft, 224
   materials, 15
   perforation, 141
   perfusion (*see perfusion balloon*)
   rupture, 141, 164, 235
Benestent trial, 124
BeStent, 104, 112
Beta-blocking drugs, 72, 76, 199
Bifurcation lesions, 31, 52, 112, 237–248
'Bigger is Better'
   Theory of restenosis, 125, 250, 253, 260
Blood transfusion, 179

Bonzel, Dr. Tassilo, 17, 25
Brachial artery, (angioplasty from), 100
Bridge collaterals, 202

C

CABG (coronary artery bypass grafting)
    Emergency, 175, 177–181, 210, 260
    Off site or On site, 70, 175, 193
Elective, 259
Calcification of vessels, 60
Calcium antagonist, 72, 76
Cardiac pacing, 70, 176
Cardiogenic shock, 193
CAT balloon, 23, 142
Catheter dawdle, 92, 259
Chronic occlusion, 125, 201–208
Chubby balloon, 15, 142, 212, 233
Circumflex artery, 81, 147, 233, 248
    Angiographic views, 47
Closure devices, 97
Coagulation check, 74
Colombo, Dr. Antonio, 2, 59, 103, 108, 127
Compliant balloon, 14
Contrast agents, 196
Contrast, (in the balloon), 95
Cordis Crossflex stent, 104, 114, 133, 174, 240, 243, 253
Core wire of balloon catheter, 151
Coronary artery,
    False aneurysm, 145
    Perforation, 30, 204, 206
    Rupture, 145
    Spasm, 30, 73, 122, 139, 152, 164, 215
Coronary flow
    reserve, 40
    TIMI grading, 191
Coronary occlusion, Acute, 189–200
    Chronic, 86, 201–208
Culprit lesion, 86, 192, 204, 260
Cumberland, Prof David, 37
    Technique, 37, 208
Cutting balloon, 25, 172
CVA (cerebro vascular accident), 191

D

Deep throating, 95
Delivery tube for hand mounted stent, 151

Dextran, 130, 216, 264
Diabetes, 72, 77, 144, 177, 194
Diagnostic catheters, 11, 208, 252
Diagonal artery, 48–54, 245
Diamorphine, 175, 264
Diazemuls, 73, 264
Diazepam, 73
Dipyridamole, 130
Discussions with patient and relatives, 68, 148, 157, 179, 186, 194
Discussions with surgeons, 70, 157, 181, 213, 244
Dissection, After PTCA, 167–176, 244
    After stenting, 141
    Risks of, 83, 155, 171
    Stenting for, 121, 174
    Treatment, 169
    Types/Severity, 167
Dog-legged bend of LCX, 91, 233
Door-to-balloon time, 191
Doppler wire, 40
Dotter, Dr. Charles, 1
Drug delivering balloon, 24
Dopamine, 216, 264

E

Ejection fraction, 82
El Gamal guide catheter, 10
Elastic recoil, 21, 124, 228, 233, 249
Embolism,
    In vein graft, 140, 165, 216
    To coronary artery, 198
Emergency CABG, 70, 175, 177–181, 191, 210, 243
Entwining of guide wires, 31, 242
Exchange devices, 34
Exchange wire, 31
Exercise test, 67, 192
Extension guide wire, 31
Extension wire, 31
Extra back-up, 30, 74, 133
Extra support guide wire (see extra back-up wire)

F

Failure to cross lesion with balloon or stent,
Faxing ECG in acute M.I., 194
Fem-stop, 75, 153

Firmness of guide wire, 29
Fixed wire balloon, 19, 224, 240
Flumazenil, 73, 264
Foreshortening, 41

G

Gastro-epiploic artery, 58, 225
Gianturco-Roubin stent, 104, 113–114, 123, 174, 240, 245
Glyceryl trinitrate (GTN), 30, 73, 100, 122, 152 195, 218, 264
Glycoprotein IIb/IIIa antagonist, 161–165, 172, 179
Gold, 30
Goose-neck snare, 135
Graft embolism, 140, 165, 214, 216
Grines, Dr. Cindy, 196
Groin complications, 132, 163
Grüntzig, Dr. Andreas, 1, 20, 67,
    Patient selection for PTCA, 67
Guide catheters, 5–12
    Back-up or stability, 81, 89, 133, 206, 214, 224 246
Guide Wire, 27
    Causing spasm, 30, 139
    Extension, 31
    Extra back-up, 30, 133
    Extra support, 30
    Firm or stiff, 29, 165, 205, 224
    Firmer section to aid tracking of balloon or stent, 29, 133, 214, 245
    Fracture, 205
    Maintain across dissection, 179
    Producing dissection, 30, 172, 205
    Radiopacity, 30, 246
    Shape, 31, 242
    Two, guide wire procedure, 31, 51, 242

H

Haemaccel, 216, 264
Haemorrhage,
    After stents, 132
    After ReoPro, 164
Haemostatic valve, 18
Hand crimping (*a stent on to a balloon*), 149
Hartzler, Dr. Geoffrey, 82, 95, 189
    Rule for primary PTCA, 189, 196, 260

Heparin, 61, 73, 75, 130, 162, 195
    ACT and PTTK measurements, 74
    Dosage, 73, 130, 163
    Flush to sheath, 163, 185
    Haemachron machine, 73
    Resistance, 72, 157
Hi Per Flex guide wire, 30
High torque floppy guide wire, 30
Hockey stick guide catheter, 10
Hydrocortisone, 164, 264
Hyperlipidaemia, 68, 76, 199, 218

I

Infection of a stent, 146
Inflation device, 17
Instent restenosis (*see stent*)
Intermediate artery, 48
Internal mammary artery, 11, 57, 221–6
Intimal hyperplasia, 124, 250
Intra Aortic Balloon Pump, 71, 86, 171, 177, 199
Iridium, 114
Isosorbide dinitrate (ISDN), 30, 218, 264
Intravascular Ultrasound (IVUS), 2, 40, 59–64, 104, 107, 127, 143, 154, 244, 250, 253, 256

J

Jail, stent, 144, 243,
Jail, surgical, 145
Jo-Stent, 104, 112, 240, 243

K

Kiemeneij, Dr. Ferdinand, 100
Kimmy radial catheter, 101
Kiss – *Keep it simple and safe*, 260
Kissing balloon technique, 241

L

LAD syndrome, 186
'Larger is better', theory of restenosis, 125
Laser, 24, 40, 206
LAST procedure, 204

Last remaining coronary artery, 156, 210, 259
Late loss, after PTCA, 124
Left Anterior Descending artery,
    Angiographic views, 48–54
    Bifurcation lesion, 237–247
Left Circumflex artery, 81
    Angiographic views, 47–48
    Dog-legged bend, 94, 233
Left Main Stem, 8, 46, 80, 94, 191, 231
Lesion
    Recoil, 21, 124, 228, 233, 249
    Types, 84, 155, 232
'Less is best',
    Theory of restenosis, 250
LIMA,
    Angioplasty, 221–5
    Graft, 11, 57, 180
Lipids, 77, 199, 218
Lorazepam, 73
Lubricant coating,
    To balloons, 15, 149
    To guide wire, 29
Lung disease, 68

M

Magnet exchange device, 35
Magnum balloon catheter, 17
Magnum guide wire, 37, 128, 206
Marco, Dr. Jean, 103
Maxolon, 175, 265
Meeting the patient, 28, 259
Meier, Prof Bernhard, 37, 183
Menu sheet, 83
Metoclopramide, 175, 265
Micro stent, 104, 108–110, 122, 128, 174, 228, 230, 231, 240, 255
Midazolam, 73, 265
Mobilization after PTCA, 76
Monorail balloon, 17
Morice, Dr. Marie Claude, 104
Mounting tube for hand mounted stent, 151
Multi-link stent, 104, 110, 133, 139, 231, 232, 253
Multipurpose guide catheters, 11, 213, 229
Multivessel PTCA, 86
Myler, Dr. Richard, 2
Myocardial Infarction,
    Complication of PTCA, 69
    Primary PTCA for, 184, 189–200

N

New lesions after PTCA/stent, 30, 122, 139, 164, 215
NIR stent, 104, 110–112, 133, 174, 228, 231, 232, 243, 253
Nitinol, 37, 106, 224
Nitrates, 72
Nitrocine, 216
No reflow phenomenon, 215
Non compliant balloon, 14, 142
Noradrenaline, 218, 265
Nurse/nursing, 41, 58, 176, 180, 200

O

Occlusion,
    acute, 155–176
    chronic, 125, 156, 201–8
Occulo-dilatory reflex, 79, 184, 261
Omnopon, 73
Open artery theory, 191
Opiate, 73
Osteal stenosis, 125, 227–232
Osteum of coronary artery, 229, 231
    of LIMA, 224
    of SVG, 213, 231
OTW, 'Over the Wire' balloon, 17
Oxygen, 73, 176

P

Pacing, temporary, 70, 176, 196, 218, 248
Palmaz-Schatz Crown stent, 108, 133, 231, 243
Palmaz-Schatz stent, 103, 104, 107, 123, 132
Perclose, 97, 153, 163
Percutaneous cardiopulmonary bypass, 71, 171
'Perfection – the enemy of good', 143, 260
Perfusion balloon, 20, 71, 93, 174, 179, 235, 254
Peripheral vascular disease, 177
Pharmacy, 200
Phenylephrine, 165, 218, 265
Pilot wire, 39
Plaque, residual after PTCA, 250
Plasma, fresh frozen, 179
Platelets, 159, 163, 179
Platinum, 30, 106, 114
PMT (*physiological measurement technician*), 41, 58, 176, 180

POBA *'plain old balloon angioplasty'*, 253
Polycythaemia, 159
Preconditioning, 92, 214
Predilatation, 95, 133, 149, 214, 224, 228, 229
Premedication, 73
Preoperative assessment for PTCA, 68
Preparation for PTCA, 67, 87, 259
Pressure wire, 40
Primary angioplasty, 189–200
Primary view for angiography, 43, 153, 206
Probing catheter, 205
Prochlorperazine, 175, 265
Profile of balloon catheter, 14
Prolonged balloon inflation, 93, 173
Protamine, 130, 265
PTCA (*see angioplasty*)

Q

Quantitative coronary angiography (QCA), 91, 149

R

Radial artery, angioplasty from, 100
Radiation exposure, 58
Radiographer, 41, 50, 180
Radiographic views, 41–58, 246
Radiopacity, 30, 106, 114, 246
Rapid exchange balloon, 17
Recoil of lesion, 21, 124, 228, 233, 249
Relatives, discussion with, 68, 69, 148, 179, 184, 195
Remodelling of artery, 250
ReoPro, 73, 128, 131, 161–164, 171, 179, 198, 265
Reperfusion arrhythmias, 196
Rescue angioplasty, 190
Residual plaque, 250
Restenosis, 69, 76, 123, 229, 244, 249–258
Restenosis,
    In vein graft, 210, 251
    Mechanisms of, 124, 249–251
    Predictions for, 252
    Time course, 251
Retrieval of dropped stent, 135
Review of angiogram prior to PTCA, 70, 79–87, 148

Rickards, Dr. Tony, 96
Right Coronary,
    Angiographic views, 43–45
    Artery, 6, 11, 43
    Bifurcation lesion, 248
    Lesion on bend, 232
    Osteal lesion, 229
Risks of PTCA, 21, 69, 155
Road map of angiogram, 92, 151
Rotablator, 2, 40, 60, 145, 164, 172, 225, 235, 256
Rotacs drill, 40, 206

S

Salvage angioplasty, 190
Saphevenous vein graft (*see vein graft*)
Schatz, Dr. Richard, 2, 103
Scopolamine, 73
Serruys, Prof. Patrick, 2, 103, 104
Sheath femoral
    Flushing, 163, 185
    Long, 86, 89, 213
    Removal, 74, 163, 184, 199
Shepherd's crook, initial course to RCA, 10, 81, 133
Short balloon, 142, 212, 233
Sigwart, Dr. Ulrich, 1, 103, 123
Simpson, Prof. John, 20, 97
Slotted-tube design for stents, 107
Sones guide catheter, 11, 99
Spasm (*see coronary artery spasm*)
Spasm, of LIMA, 224
Spider view for angiography, 52
Stack, Dr. Richard, 20
Standard guide wire, 30
Statin drug, 77, 199
Stemetil, 175, 265
Stent,
    Balloon rupture, 141
    Bare, 149
    causing dissection, 141, 215
    Causing embolism, 140
    Complications, 127–146
    Delivery system, 105
    Dropped, 133
    For acute M.I., 198
    For bifurcation lesion, 240
    For chronic occlusion, 208
    For osteal lesion, 228

Groin complication, 132
Haemorrhage, 132
Inadequate deployment, 62, 127, 142
Infection, 146
instent restenosis, 62, 144, 256
Jail, 117, 144, 243
Leading to spasm, 139
Persistent lesions, 143, 162, 198
Placement problems, 132, 228
Radiopacity, 106
Retrieval, 135
Second generation, 110
Shortening, 116
Surgical jail, 145
Thrombosis, 127, 211
To treat dissection, 121, 174
Types, 103–119
Uncoiling, 144
'Stent-like result', after PTCA, 22, 198, 256
Stentomania, 104
Streptokinase, 131, 161, 265
Stress trial, 124
Stylet of balloon catheter, 151
Surgical cover for PTCA, 70, 86, 157, 175, 184

T

Tantalum, 106, 113, 114
Telephone, patient contact, 69, 131, 154, 157, 195
Terumo wire, 38, 206, 224
Thallium scan, 67, 193
Thrombolytic drugs, 179, 189
Thrombus/Thrombosis,
    After PTCA, 157
    Embolism, 198
    In a stent, 127
    Types at angioscopy, 65
    Within coronary artery, 60, 242
Ticlopidine, 73, 76, 104, 130, 154, 199, 265
TIMI grading of coronary flow, 191
Torquer, 29, 244
tPA, 133, 161, 190, 198, 266
Tracking of balloon or stent, 30, 132, 214

Tranexamic Acid, 179, 266
Trapper balloon, 34
Trasylol, 179
Tuohy-Borst adaptor, 19
Two wire technique, 31, 51, 242
Type A personality, 93

U

Undilatable Lesion, 235
Uren, Dr. Neal, 62

V

Varicose veins, previous stripping of, 68, 177
Vasoseal, 97
Vein graft, 11, 56, 123, 125, 180, 209–219, 228, 251
    Embolism, 140, 165, 215
Verapamil, 164, 216, 266
Vessel rupture, 145
Voda guide catheter, 9, 81, 133, 232, 244

W

Wallstent, 104, 114–119, 123, 174, 217
Warfarin, 131, 219
Wholey wire, 222
Wiktor stent, 104, 113, 123, 139, 144, 232, 240, 243
Wire introducer, 29, 244

X

X-T stent, 104, 112

Y

Y-Connector, 18, 89, 151, 244
Yock, Prof. Paul, 250